Drug and Alcohol Abuse

A Clinical Guide to Diagnosis and Treatment

Sixth Edition

Drug and Alcohol Abuse

A Clinical Guide to Diagnosis and Treatment

Sixth Edition

Marc A. Schuckit

University of California Medical School and
Veterans Administration Hospital
San Diego, CA, USA

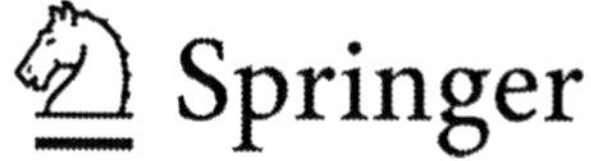

Library of Congress Control Number: 2005924429

ISBN-10:0-387-25732-2 0-387-25733-0 (eBook)
ISBN-13:978-0387-25732-7

Printed on acid-free paper.

Printed in the United States of America. (SPI/SBA)

9 8 7 6 5 4 3 2 1

springeronline.com

Preface

This book uses a clinically oriented approach for working with patients and clients with substance-use disorders. The material represents a blending together of my three major professional roles as a clinician, teacher, and researcher. The overall goal is to help the busy clinicians feel comfortable with their level of understanding of alcohol and other drug-related disorders, and to offer the best clinical care possible.

The first edition of this text, published in 1979, grew out of my need to place the 200 or so drugs of abuse into a clinically useful perspective. There was no way I could remember each and every drug, and I faced a challenge when a new drug (or perhaps an old substance with a new name) was introduced. I learned that I can place these substances into a limited number of categories based on the usual clinical effects, thereby creating groups similar in the quality of intoxication, associated physiological changes, and patterns of problems likely to be observed in the context of intoxication and withdrawal. This clinically oriented and pragmatic approach remains the core of this book, continuing to be as useful to me today as when the first volume was published.

Of course, over the years, many details have changed. First, the diagnostic criteria have evolved from DSM-II to DSM-III in 1980, DSM-III-R in 1987, and DSM-IV in 1994. I was fortunate to hold the Chair of the DSM-IV Substance Use Disorders Workgroup, and to participate in one of the committees leading to DSM-V. Therefore, each edition of the text has had the opportunity to offer some perspectives on the most recent diagnostic systems. Over the years, the patterns of substance use in populations have gone up, come down, and sometimes gone up again, while our understanding of pharmacology, physiology, and genetic influences has continued to expand at a rapid rate. These historical issues and background on epidemiology and physiology have formed the basis for the first half of each chapter dedicated to a category of drugs (e.g., depressants, opioids, stimulants, cannabinoids, and so on) and have been updated with each new edition. The second half of each current substance-oriented chapter offers a clinically oriented presentation of recent developments in the treatment of substance-related conditions, many of which represent expansions of our understanding of the cognitive behavioral core of treatment, along with the development of new pharmacological approaches. Chapter 14 is dedicated to reviewing the current status of rehabilitation approaches in an effort to pull together much of the information presented within the previous drug category-oriented chapters.

Therefore, the structure of the book reflects my background as both a clinician and teacher. The specifics, however, rest with my training as a researcher. About 80% of the references in this sixth edition have been published since 2000. The Refrences for each chapter give the reader the opportunity to learn more about specific topics offered within the text, with references given as more of a general background, rather than a highly linked statement based on each reference.

In addition to a thorough updating of the References, the sixth edition incorporates another important change. In the course of developing the five previous editions, and as a consequence of the consistent and impressive increase in knowledge in our field, the number of chapters and pages increased across the five editions. As I looked at the version of this book published in 2000, I felt that if the length of the text continued to expand, it would do so at the potential cost of limiting the usefulness and clinician-oriented emphasis of the work. Therefore, the sixth edition has been streamlined by deleting two previous chapters (the section on phencyclidine has been folded into the overall chapter on hallucinogens and the thoughts on prevention have now been incorporated into Chapter 1). At the same time, efforts have been made to shorten each of the remaining chapters whenever possible.

Finally, this remains a single-author text. This facilitates consistency across chapters in both philosophy and writing style. Having said that, this work has been strongly influenced by many people in this field, including, but not limited to, authors cited in the References for the various chapters. In addition, this text could not have been accomplished without the help of the wonderful people in my office. Emily Wick worked day and night to help me place the chapters into a final form, and has been indispensable regarding pinning down references. Lynnette Fleck transcribed the initial changes in the first several drafts of the updated chapters, putting up with my awful handwriting and, at times, my inability to sit still long enough explaining things. Finally, everything that comes out of my office reflects the dedication, warmth, and support of Marcy Gregg and Tom Smith. I would be lost without any of them.

Marc A. Schuckit, M.D.

Contents

CHAPTER 1

An Overview

1.1. INTRODUCTION

1.1.1. Some General Thoughts About Alcohol and Drugs

People have used mind-altering substances (from nicotine to heroin and beyond) for thousands of years.[1,2] These drugs (using that term to include alcohol as well) help us to concentrate, offer a diversion from our usual way of feeling (even if the change is from good to just different, not always from bad to good), and help us to feel as if we fit in with those around us. Some substances, like alcohol, have distinct healthful effects at low doses, including increased appetite, lowered risks for some forms of heart disease and stroke, and possibly even a mild protective effect against some forms of dementias.[3,4] Other drugs (e.g., cannabinols, cocaine, amphetamines, and opioids) have medicinal properties that can be useful in treating a variety of medical conditions.[5]

So, it is not surprising to discover that a large proportion of men and women in western countries have used such substances. For example, in 2002 and 2003, 51% of high school seniors and 59% of young adults admitted to ever having used an illicit substance, including about 45% of each who had used a cannabinol (e.g., marijuana), 11 and 20%, respectively, who have ever taken a hallucinogen and, almost 15% of each who have ever taken amphetamines.[6] While the rates of substance-use disorders (e.g., abuse and dependence) are harder to determine, these figures are also substantial. It has been estimated that approximately 25% of men and women in the United States regularly smoke cigarettes (and presumptively have dependence), while the lifetime risk for abuse or dependence on alcohol is at least 15% for men and 8% for women, with an estimated 10 and 5% of the two sexes ever having met criteria for abuse or dependence on an illicit drug.

As described later in this chapter, repeated heavy use of substances has serious implications for health, interpersonal functioning, legal difficulties, as well as job and school performance.[7,8] Intoxication or withdrawal from many substances can temporarily mimic almost any major psychiatric syndromes, most drugs of abuse can exacerbate preexisting medical conditions, and almost all of these substances are metabolized by the liver where they can interfere with the breakdown and subsequent blood levels of most prescribed medications.[2,9] Therefore, healthcare deliverers need to understand the impact that these substances and associated substance-use disorders are having on the symptoms, syndromes, and treatment of disorders in their clients and patients.

Unfortunately, schools that teach clinicians how to deliver optimal treatment rarely include substance-related topics in their busy schedules. The emphasis tends to be on the more straightforward medical and psychiatric disorders, with little time reserved in the curriculum to teach about the highly prevalent conditions associated with substance use.[10,11] In one recent survey, 40% of general medical practitioners could not remember having received any training regarding substance-use disorders, and an additional quarter (i.e., adding up to almost three quarters of those surveyed) noted having received less than 4 h of continuing education regarding these conditions.[11] It has been estimated that the average medical school graduate has received less than 1 h per year of substance-use disorder training. The end result is that few of us enter healthcare-related practices having been adequately educated to understand how the use of both legal and illicit substances might impact those we treat, and even fewer have received adequate training on how to recognize and treat related abuse and dependence conditions.

Recently, a series of papers have offered important insights into how the basic elements of treatment of substance-related conditions are similar to approaches used for other long-term disorders that tend to wax and wane over time, including optimal steps required in the treatment of diabetes and hypertension.[12,13] Using adult onset diabetes as an example, while useful medications have been identified, their effectiveness depends upon helping the patient to develop and maintain relatively high levels of motivation regarding compliance with prescriptions, as well as changes in diet, improvement in exercise, and cessation of smoking. Elements similar to those used in the treatment of substance-related conditions are also employed in medicine to enhance levels of motivation, and to help patients recognize and address their disorder and associated treatments on both emotional and cognitive levels.[14,15] When these techniques are applied appropriately to substance-related conditions, one can expect a high proportion of patients to modify their behaviors, with absolute abstinence from substances for extended periods of time likely to be seen in as many as 70% of patients who have relatively stable life styles, and more than 50% for those without immediate resources regarding jobs and families.[16]

This book has been written to help to bridge the gap that exists in most healthcare providers regarding substances of abuse and related problems. It is written for the medical student, the physician in practice, the psychologist, the social worker, and other health professionals or paraprofessionals who need a quick, handy, clinically oriented reference on alcohol and other drug problems. A parallel text, entitled *Educating Yourself About Alcohol and Drugs*, presents a similar message in terms useful to patients and clients and their friends and families.[17] Similar to the approach used in major diagnostic manuals, the emphasis here is on substances of abuse and related disorders, and does not include discussion of "compulsive" behavioral syndromes such as gambling and compulsive shopping.[18]

1.1.2. Changes Incorporated into this Sixth Edition

The first edition of this text was published in 1979, and received complimentary reviews. Each subsequent edition has incorporated new developments in the field, and updated more than half of the references.

This sixth edition is the first to use information from the new millennium. In addition, it is the first being developed entirely under the auspices of our current publisher. Both transitions (i.e., time and publisher) contributed to the decision to thoroughly revise what is offered here. This has involved a number of changes.

First, an effort has been made to update about 80% of the references so as to primarily reflect citations published since 2000. Second, in order to optimize the ease of use for the reader, and to keep the cost of the text as low as possible, the material has been streamlined. This includes attempts to list key, most salient references, and keeping the length of each chapter as short as possible while still covering all the material that needs to be presented.

A third, related step has been to combine chapters whereever appropriate. For example, prior editions of the text were based on the increasing prevalence of the use of phencyclidine (PCP) and related drugs such as ketamine. However, in recent years the prevalence of use of these substances has remained relatively low and stable, and their pattern of use on the streets has continued to greatly overlap with the more classical hallucinogens. Therefore, what was previously known as Chapter 9 on PCP has been combined with the traditional hallucinogens in Chapter 8. As a result, Chapter 10 from the prior texts has become Chapter 9, Chapter 11 has become Chapter 10, and so on.

The previous edition was the first to prepare a separate section (Chapter 16) dealing with prevention. While I recognize the great importance of this topic, the feedback we received regarding the fifth edition indicates that readers have focused primarily on the specific drug-related chapters, as well as the descriptions of treatment approaches, but may have found the information on prevention less directly useful to their clinical work. Therefore, Chapter 16 has been deleted and the most salient information incorporated into a subsection of Chapter 1.

Another important development in recent years is the beginning of the process of planning for the fifth edition of the *Diagnostic and Statistical*

Manual of the American Psychiatric Association, which will probably be published sometime soon after 2010. I have been fortunate to be involved in the process, and have used my experience as Chair of the DSM-IV Substance Use Disorders Workgroup and my efforts to date on developing information for DSM-V to update and better focus the material on diagnostic-related issues.

The resulting text deals primarily with the most recent information available, and is a bit slimmer and more directly clinically -focused than was true for the fifth edition.

1.1.3. The Structure of the Book

While changes have been made, this edition of *Drug and Alcohol Abuse* maintains the same basic structure that has worked so well in the past. This first chapter addresses the need to learn the drug *classes* and the relevant problem areas from which generalizations can be made. Chapters 2–11 deal with a specific class of drugs each. The discussion in each of these chapters is subdivided into general information sections on the drugs in that class and sections covering the problems faced in emergency situations. Chapter 12 deals with multidrug misuse, Chapter 13 briefly outlines an approach to treatment in emergency situations, and Chapter 14 presents most of the material on rehabilitation.

The text can be used in at least two basic ways:

1. *If you are treating an emergency problem* and know the probable class of the drug involved, you will turn to the emergency problem section of the relevant chapter. If you do not know the drug and need some general emergency guidelines, you will use the appropriate subsections of this chapter and Chapter 13. Emphasis is placed on the most relevant drug-related material, and it is assumed that the reader already has some working knowledge of the more general issues such as counseling techniques and/or physical diagnosis, laboratory procedures, and the treatment of life-threatening emergencies.

   Once the emergency has been handled, you will want to read the information available on that class of drugs. At your leisure, then, you might review the general information presented in this chapter and go on to read the first section and some of the new and updated references cited in the bibliography of the relevant chapter.
2. *If you are interested in learning about drug classes* and their possible emergency problems, you should begin by skimming all the chapters. After gaining some level of comfort with the general thrust of the material, you can then reread in detail those sections of most interest to you, going on to the more pertinent references. The first section of each chapter contains as little medical jargon as possible.

To address these goals and to make each chapter as complete in itself as possible (in the emergency room you do not want to have to jump too much from chapter to chapter), there is some redundancy in the sections of the various chapters that deal with the same subjects. The misuse of drugs of different classes, for example, may give rise to problems that require similar treatment. I have tried, however, to strike a balance between readability and clinical usefulness.

No handbook can answer all questions about every drug. The emergency-oriented nature of this text also tends to lead to oversimplification of rather complex problems. So, it is important to remember that I give general rules that will need to be modified in specific clinical situations. Although you will not know everything about drugs after finishing the book, it is a place to start learning.

To present the material in the most efficient way, I have used a number of shortcuts.

1. In giving the generic names of medications, I have deleted the suffixes that indicate which salt forms are used [e.g., *chlordiazepoxide hydrochloride* is noted as *chlordiazepoxide* (Librium)] because they provide relatively little useful information.
2. The specific medications recommended for treatment in the emergency room setting represent the idiosyncrasies of my personal experience as well as those of other authors in the literature. The physician will usually be able to substitute another drug of the same class so that he or she can use a medication with which he or she has had experience [for example, when I note the use of haloperidol (Haldol), the physician might substitute *comparable* doses of trifluoperazine (Stelazine) or of risperidone (Risperdal).
3. *Treatment of emergency medical situations is complex and beyond the scope of this book*. Very general guidelines are offered in relevant chapters, but the reader is strongly encouraged to consult established medical texts (e.g., Kasper et al.'s *Harrison's Principles of Internal Medicine*) or emergency texts (e.g., Ma and Cline's *Emergency Medicine Manual*).[19,20]
4. The dose ranges of medications recommended for treatment of emergency situations are *approximations only* and will have to be modified for the individual patient based on the clinical setting and the patient's characteristics.
5. Although the treatment discussions are frequently offered as a series of steps (as seen in most of the discussions of toxic reactions or overdose conditions), the order offered is a general guideline that may be modified for the particular clinical setting.
6. It must be noted that the appropriate place for treating most emergency problems such as toxic reactions (overdoses) is in a hospital. However, many other problems can be handled in outpatient settings.

I have attempted to use the limited space I have in a manner that reflects the frequency with which the nonspecialist clinician encounters substance-related problems. Therefore, the greatest amount of material is presented for the substance most likely to be noted clinically, alcohol. Also, alcohol and opioids, drugs for which the most data on rehabilitation are available, are used as prototypes for the other discussions of rehabilitation.

The genesis of most alcohol and drug problems rests with a complex interaction between biological and environmental factors.[21] Regarding the former, there is evidence that genetic factors may influence smoking and other drug-taking behaviors, and there is excellent evidence, which is briefly mentioned in Chapter 3, that genetic factors contribute to the genesis of alcoholism. However, consistent with the clinical focus of this book, etiology is not typically covered in depth.

Two final notes that reflect the sensitivities of our times are needed. To save time and space, male pronouns are used in the text for the most part but are meant to refer to both genders. For similar goals of efficiency, the terms *client*, *patient*, and *subject* are used interchangeably.

1.2. SOME DEFINITIONS

Before we can begin, it is important to set forth some clinical concepts central to the discussion of substance-related problems. The definitions that follow might not always be the most pharmacologically sophisticated, but they are useful. To arrive at these terms, I have borrowed from a variety of standard texts and published studies, attempting to blend them into a clinically relevant framework.

1.2.1. Drug of Abuse

A drug of abuse is any substance, taken through any route of administration, that alters the mood, the level of perception, or brain functioning.[17,22] These include some prescribed medications, alcohol, inhalants, and all the categories of substances described below. All are capable of producing changes in mood and altered states of learning.

There are a number of other clinical problems I considered to include. For instance, there are parallels between some forms of obesity and the misuse of drugs. Similarly, compulsive gambling has much of the "feel" of the "obsessive" behavior observed during substance dependence.[17] However, these problems are not listed with the substance-use disorders in the fourth edition of *Diagnostic and Statistical Manual of Mental Disorders* (DSM-IV-TR), and it is not possible for one text to cover everything.[23] Expansion into these topics, interesting as they might be, could jeopardize my attempt to cover clinically related topics succinctly and thereby help the clinician in his or her day-to-day practice.

1.2.2. Substance-Related Disorders

The majority of people in Western societies are current or past users of at least one psychoactive drug (e.g., caffeine, nicotine, alcohol, marijuana), and a large proportion of users have had some adverse experience related to a substance (e.g., heartburn or anxiety from coffee, a cough from smoking cigarettes, driving with someone impaired with alcohol). Although use and temporary problems should be noted for any individual, these are not synonymous with diagnosable disorders.

As used in this text, a label or diagnosis is a guide to determine when it is appropriate to intervene and which treatment has the best chance of doing the best with the least harm. Whenever possible, criteria (e.g., abuse, dependence, intoxication, withdrawal, or a substance-induced disorder) should be stated in objective terms, with studies demonstrating the usual clinical course and response to treatment for individuals who meet criteria for that diagnosis.[24] Thus, the overall emphasis in this book is on the DSM-IV. The criteria for abuse and dependence are briefly presented in Table 1.1.

1.2.2.1. Intoxication and Withdrawal

The diagnostic criteria for *intoxication* are straightforward. There must be evidence of recent ingestion of the substance, clinically relevant behavioral and psychological changes must be observed, and a variety of specific signs (which differ for different types of drugs) must be documented.

The criteria for *withdrawal* are most relevant to the depressants (including alcohol), stimulants (e.g., all forms of cocaine and amphetamines as well as many weight-reducing drugs), and opioids (e.g., heroin, methadone, and prescription pain pills). Here, the diagnostic criteria require evidence that a person has used that substance regularly and heavily, has recently decreased or stopped use, and now demonstrates a pattern of signs and symptoms that in general are the opposite of the acute effects of the drug.

1.2.2.2. Substance Dependence: The "Official Definition"

Dependence may be a more reliable and valid (regarding predicting outcome) diagnosis than abuse.[25,26] DSM-IV uses a broad concept of dependence to indicate a central role that the substance has come to play in the individual's life, evidence of problems relating to controlling intake, and the development of difficulties (especially physical and psychological problems) despite which the individual continues to return to the substance. DSM-IV requires that a minimum of three of seven substance-related items occur and cluster together within the same 12-month period. Once a patient has been diagnosed as having dependence on a particular substance, the clinician knows that he or she is highly likely to have significant problems with this substance in the future if use continues or resumes.[27] The 10th edition of the

Table 1.1
DSM-IV Criteria for Abuse and Dependence

Abuse

A. A maladaptive pattern of substance use leading to clinically significant impairment or distress, as manifested by one or more of the following occurring at any time during the same 12-month period:
   1. Recurrent substance use resulting in a failure to fulfill major role obligations at work, school, or at home (e.g., repeated absences or poor work performance related to substance use; substance related absences, suspensions, or expulsions from school; neglect of children or of household).
   2. Recurrent substance use in situations in which it is physically hazardous (e.g., driving an automobile or operating a machine when impaired by substance use).
   3. Recurrent substance-related legal problems (e.g., arrests for substance-related disorderly conduct).
   4. Continued substance use despite having persistent or recurrent social or interpersonal problems.

B. Has never met the criteria for Substance Dependence for this class of substance.

Dependence[a, b]

A maladaptive pattern of substance use leading to clinically significant impairment or distress, as manifested by three or more of the following occurring at any time in the same 12-month period:

1. Tolerance, as defined by either of the following:
   (a) Need for markedly increased amounts of the substance to achieve intoxication or desired effect.
   (b) Markedly diminished effect with continued use of the same amount of the substance.
2. Withdrawal, as manifested by either of the following:
   (a) The characteristic withdrawal syndrome for the substance.
   (b) The same (or closely related) substance is taken to relieve or avoid withdrawal symptoms.
3. The substance is often taken in larger amounts or over a longer period than was intended.
4. A persistent desire or unsuccessful efforts to cut down or control substance use.
5. A great deal of time is spent in activities necessary to obtain the substance (e.g., visiting multiple doctors or driving long distances), use the substance (e.g., chain smoking), or recover from its effects.
6. Important social, occupational, or recreational activities given up or reduced because of substance use.
7. Continued substance use despite knowledge of having had a persistent or recurrent physical or psychological problem that was likely to have been caused or exacerbated by the substance (e.g., current cocaine use despite recognition of cocaine-induced depression, or continued drinking despite recognition that an ulcer was made worse by alcohol consumption).

[a]If tolerance and/or withdrawal have been documented as part of the dependence syndrome, the appropriate diagnosis is dependence with a physiological component.
[b]Abuse is not to be diagnosed if the person meets criteria for dependence on that substance.

International Classification of Diseases (ICD-10) uses similar criteria, although six rather than seven items are listed.[28]

1.2.2.3. Substance Abuse

The DSM-IV diagnostic criteria for *abuse* require evidence of repeated occurrences within a 12-month period of any of four possible social, legal, or interpersonal problems related to the substance. This expanded diagnostic list for abuse in DSM-IV was developed because the definition of abuse in the third revised edition of the *Diagnostic and Statistical Manual* (DSM-III-R) and its companion, "harmful use" in the ICD-10, were not likely to identify the same individuals and they were unreliable. Abuse appears to be reliable and it predicts the course of future problems fairly well.[24,29]

1.2.2.4. Other Meanings for Dependence

Dependence can also refer to a psychological and/or physical "need" for the drug. Furthermore, it can be important to distinguish between physical and psychological dependence.

1. *Psychological dependence* is an attribute of all drugs of abuse[21,22] and centers on the user feeling that he or she needs the drug to reach a maximum level of functioning or well-being. This is a subjective concept that is difficult to quantify and, thus, is of limited clinical use.
2. *Physical dependence* indicates that the body has adapted physiologically to the chronic use of the substance, with the development of tolerance or, when the drug is stopped, of withdrawal symptoms.
   a. *Tolerance* is the toleration of higher and higher doses of the drug or the need for higher doses to achieve the same effects. The phenomenon occurs both through alterations in drug metabolism by which the liver destroys the substance more quickly (*metabolic tolerance*), and via physiological changes in the functioning of the target cells (usually in the nervous system) in the presence of the drug (*pharmacodynamic tolerance*). Tolerance is not an all-or-none phenomenon, and an individual may develop resistance to one aspect of a drug's action and not another. The development of tolerance to one drug of a class usually indicates *cross tolerance* to other drugs of the same class.[22]
   b. *Withdrawal* or an *abstinence syndrome* is the appearance (when the drug is decreased or stopped quickly) of physiological symptoms that are the opposite of the usual acute effects. This phenomenon was described most completely for opioids, depressants, or stimulants, substances that depress or enhance the action of the central nervous system (CNS) or brain. Like tolerance, withdrawal is not an all-or-none phenomenon and usually consists of a syndrome

comprising a wide variety of possible symptoms, with patterns that are different for opioids, depressants, and stimulants.

DSM-III-R in 1980 was the first of the major diagnostic manuals to fail to emphasize a special relevance for tolerance and/or withdrawal in defining dependence. While there were good theoretical reasons for this move, there was insufficient research evidence to evaluate the clinical implications of the paradigm shift. Therefore, the framers of DSM-IV requested that clinicians and researchers subdivide individuals with dependence into those with and without a physiological component. Recent papers continue to support this distinction indicating that the presence of those physiological symptoms, especially a history of withdrawal from a substance, are associated with more intense substance use and related problems.[30,26] These data support the usefulness of the distinction between dependence with and without a physiological component, findings which might be useful for DSM-V which is in the early planning phases.

1.3. GENERAL COMMENTS ABOUT DRUG MECHANISMS

All of the drugs described in this text cross relatively easily from the blood to the brain and affect how an individual feels.[22] These changes are usually perceived as pleasurable or rewarding, with the result that many people continue to take the substances even in the face of serious consequences.

The mechanisms through which this "reinforcement" occurs differ across drugs. This sixth edition of the text offers detailed and expanded discussions of these mechanisms in the "Pharmacology" subsections of each relevant chapter, with an emphasis on papers published since 2000. Examples of some of these mechanisms include the ability of stimulants (both amphetamines and cocaine) to cause the release of the brain chemicals dopamine and norepinephrine and to affect the dopamine transporter, and the actions of opioids on the opioid receptor systems. In addition, a variety of overlapping mechanisms of action can be described for the cannabinoids, hallucinogens, inhalants, and so on.

These relatively diverse mechanisms of action all share an ability to produce a false sense of satisfaction, or fitness.[31,32] This is thought to be "false" in that the feeling of reinforcement did not occur in response to any essential activity of the body such as the satisfaction of thirst, supplying of nutrients, sleep, or sex. Nonetheless, these drug-related physiological changes are perceived as rewarding and contribute to subsequent feelings of craving or "wanting" for the substance while interfering with the ability of the body to function and to appropriately respond to important cues in the environment.

In addition to the divergent neurochemical actions that are a bit more substance specific (e.g., cocaine and the dopamine transporter and cannabinols and their related receptors), there are also some important shared mechanisms across substances. Prominent among these is the ability of most drugs of abuse to change the level of adaptation of the coupling of G proteins to receptors, and to upregulate the activity of adenosine 3*N*, 5*N*-monophosphate (cAMP).[33] Drugs of abuse also share important direct or indirect effect on the activity of the neurotransmitter dopamine in the nucleus accumbens and broader ventral tegmental area of the brain.[34,30] This mesolimbic area is involved in feelings of reinforcement or reward from a wide range of sources including food and sex, and play a role in the perception of pleasure. Alcohol, nicotine, opioids, stimulants, and many other drugs increase the amount of dopamine in these areas, with evidence that these changes parallel the feeling of intoxication or high.[35,36] Thus, it is hypothesized that the "dopamine reward system" might serve as a final common pathway for some drug effects. However, it is important to remember that no single mechanism is likely to explain the majority of drug actions, and careful study of the pharmacological effects relevant to each drug is needed.

The problems of understanding what to expect with a specific drug are even more complex for drugs bought "on the street." Most of these substances are not pure, and many [almost 100% for such drugs as tetrahydrocannabinol (see Section 1.5.4)] do not even contain the purported major substances.[37] Thus, one must apply the general lessons discussed in this text carefully, staying alert for unexpected consequences when treating drug abusers.

Specific drug actions depend on the route of administration, the dose, the presence or absence of other drugs, and the patient's clinical condition. Disposition, metabolism, and sensitivity to substances are also affected by genetic mechanisms, probably both through levels of end-organ sensitivity (e.g., in the CNS) and through the amount and characteristics of the enzymes of metabolism and the amount of protein binding. One important factor to consider in predicting reactions to drugs is age, as growing older is accompanied not only by increased brain sensitivity but also by a reduction in total drug clearance for many substances, especially for the depressants.

In summary, a clinically oriented text such as this can make generalizations about the mechanisms of drug actions, but there are important, specific differences between drugs. The reader is referred to general pharmacology texts, including Goodman and Gilman's *Pharmacological Basis of Therapeutics*, for more details.[9]

1.4. SOME THOUGHTS ON EPIDEMIOLOGY

Two out of three men and women in the United States are drinkers at some point in their lives, even higher numbers have consumed caffeinated beverages, and many have used tobacco products. In fact, the pattern of substance use in most parts of the world is prodigious, even without considering the intake of illegal substances.

Regarding the latter, data are available from interviews carried out yearly with Americans of age 12 and above.[38] However, it is also important to remember that a third of 10- to –12-year olds in some studies have been offered drugs or were in situations where illicit substances are being used.[39] Regarding the U.S., overall about 36% admitted to ever having had experience with an illegal substance, including 40% of men and 31% of women. More than 11% had taken an illicit substance in the prior year (14% of men and 8% of women), along with 6% (8 and 4% across the genders) who had ingested such substances in the prior month. The ages with the highest lifetime rates of consumption of illegal substances (51%) was 26–34 years, including 56% of men and 46% of women. The 18–25-age range had the highest prevalence of illicit drug taking in the prior year (25% overall, including 31% of men and 20% of women), as well as in the prior month (15% overall, 20% in men, and 10% in women). Other studies confirm the higher rates in men, as well as the still substantial risks for use in women.[40–42] Illicit substance use was observed in all parts of the country, all socioeconomic strata, and in all ethnicities. The lifetime history of intake was slightly higher in the West (41%) and in the North Central areas (37% in the lifetime) as compared to the South (33%) and the Northeast (33%). Regarding racial groups, 42% of white men, 39% of Black men, and 32% of Latino men reported ever having consumed any illicit substance. For women, the lifetime histories across the three racial groups were 34%, 25%, and 19%, respectively. Across the three groups, a history of ever having consumed an illicit drug through a needle was about 1% for each group.

The relatively high lifetime rates for exposure to illicit substances among younger cohorts was also investigated by the yearly Monitoring the Future Survey of high school students.[6] In 2003, 51% of 12th grade students admitted to ever having consumed an illicit drug, compared to 41% of 10th graders, and 23% of those in the 8th grade. Focusing on the consumption of illicit substances in the prior year, the rates were 39, 32, and 16% across the three grades.

Most other countries tend to report lower levels of experience with illicit drugs. However, a survey of more than 3,000 university students in the United Kingdom revealed that 60% of the men and 55% of the women admitted to ever having used marijuana, including 20% who consumed the drug weekly,[43] and a survey of secondary school students in that country reported that 65% of such students admitted to ever having taken an illicit drug.[44] The proportion of individuals who have consumed drugs was lower in Latin America as demonstrated by surveys in Mexico, Brazil, Uruguay, and Peru, and was also significantly lower in Spain.[45,46] These included a lifetime rate of use of about 10% in northern Mexico, and a rate of experience with illicit drugs among 15–65-year olds in Uruguay of 4.5%.

Studies from the United States, with their high rates and more detailed data, offer some insights about how rates have changed over the years.[6] Most studies reveal that the highest figures of drug intake occurred in the mid-1970s to mid-1980s, after which rates for most substances decreased until the early 1990s. Unfortunately, the lifetime history of exposure to several types of illicit drugs has slowly increased since the mid-1990s to around 2000 when rates began to plateau. For example, among high school seniors, the proportion who ever took an illicit substance decreased from 47.9% in 1990 to a low of 40.7% in 1992, after which figures rose to 48.4% in 1995, 50.8% in 1996, and 54.3% in 1997.

Diagnoses of abuse or dependence are, unfortunately, also quite common.[47,48] These substance-use disorders are among the most often observed diagnoses from the DSM-IV. The lifetime risk for alcohol abuse or dependence is between 15 and 20% for men, with lower but still substantial figures for women. However, overall, a recent study of students at U.S. universities revealed about 30% ever met criteria for alcohol abuse, with 6% for alcohol dependence.[47] Repetitive use of alcohol and other drugs contributes to problems in the workplace, can cause a wide range of psychiatric symptoms, is a substantial factor in a large proportion of fatal accidents, and exacerbates almost all major medical problems. The conditions described in the chapters that follow have great relevance in any clinical practice setting.

The pattern of use for each specific group of drugs in the mid to late 1990s is discussed in more detail in each of the relevant chapters that follow. In general, for most substances the period of highest prevalence of use as well as the highest likely quantity of intake occurs between the mid-teens and mid-20s. Most people begin with caffeine or nicotine, move on to alcohol, and, if experimentation with drugs continues, progress on to cannabinols, then any mixture of stimulants, depressants, and/or hallucinogens, and on to opioids. The proportion of the population continuing to use and the intensity of intake both decrease with each subsequent decade of adult life. In general, most substances are more likely to be taken by men than women, though among those men there are few large ethnic differences in substance-use disorders.

Of course, there are some subgroups of the population that appear to be more vulnerable to the development of problems with some substances. One group at high risk are young people with conduct disorder.[49] Another involves health care workers, including physicians, medical students, and nurses. They have rates of alcohol dependence that resemble those of the general population, but their risk for abuse or dependence on some other substances is substantially higher.[50,51] Among these, dependence appears to be highest for physicians in general practice, in anesthesiology, and in psychiatry, in decreasing order. The risk appears to be highest for prescription substances, especially opioids (e.g., prescription pain pills) and brain depressants (e.g., the Valium-type drugs and the barbiturates drugs used for the treatment of anxiety or insomnia). There are many theories about the potential role of job stress, fear of making mistakes, and long hours of work as contributors toward this vulnerability for problems with drugs, but it is equally likely that the major difficulty involves the ease of access to drugs of abuse.

1.5. ONE APPROACH TO DRUG CLASSIFICATION

It is possible to learn the characteristics of a drug class and then to apply the general rules to the specific case. While there are many possible classifications, I present a breakdown of drugs into classes that have particular usefulness in clinical settings and in which the drug class is determined by the most prominent CNS effects at the usual doses.[21,52]

This drug classification is presented in Table 1.2, along with some examples of the more frequently encountered drugs of each class. The classes are discussed in the following sections.

1.5.1. The Depressants

The most prominent effect of these drugs is the depression of tissues at all levels of the brain, along with relatively few analgesic properties at the usual doses.[52] The depressants include most sleeping medications, antianxiety drugs (also called *anxiolytics or minor tranquilizers*), and alcohol. The antipsychotic drugs (also called *major tranquilizers* or *neuroleptics*), such as chlorpromazine (Thorazine), risperidone (Risperdal), or haloperidol (Haldol), are *not* depressants, do not resemble the antianxiety drugs in their structures or predominant effects, do not cause physical dependence, and are rarely used to induce a "high."

Table 1.2
Drug Classification Used in This Text

Class	Some examples
Depressants	Alcohol, hypnotics, most antianxiety drugs (benzodiazepines)
Sympathomimetics or stimulants	Amphetamine, methylphenidate, all forms of cocaine, weight-reducing products
Opioids	Heroin, morphine, methadone, and almost all prescription analgesics
Cannabinols	Marijuana, hashish
Hallucinogens	Lysergic acid diethylamide (LSD), mescaline, psilocybin, ecstasy (MDMA)
Inhalants	Aerosol sprays, glues, toluene, gasoline, paint thinner
Over-the-counter drugs	Contain: atropine, scopolamine, weak stimulants, antihistamines, weak analgesics
Others	Phencyclidine (PCP)

1.5.2. Sympathomimetics or Stimulants

The predominant effect of these drugs at the usual doses is the stimulation of brain tissues. Some of these drugs block removal of some stimulatory neurotransmitters (chemicals released from one brain cell to stimulate the next cell) from the space between nerve cells (the synapse). Other substances also enhance actions of stimulatory systems by the release of transmitters from the cells or by direct action on the cells themselves. The substances most relevant to clinical situations include all the amphetamines, methylphenidate (Ritalin) or similar drugs, many prescription weight reducing medications, and all forms of cocaine. The related substances nicotine and caffeine are discussed separately in Chapter 11, as their pattern of associated problems is limited and their actions quite different from the classical stimulants.

1.5.3. Opioids

These drugs, also called *narcotic analgesics*, are used clinically to decrease pain, cough, or diarrhea. They include morphine and other alkaloids of opium as well as synthetic morphine-like substances and semisynthetic opium derivatives. Prominent examples include almost all pain-killing medications, ranging from propoxyphene (Darvon) to methadone (Dolophine) along with oxycodone (Percodan) and pentazocine (Talwin) and, for all practical purposes, tramadol (Ultram) and similar medications.

1.5.4. Cannabinols (Principally Marijuana)

The active ingredient in all these substances is tetrahydrocannabinol (THC), which has the predominant effects of producing euphoria, an altered time sense, and, at doses higher than those usually found in clinical situations, hallucinations. This is a "street" drug sold in the United States primarily as marijuana or hashish, as pure THC is almost never available on the "black market."

1.5.5. Hallucinogens (Ketamine and Phencyclidine or PCP)

The predominant effect of these substances is the production of enhanced sensory perceptions. At higher doses the classical hallucinogens can also produce hallucinations, usually of geometric shapes and colors or flashing lights. The hallucinogens have no accepted medical usefulness and are a second example of "street" drugs. PCP is misused as a hallucinogen but, here, hallucinations are only likely to be observed in the context of an agitated, confused state (a delirium).

1.5.6. Inhalants: Glues, Solvents, and Aerosols

These substances include various fuels, aerosol sprays, glues, paints, and industrial solutions. They are used as drugs of abuse in attempts to alter the state of consciousness, producing primarily light-headedness and confusion.

1.5.7. Over-the-Counter and Some Prescription Drugs

A variety of substances are sold without prescription for the treatment of constipation, pain, cold symptoms, nervousness, insomnia, and other common complaints. The sedative or hypnotic medications are the most frequently misused, contain antihistamines, and can be taken to produce feelings of light-headedness and euphoria. There are also a number of other prescription drugs that are less likely than the substances listed above to be misused, including diuretics, antiparkinsonian drugs, laxatives, and some antipsychotics.

1.6. ALTERNATE CLASSIFICATION SCHEMES

An additional breakdown of these substances, addressing a series of "schedules" developed by the Federal Drug Enforcement Administration (DEA), is presented in Table 1.3.[53] The classification is based on both the degree of medical usefulness and the misuse potential of the substance, ranging from Schedule I, which includes those drugs with few accepted medical uses and a high probability of misuse (e.g., heroin), to Schedule V, drugs that have a high level of medical usefulness and relatively little misuse potential. Unfortunately, it is not always possible to generalize from the schedule level to the actual drug dangers, as exemplified by the classification of marijuana and heroin at the same level.

Table 1.3
DEA Drug Schedules with Examples

Schedule	Examples
I. (High potential for misuse, low usefulness)	Heroin
	Hallucinogens
	Cannabinols
	Methaqualone (Quaaludes)
II.	Opium
	Codeine
	Morphine
	Most prescription opioids (e.g., fentanyl)
	Methadone and LAAM
	Amphetamines, methylphenidate (Ritalin), phenmetrazine (Preludin)
	Most barbiturates [e.g., secobarbital (Seconal)]
	Glutethimide (Doriden)
	PCP
	Dronabinol (Merinol)

(*Continued*)

Table 1.3
DEA Drug Schedules with Examples—Cont'd

Schedule	Examples
III.	Most barbiturates as combination drugs
	Methyprylon (Noludar)
	Medications with limited opioids in combinations (e.g., aspirin with codeine)
	Anabolic steroids
	Ketamine
IV.	Propoxyphene (Darvon)
	Phenobarbitol (Luminol)
	Chloral hydrate (Noctec)
	Benzodiazepines
	Ethchlorvynol (Placidyl)
	Fenfluramine (Pondimin)
	Phentermine (Fastin)
	Pemoline (Cylert)
	Diethylpropion (Tenuate)
V. (Low potential for misuse, very high usefulness)	Low dose opioid mixtures
	Buprenorphine (Buprenex)

Another approach is to classify them by their "street" names (Table 1.4). These differ from one locale to another and at the same place over time; therefore, this table contains only a brief list of some of the more relevant street names that are *usually* used. It is important to learn the specific drug names in your vicinity. In the table, drugs are divided into the major classes outlined in this chapter, and the street names are given alphabetically within

Table 1.4
A Brief List of "Street" Drug Names

Depressants[a]			
Amies	Downs	Quads	T-bird
Blue birds	Fours and Dors (glutethimide plus codeine)	Rainbows	Ts and Ds (glutethimide plus codeine)
Blue devil	Goofballs	Red birds	Tooies
Blue heaven	Green and whites (Librium)	Red devils	Toolies
Blues	Greenies	Roaches (Librium)[b]	Tranqs (Librium-type)
Bullets	Ludes	Roofies (Robypnol)	Wallbangers
Candy	Mickey Finn (chloral hydrate and alcohol)	Roshay (Robypnol)	Yellow jackets
Christmas trees	Nebbies	Seccy	Yellows
Dolls	Nembies	Seggy	Zim Zims (Zopiclone)
Double trouble	Peanus	Sleepers	
Downers	Peter (chloral hydrate)	Soapers	

(*Continued*)

Table 1.4
A Brief List of "Street" Drug Names—Cont'd

Stimulants					
Amphetamines			Cocaine		Other
Bennies	Double cross	Pinks	Blow	Lady	Khat
Blue angels	Footballs	Pink and green	C	Nose	Ma-Huang (ephedrine)
Blue beauties	Green and clears	Roses	Coke	Nose candy	Iceberg (benzocaine and/or procaine)
Chris	Greenies	Speed	Crack	Rock	Snort (benzocaine and/or procaine)
Christine	Hearts	Truck drivers	Dust	Snow	Cocaine snuff (caffeine)
Christmas tree	LA turn-arounds	Turnarounds	Dynamite	Speedball (cocaine plus heroin)	Coca snow (caffeine)
Coast to coast	Lip poppers	Uppers	Flake	Toot	Incense (caffeine)
Copilot	Meth	Ups	Gold dust	White	Zoom
Crisscross	Oranges	Wake-ups	Heaven dust		
Crossroads	Peaches	Whites			
Crystal (IV methamphetamine)[b]	Pep pills	Yellow Jackets			

Opioids			
Heroin		Other	
Bomb	Junk	Black (opium)	PG or PO (paregoric)
Brother	Mexican mud	Blue velvet (paregoric plus antihistamine	Pinks and grays (Darvon)
Brown	Scat	Dollies (methadone)[b]	Poppy (opium)
Cat	Shit	Fours and Dors (codeine plus glutethimide)	Tar (opium)
Chinese white	Skag	M (morphine)	Terp (terpin hydrate or cough syrup with codeine)

Analgesics			
Heroin		Other	
Dogie	Smack	Microdots[b]	T's and blues (Talwin and antihistamine)
Duji	Snow	Miss Emma (morphine)	Ts and Ds (codeine plus glutethimide)

(*Continued*)

Table 1.4
A Brief List of "Street" Drug Names—Cont'd

Duster (cigarette)	Speedball (heroin plus cocaine	Morphy (morphine)
H	Stuff	O (opium)
H and stuff	Tango and cash	Pellets (opium)
Horse		

Cannabinols

Marijuana			Hashishlike (more potent)		
Acapulco gold	Gold	Lid	Rope	Bhang	Hash
Afgani	Grass	Locoweed	Sativa	Charas	Rope
A stick	Hay	Mary Jane	Stick	Gage	Sweet Lucy
Boo	Hemp	Mexican	Stuff	Ganja	THC
Bomb	J	MJ	Tea		
Brick	Jane	Muggles	Texas tea		
Buddah sticks	Jive	Pot	Thai sticks		
Columbian	Joint	Reefer	Weed		
Dope	Key or kee	Roach[b]	Yesca		

Phencyclidine (PCP)

Angel	Cosmos	Guerrilla	Mauve	Rocket fuel	Supergrass
Angel dust	Criptal	Hog	Mist	Shermans	Superjoint
Aurora	Dummy mist	Jet	Mumm dust	Special L.A. coke	Trangs
Busy bee	Goon	K	Peace pill	Superacid	Tranq
Cheap cocaine	Green	Lovely	Purple	Supercoke	Whack

Hallucinogens

Acid (LSD)	D (LSD)	Magic mushroom (psilocybin)	Pearly gates (morning glory seeds)
Blue dots (LSD)	Deaths head (psilocybin)	Mellow drug of America (MDA)	Psilocyn (psilocybin)
Blue heaven (LSD)	E (MDMA)	Mesc (mescaline)	STP (DOM)
Businessman's LSD (DMT)	Ecstasy (MDMA)	Mescal (mescaline)	Sugar (LSD)
Buttons (peyote)	Eve (MDA)	Mexican mushroom (psilocybin)	White lightening (LSD)
Cactus (mescaline)	Heavenly blue (LSD or morning glory seeds)	Microdots (LSD)	XCT (MDMA)
Crystal[b]	Love drug (MDMA)	Mushroom (psilocybin)	25 (LSD)
Cube (LSD)	Lysergide (LSD)	Owsleys (LSD)	

Other

Rush (amyl/butyl nitrate)	Belt (amyl/butyl nitrate)
Kick (amyl/butyl nitrate)	Nitrous (nitrous oxide)

[a]Most have a moderate length of action like secobarbital.
[b]Many drugs have the same name.

each class. For ease of reference, this is one of the few places in this text where trade names rather than generic names are used.

1.7. A CLASSIFICATION OF DRUG PROBLEMS

All drugs of abuse cause intoxication, *all induce psychological dependence* (feeling uncomfortable without the drug), and all are self-administered by an individual to change his level of consciousness or to increase psychological comfort. Indeed, if people did not begin to feel at least a psychological need for the drug, the substance would be unlikely to have caused a problem. Each class of drugs has its dangers, with patterns of problems differing among classes. In this section, I present some general concepts that will be discussed in greater depth in each chapter.

There is a limited range of adverse reactions to the drugs of abuse, and it is possible to summarize the drug classes and the problems most prominent for each (Table 1.5). In each chapter, for most types of problems (e.g., a psychosis), I first discuss the most common history, then note the usual physical signs and symptoms and the most prominent psychological difficulties, and, finally, give an overview of relevant laboratory tests. The generalizations presented for psychoses, states of confusion (e.g., a delirium), and so on are relatively consistent among drug categories, and only a brief discussion of the clinical picture is presented in each relevant chapter. On the other hand, the overdose or toxic reactions and the withdrawal pictures seen with the different drug classes differ enough that more detailed information is presented.

It is important at this juncture to note that, with the exception of some blood tests associated with recent heavy drinking, toxicological screens of

Table 1.5
Clinically Most Significant Drug Problems by Class

	Toxicity or overdose	With-drawal	Delirium or dementia[b]	Psychosis	Flash-backs	Depression or anxiety
Depressants	++[a]	++	++	+	–	++
Stimulants	++	+	–	++	–	++
Opioids	++	++	–	–	–	+
Cannabinols	–	–	–	++	+	–
Hallucinogens	+	–	–	–	++	+
Inhalants	++	–	++	–	–	–
Phencyclidine (PCP)	+	–	++	–	–	–
Over-the-counter	+	–	+	–	–	+

[a]++ means a likely and dramatic syndrome for that drug; + indicates that problems might occur but are not likely to be dramatic; – connotes lack of substantial evidence that this problem is likely to be seen for this drug, but does not mean the problem has been proven to never occur.
[b]A delirium or dementia is expected with any toxic reaction to a drug. As used here, however, a + or ++ indicates the likelihood of confusion during intoxication.

the urine (to determine *if* the drug has been taken in the last day perhaps the recent week or so) and blood toxicology tests (to determine *how much* of the substance, if any, is in the blood), there are few laboratory tests that help to establish a drug diagnosis. The normal laboratory result for each of the toxicological screens is at or near zero.

In the material that follows, a hierarchy has been established to help you address the most clinically significant problem first.

1. Any patient who has taken enough of a drug to seriously compromise his vital signs (e.g., blood pressure and respiration) is regarded as having an overdose or a *toxic reaction*. In this instance, any associated symptoms of confusion and/or hallucinations/delusions can be expected to clear as the overdose is properly treated.
2. Patients who demonstrate a drug-related clinical syndrome with relatively stable vital signs but show strong evidence of any of the three classical drug withdrawal states (even if the syndrome includes confusion or psychotic symptoms) are labeled withdrawal.
3. Patients with stable vital signs and no evidence of withdrawal, but with levels of drug-induced confusion, are regarded as having a substance-induced delirium or dementia, even if hallucinations or delusions are part of the clinical picture. In this instance, the psychotic symptoms can be expected to clear as the confusion lifts.
4. Patients who show stable vital signs, no evidence of clinically significant confusion, and no signs of withdrawal, but who show hallucinations and/or delusions without insight (i.e., resemble cases of schizophrenia), are regarded as having a *psychosis*.
5. Most remaining patients with clinical syndromes are likely to show evidence of intoxication or have a flashback or a drug-induced depression or anxiety state.

1.7.1. Toxic Reaction

A toxic reaction is an overdose that occurs when an individual has taken so much of the drug that the body support systems no longer work properly. Clinically, this reaction is most frequently seen with the depressants, stimulants, and opioids. Detailed discussions of these phenomena are given in each relevant chapter, as the picture differs markedly between drug classes. This diagnosis takes precedence even if signs of confusion or psychosis are present. This syndrome is discussed in detail in the relevant chapters (e.g., Chapters 2, 4–6, and 13).

1.7.2. Withdrawal or Abstinence Syndrome

The withdrawal or abstinence syndrome consists of physiological and psychological symptoms when a relevant drug is stopped too quickly.

The symptoms are usually the opposite of the acute effects of that same drug. For instance, for drugs that induce sleep, that can be used to help achieve relaxation, and that acutely decrease the heart rate and blood pressure (e.g., the depressants), withdrawal consists of insomnia, anxiety, and increase in pulse and blood pressure rate. The duration of the withdrawal syndrome varies directly with the half-life of the specific drug being misused (the time necessary to metabolize one-half of the drug), and the intensity increases with the usual dose taken and the length of time over which it was consumed. Treatment consists of a good medical evaluation, offering general support (e.g., rest and nutrition), and, for some classes, addressing the immediate cause of the withdrawal symptoms by administering enough of the substance (or any other drug of the same class) to markedly decrease symptoms on day 1 of treatment, and then decreasing the dose over the next 5 days or so (or longer for drugs with very long half-lives).

Clinically significant withdrawal syndromes are seen with the depressants, the opioids, and the stimulants. Because these syndromes differ for each specific kind of drug, the reader is encouraged to review each relevant chapter, and the symptoms are described in detail in Chapters 2, 4–6, and 13.

1.7.3. Delirium, Dementia, and Other Cognitive Disorders

These pictures consist of confusion, disorientation, and decreased intellectual functioning along with stable vital signs in the absence of signs of withdrawal.

1.7.3.1. Typical History

Any drug can induce confusion and/or disorientation if given in high enough doses, but at very high levels, the physical signs and symptoms of a toxic overdose predominate. There are a number of drugs, including the inhalants, the depressants, and PCP, that can produce confusion at relatively low doses. There are, in addition, some factors that predispose a person to confusion, including physical debilitation (e.g., hepatitis), Alzheimer's disease, a history of prior head trauma, or a long history of drug or alcohol dependence. These factors combine to explain the varied types of onset for confused states ranging from a very rapidly developing picture after PCP in a healthy young person, to a slow onset (e.g., over days to weeks) of increasing confusion for an elderly individual taking even therapeutic levels of depressants.

1.7.3.2. Physical Signs and Symptoms

As defined in this text, the confused patient most often presents with relatively stable vital signs and a predominance of mental pathology. However, because confusion is more likely to be seen in an individual with a physical problem, any mixture of physical signs and symptoms can be seen.

1.7.3.3. Psychological State

The patient demonstrates confusion about where he is, what he is doing there, the date and time, or who he is. He has trouble understanding concepts and assimilating new ideas, but usually maintains some insight into the fact that his mind is not working properly. This, in turn, may result in anxiety or irritability. These symptoms and signs may be accompanied by visual or tactile (i.e., being touched) hallucinations.

1.7.3.4. Relevant Laboratory Tests

The first step in treating any state of confusion is to rule out major medical problems. Although the delirium or dementia may continue beyond the length of action of any drug (especially in the elderly), a blood or urine toxicological screen may be helpful. It is also important to aggressively rule out all potentially reversible nondrug causes of confusion. Thus, in addition to a good neurological examination, blood tests should be drawn to determine the status of the electrolytes [especially Na, Ca, and K (see Table 1.6)], blood counts (especially the Hct and Hgb levels, as shown in the table) and liver and

Table 1.6
A Brief List of Relevant Laboratory Tests and Usual Norms

Abbreviation	Name	Usual value
	Serum chemistry	
—	Amylase	0–100 μ/l
—	Bilirubin	Total < 1.2 mg/dl Direct ≤ 0.2 mg/dl
BUN	Blood urea nitrogen	8–23 mg/dl
Ca	Calcium	8.4–10.2 mg/dl
CDT	Carbohydrate deficient transferrin	≤20 U/l
—	Creatinine	0.4–1.2 mg/dl
CPK	Creatine phosphokinase	0–175 IU/l
GGT	Gamma glutamyl transferase	≤35 U/l
—	Glucose	70–110 mg/dl
LDH	Lactic dehydrogenase	25–200 IU/l
Mg	Magnesium	1.6–2.5 mg/dl
K	Potassium	3.5–5.0 mMol/l
SGOT (AST)	Serum glutamic oxalacetic transaminase	15–65 IU/l
SGPT(ALT)	Serum glutamic pyruvic transaminase	17–67 IU/l
Na	Sodium	135–145 mMol/l
	Blood counts	
Hgb	Hemoglobin	Men: 14–18 g/dl Women: 12–16 g/dl
Hct	Hematocrit	Men: 42–52% Women: 37–47%
MCV	Mean corpuscular (RBC) volume	82–92 μ^3
WBC	White blood count	4.8–10.8 × 10^3 cells/μl

kidney function (including the BUN and creatinine for the kidney and the SGOT or AST, SGPT or ALT, and LDH for the liver). It is also necessary to consider the need for skull x-rays (to look for fractures and signs of internal bleeding), a spinal tap (to rule out bleeding, infection, or tumors of the CNS), and an EEG (to look for focal problems as well as general brain functioning).

1.7.4. Psychosis

A *psychosis*, as used here, occurs when an awake, alert, and relatively well-oriented individual with stable vital signs and no evidence of withdrawal experiences hallucinations or delusions *without insight*. The latter means he or she believes the hallucinations and "crazy thoughts" are real.

1.7.4.1. Typical History

Drug-induced psychoses are usually seen in individuals who have consumed higher doses of stimulants. They also develop in less than 5% of depressive dependent persons, and can be seen after consumption of extremely potent cannabinols. The onset of symptoms is usually abrupt (within hours to days) and represents a gross change from the person's normal level of functioning. The disturbance is dramatic and may result in the patient's being brought to a psychiatric facility or to the emergency room by police.

1.7.4.2. Physical Signs and Symptoms

There are few physical symptoms that are typical of any particular psychotic state. It is the loss of contact with reality beginning during intoxication that dominates the picture. However, during the psychosis, an individual may be quite upset and may present with a rapid pulse or an elevated blood pressure.

1.7.4.3. Psychological State

A psychosis occurs with the development of either hallucinations (an unreal sensory input, such as hearing things) or a delusion (an unreal and fixed thought into which the individual has no insight). In general, the drug-induced psychotic state begins during intoxication and lasts for several days to weeks of abstinence. Thankfully, it is usually totally reversible. As discussed in greater depth in the appropriate chapters, there is little, if any, evidence of permanent psychoses being induced in individuals who have shown no obvious psychopathology antedating their drug experience.

1.7.4.4. Relevant Laboratory Tests

No specific laboratory findings are associated with the psychosis, as the patient may be drug-free for several days or weeks but still out of contact with reality. For patients who misuse drugs intravenously, the stigmata of infection (e.g., a high WBC) and hepatitis (e.g., elevated SGOT or AST,

SGPT or ALT, CPK, and LDH) may be seen. It is also *possible* that a urine or blood toxicological screen will reveal evidence of a drug.

1.7.5. Flashbacks

A flashback, most frequently seen with the cannabinols and the hallucinogens, is the unwanted recurrence of drug effects. This is probably a heterogeneous group of problems, including the presence of residual drug in the body (e.g., with cannabinols), psychological stress, a behavioral "panic," or the possibility of a temporary alteration in brain functioning.

1.7.5.1. Typical History

This picture is most frequently seen after the repeated use of marijuana or hallucinogens. The typical patient gives a history of relatively recent drug use with no current intake to explain the episode of feeling "high."

1.7.5.2. Physical Signs and Symptoms

These depend on how the patient responds to the flashback, including his degree of "panic." Physical pathology is usually minimal and ranges from no physical symptoms to a full-blown panic.

1.7.5.3. Psychological State

The patient most typically complains of an altered time sense, feelings of unreality, or visual hallucinations (e.g., bright lights, geometric objects) or a "trailing" image (palinopsia) seen when objects move. Symptoms are most common when the subject enters darkness or before going to sleep. The emotional reaction may be one of perplexity or a panic like fear of brain damage or of going crazy.

1.7.5.4. Relevant Laboratory Tests

Except for the unusually intense or atypical case in which actual brain damage might be considered [which would require a brain-wave tracing or electroencephalogram (EEG), an adequate neurological examination, x-rays of the skull, and so on], there are no specific laboratory tests. The patient will probably be drug-free, and it is likely that even toxicological screens will not be helpful.

1.7.6. Anxiety and Depression

1.7.6.1. Typical History

Symptoms of sadness and nervousness are quite common in society and relate to personalities, situations, and reactions to stress. Even more strictly defined major depressive episodes and major anxiety disorders are seen in 15% or more of the general population at some time during their lives. Not only can symptoms of sadness and nervousness temporarily develop in the context of substance use, but even severe depressive episodes and symptoms resembling major anxiety syndromes (such as panic disorder, social phobia, and so on) can occur with heavy and repeated intake of substances.[54,55] Major depressive-like syndromes are likely to be seen with severe repeated *intoxication* with depressant drugs, whereas *withdrawal* from depressants is usually associated with temporary anxiety syndromes. *Intoxication* with stimulants can cause pictures that resemble major anxiety syndromes, whereas *withdrawal* from the stimulants resembles depression.

The high prevalence of substance-related symptoms of psychiatric syndromes, the high rate of actual major anxiety and depressive disorders in the general population, and the high prevalence of substance-use disorders require that all patients presenting with anxiety or depressive syndromes be considered as potentially having a substance-use disorder.[56] Thus, it is hard to pinpoint a "typical" history, but a high level of suspicion for potential substance-use disorders, especially those involving brain depressants or stimulants, must be kept in mind when evaluating patients with anxiety or depressive syndromes.

1.7.6.2. Physical Signs and Symptoms

Anxiety conditions are accompanied by multiple signs of increased adrenaline like activities. Conditions can range from general feelings of nervousness to insomnia to full-blown panic attacks characterized by palpitations, shortness of breath, and a fear that a heart attack is occurring. In addition, heightened levels of anxiety that can accompany stimulant intoxication and depressant withdrawal are likely to be associated with a feeling of intolerance of noise and discomfort with high levels of activity, with a resulting avoidance of social situations or crowds, which can be misdiagnosed as social phobia or agoraphobia.

Temporary depressive episodes occurring in the context of stimulant withdrawal and depressant intoxication, however, have few specific physical signs and symptoms.[56] Here, individuals are likely to complain of insomnia, a lack of ability to concentrate, and a loss of appetite but are not likely to demonstrate specific symptoms different from those seen in independent major depressive episodes.

1.7.6.3. Psychological State

Although the conditions that occur in relation to substance intoxication and withdrawal can closely resemble the psychiatric syndromes described in the DSM-IV as major depressive or major anxiety conditions,[23,57] it is important to remember that psychiatric pathology only observed in the context of intoxication or withdrawal from substances is likely to disappear within a month of abstinence without major intervention. These substance-induced conditions, therefore, improve more rapidly than the time antidepressant medications require to take effect. Hence, there are not data to support the usefulness of antidepressants, for example, in treating substance-induced conditions such as depressions.

1.7.6.4. Relevant Laboratory Tests

Depending on the patient's clinical picture, steps must be taken to rule out any obvious physical pathology. Thus, in addition to establishing the vital signs, it is necessary to evaluate the need for an electrocardiogram (EEG) and to draw routine baseline laboratory studies [e.g., red blood cell count, glucose, liver function, and kidney function tests, white blood cell count (WBC), and tests of skeletal or heart muscle damage, such as creatinine phosphokinase (CPK)]. Some of the more relevant tests, along with their abbreviations and *most usual* normal values, are presented in Table 1.6. Of course, when a drug-related condition is suspected but no adequate history can be obtained, urine (approximately 50 ml) and/or blood (approximately 10 cc) or hair samples should be sent to the laboratory for a toxicological screen to determine which, if any, drugs are present.

1.8. A GENERAL INTRODUCTION TO EMERGENCY AND CRISIS TREATMENT

The emergency care of the substance-dependent patient is covered within each chapter, and in a general review in Chapter 13. The treatment approaches represent common-sense applications of the lessons learned about the particular drug category, the probable natural course of that class of difficulty, and the dictum, "First, do no harm."

1.8.1. Acute Emergency Care

One must first address the life-threatening problems that may be associated with toxic reactions, psychoses, states of confusion, withdrawal, and medical problems. The approach to emergency care begins with establishing an adequate airway, supporting circulation and controlling hemorrhage, and dealing with any life-threatening behavior.

1.8.2. Evaluation

After the patient has been stabilized, it is important to evaluate other serious problems by gathering a good history from the patient and/or a resource person (usually a relative), doing careful physical and neurological examinations, and ordering the relevant laboratory tests.

1.8.3. Subacute Care

1. It is then possible to begin the more subacute care, attempting to keep medications to a minimum, especially for symptoms of *anxiety* and *flashbacks*, which tend to respond to reassurance.
2. For *toxic reactions*, the subacute goal is to support the vital signs until the body has had a chance to metabolize the ingested substance adequately.
3. The transient nature of the *psychoses* indicates that the best care is suppression of any destructive behavior during the several days to weeks necessary for the patient to recover. This often requires prescription of antipsychotic medications for a few days to a few weeks.
4. Evaluation of a delirium or dementia requires careful diagnosis and treatment of all life-threatening causes.
5. *Withdrawal* is usually treated by conducting an adequate physical evaluation to rule out associated medical disorders, giving rest and good nutrition, and, for depressants, slowly decreasing the level of the substance of abuse.
6. *Medical problems* are handled based on the specific syndrome observed.

1.9. THE ROLE OF DRUG TESTING

Over the 25 years since the publication of the first edition of this text, Western societies have become increasingly sophisticated regarding the dangers of substances in the workplace. Approaches to treatment and to monitoring of abstinence following rehabilitation efforts have also become more systematic and test oriented.

These thoughts relate to the use of drug testing both in the workplace and as a part of aftercare following treatment. A new industry has developed, and fine guidelines have been produced regarding the assets and liabilities of drug-testing procedures as well as their proper application.[58,59] The specific method to be used depends greatly on the goals of the testing (e.g., to monitor abstinence or to make sure that employees such as pilots are in optimal condition).

Regardless of the reasons for testing or the actual technical laboratory procedures, steps must be taken to optimize the validity of the sample obtained. Thus, the blood or urine sample must be taken under direct observation, the specimen must be carefully labeled, handling must be closely monitored, and all possible steps must be observed to be certain that the specific specimen delivered to the laboratory actually relates to the person named on the label on the test tube or vial.

With the exception of alcohol, for which breath samples can be taken, the determination of the amount or quantity of the substance in the body requires blood samples. Unfortunately, these quantitative methods can be too expensive for use in workplace screening or usual posttreatment monitoring. Thus, the majority of drug testing occurs through urine samples. Here, the results are often discussed in terms of sensitivity (the chances that a drug, if present, will be identified) and specificity (the proportion of substance-free samples that were accurate). The analytical approaches with high levels of both sensitivity and specificity are very costly. Therefore, the initial testing of a sample is usually carried out with several approaches that are highly sensitive (usually 98% or higher) but not as specific as one would like, with false-positive rates as high as 30–35%.

These less specific screening procedures usually utilize one of several forms of immunoassay.[57] In the enzyme immunoassay, animals are used to develop a specific antibody for a specific drug. Then, samples of the urine are mixed with samples of antibodies attached to an enzyme taken from animals. If the substance is present in the sample, the antibody, along with its attached enzyme, sticks to the drug. Subsequently, the presence (not the quantity) of the enzyme can be detected through a variety of chemical reactions, usually involving a change in color. Similar procedures involving mixing of antibodies related to specific drugs with samples of urine can also be carried out using radioactively labeled antibodies. Here, the amount of radioactivity in a sample will be related to the presence of the drug in that test tube of urine. The radioimmunoassay is even more sensitive than the enzyme approach but does involve greater expense and the additional safety problems associated with handling of radioactive materials.

No matter which of the less expensive but less specific assays is used for the initial screen, a positive result *must* be confirmed by a more expensive but more specific second analysis. Therefore, all samples determined to be positive for the presence of a drug by the first analysis must be saved and reanalyzed by the more expensive second methodology. The confirmatory evaluations usually involve some form of chromatography. In the thin-layer chromatography approach, the sample goes through a series of chemical steps to increase its purity, after which the prepared sample is placed on a thin glass plate where a small electric current causes migration, or movement, of the contents. Then, the subsamples of materials that have migrated or moved various distances in the electric current can be tested to determine whether these highly purified substances contain the drug.

A related confirmatory approach, called gas–liquid chromatography (GLC), also uses a purified preparation from the sample, which is injected into a glass or metal column in a machine. Subsequently, the material moves through the entire length of the column, and the time of movement or migration can be measured by the appearance of the substance at the far end where it is burned and the ignition noted on graph paper. Knowledge of the contents of the column and the time of appearance of the peak on a graph can be compared with samples of known substances in order to determine the presence of a specific drug. The gas chromatograph/mass spectrometer

(GC/MS), often considered the most sensitive and specific approach, is a variation of the GLC. Here, instead of being burned, the substance in the column is broken apart into fragments through the actions of electrons, producing a specific fingerprint unique to each drug, which can be detected by the machine.

Whichever combination of initial screens and confirmatory analyses is done, interpretation of the results must be carried out with care. One problem relates to the fact that a number of substances can cause false-positive initial screening results. For example, many over-the-counter decongestants and diet pills can result in positive initial screens for amphetamines. The antiepileptic drug, phenytoin (Dilantin), can produce a false-positive response for barbiturates, and it must be remembered that many substances (e.g., codeine) are actually metabolized to other substances (e.g., morphine) so that even confirmatory analyses can report what appear to be multiple drugs of use when only one substance was actually taken.

An additional important caveat is to recognize that many substances remain in the body for days to even weeks after their ingestion. Therefore, the qualitative analyses that are carried out in urine (telling you *if* the drug is present, not *how much* is there) cannot tell you how recently a drug was taken. Table 1.7 briefly describes how long after self-administration of a substance the particular group of drugs is likely to remain in the urine. However, these figures are only approximations, and the reader should go back to the cited references for more details.[60]

Street lore cites a number of steps that people can take to try to diminish the possibility that a recently ingested drug of abuse will be accurately identified in a sample. Prior to giving the sample, people have consumed aspirin, ibuprophin, vinegar, vitamin C, table salt and an herb known as

Table 1.7
Length of Time Urine Toxicology Screens Are Likely to Remain Positive after Abstinence

Substance	Usual time positive
Amphetamines	48 h
Barbiturates	
Short-acting	24 h
Long-acting	7+ days
Benzodiazepines	3+ days
Cannabinols	5+ days[a]
Cocaine	3+ days[a]
Codeine	48 h
Morphine	48 h

[a]Positive tests can be seen for longer periods of time following regular use up to 31 weeks for cannabinols and perhaps several additional days for cocaine.

"Golden Seal" which is usually taken as a capsule or tea. While changing the urinary pH can have a modest effect on some types of assays, in general these in vivo steps rarely mask the presence of a drug of abuse.[60] Drug users have also attempted many maneuvers to switch urine samples or to add contaminants to the urine, such as detergents, bleach, and Drano. These in vitro steps can interfere with some laboratory tests, and it is essential that the urine sample be obtained immediately after a directly observed micturition.[60]

Another qualitative analytical approach is worthy of brief mention here.[58,59,61] Urine drug testing, although positive for hours to days, cannot tell you whether a person has ingested most substances in the last month or two. However, most drugs are carried to hair follicles through the blood circulation. The hair roots incorporate the substance into the follicle. Because hair grows at a specific rate, it is possible to harvest 10–20 hairs from a spot approximately 1–2 in. back from an imaginary line going across the head from top of the ear to top of the ear, analyze separate sections of the length of hair, and know when an individual had experience with any of several drugs. The knowledge that most hair grows 1.3 cm/ month makes it possible to estimate the month in which the drug was taken.

The samples of hair are carefully washed, cut into segments, dissolved through a series of steps, and analyzed through reactions with specific antibodies using methods similar to the screening test reported above. As recently discussed in a series of articles, this approach is qualitative, with little evidence that it can be used as a quantitative analysis. There is also disagreement in the literature regarding the specificity and sensitivity of hair follicle analysis.

1.10. SOME BRIEF THOUGHTS ON PREVENTION

This section was developed specifically for the streamlined approach used in the sixth edition. The goal is to highlight a few major issues on prevention by focusing on recent publications that will give you a place to start if you want to read more about this important area. The material presented here is based on the thoughts developed in more detail in Chapter 16 of the fifth edition.

1.10.1. A Bit of History

Attempts at controlling alcohol and drug use date back hundreds of years. These include the longstanding recognition of the potential dangers of tobacco with resulting efforts to decrease use by increasing taxes, and efforts to develop less dangerous drugs to replace those recognized by society as more problematic (e.g., the misdirected effort to replace the dangers of morphine by substituting heroin). A massive international experiment with *primary prevention* (efforts aiming at decreasing the risk for problems before they began) was seen soon after World War I through prohibition of the sale of alcohol.[62]

The modern era of world wide efforts to control opioids and other drugs of abuse began with the Hague Opium Convention in 1912.[63] The subsequent Harrison Act in the United States in 1914 required registration of individuals engaged in the sale of narcotic drugs, the restriction of opioid use to legitimate medical purposes, and the criminalization of individuals engaged in the illicit use of this drug. Thus, the road was set toward the Volstead Prohibition act of 1919 regarding alcohol. The philosophy of the need to restrict substances that can be misused continued forward even after the repeal of prohibition, contributing to the 1936 International Collaboration on Drug Trafficking. Additional relevant legislation included the 1937 Marijuana Tax Act, and the 1946 Robertson Bill which extended restrictions to any synthetic drug similar to morphine and cocaine.

1.10.2. Typical Components of Prevention Approaches

One way to subdivide such efforts is to distinguish between *primary* and *secondary prevention.* The former seeks to stop substance use before it begins, while the latter deals with ways to decrease the levels of damage once intake is initiated.[64] Alternatively, prevention efforts can be simplistically described through the approaches listed below.

1. First are *efforts to limit availability of the substance through increasing price or limiting the numbers or hours of operation of alcohol outlets*,[65–68] or access can also be limited through restrictions that dissuade people from traveling from a more restrictive area (e.g., San Diego) to a location where alcohol is more readily available (e.g., Tijuana).[69]
2. Legal interdiction is a related, but debated, step to decrease the availability of substances, and, thus, increase the price. This follows upon the logic that scarcity enhances cost, which decreases use, while relevant laws[70] educate the population regarding the risks associated with use of illicit drugs. While there are no definitive data regarding a relationship between illegal seizures of street drugs and subsequent purity or cost, interdiction and the control of sales is a natural consequence of decisions to restrict drug use to youth under the age of 21.[71] However, the United States and most other countries are philosophically and politically committed to attempting to decrease availability to limiting supply from sources outside their borders.
3. A third approach is to *dissuade people from using the substance*, or to limit their intake to lower levels. This can include school and family-based education programs,[71–73] education efforts offered in high risk groups such as fraternities and sororities[74] education through the internet or mail,[75] and efforts based on limiting alcohol and tobacco

advertising along with increasing antidrug pieces in newspapers, television, and radio.[76,77] Variations on this approach can include programs (and, sometimes laws) that require that alcohol beverage servers be educated to identify and withhold liquor from individuals who are consuming large amounts,[78,79] as well as educating students regarding the actual alcohol intake patterns at their universities, which are often a good deal less than what they think.[80] However, not all researchers agree that these approaches are generally effective.[81,82]

4. *General community projects* include antidrug or antialcohol advertisements, and limitations in pro-smoking and drinking ads. These efforts influence attitudes toward drinking, smoking, and drug use in the general society in a manner similar to those used in increasing awareness of cancer risks, dangers of high blood pressure, the importance of a good diet, and so on. Regarding the efficacy of these approaches, people do remember information regarding alcohol and nicotine advertising, and these appear to influence their attitudes toward use.[83] While developing appropriate research methods for evaluating the impact of advertising is a daunting task, there does seem to be a significant relationship between advertising and substance use, at least when studied on the local level.[84]
5. *Punishment* is also viewed as a mode of prevention, including programs that seize drivers licenses from teenagers caught driving with any measurable alcohol level, fines, and jail time for use of illicit substances. A variation that spans between education and punishment is the use of victim impact panels so that users who have developed problems such as drunk driving can learn more about the impact of their behaviors.[85–87]
6. An interesting and potential approach involves *harm reduction*. The goal is to decrease the risk for life-threatening consequences of substance use. Examples include needle-exchange programs to diminish the risk for spreading AIDS and other conditions, the addition of nutrients to alcoholics beverages, offering hepatitis vaccinations for IV drug users, encouraging people to take taxis rather than drive while intoxicated, the use of ignition devices sensitive to alcohol, and so on.[88,89]
7. Additional relevant approaches include *Employee Assistance Programs* (EAPs). Many businesses incorporate education, supplying alternative activities to replace drinking and drug use, early identification, and treatment. These have been found to be cost effective regarding decreases in costs associated with missed work time, early retirements, and treatment of substance-related physical and psychological problems.[90]

Another general community approach that, while promising, is difficult to evaluate involves neighborhood action groups. These include neighborhood campaigns to drive out drug dealers, improve street lighting and to discourage drug use, such as the Miami-based Push Out the Pusher program.[91] A general population group worthy of special efforts are pregnant women. Thus, educational and cognitive techniques have been incorporated in maternity programs and obstetrician clinics.[92]

Finally regarding this brief review of efforts to change community attitudes toward either the use or heavy intake of substances, there are some data on the effectiveness of warning labels on legal substances such as alcohol and cigarettes.[93] Thus, while it is difficult to be certain that warning labels are helpful, they do make an important philosophical and political statement, are unlikely to do harm, and indirect evidence indicates that they might have an impact.

8. *Treatment can be viewed as a form of secondary prevention*. Chapter 14 focuses on identifying people who are having difficulties related to substances, appropriately evaluating them, and facilitating their treatment. These efforts can be viewed as secondary prevention in that successful treatment, by definition, results in lower levels of social, occupational, and physical morbidity and a diminished risk for premature death.
9. *A Community-Based Integration of Multiple Prevention Strategies*. If most of the approaches outlined above have potential beneficial effects on substance use and associated problems, their combination might be even more effective. In fact, the discussion of each prevention component as an individual entity is misleading, as most locales simultaneously offer multiple approaches as part of community based programming.[91] This is important because substance use and associated problems are complex and multifactorial processes that are best addressed through a combination of decreasing availability, changing attitudes toward substance use, improving access to treatment, and so on. There are several examples of the potential effectiveness of community-wide programming.[94,95] The Midwest Prevention Project contained five components focusing on the communication media, school programs, and general community education in an attempt to decrease adolescent use of alcohol, tobacco, and other drugs. An evaluation of the program revealed a decrease in tobacco use in youth as well as a lower proportion of individuals who used marijuana compared to a control population.

A second example comes from a Massachusetts based program that combined announcements through the public media, information to businesses, drunk driving awareness, police training, and alcohol-free alternative activities to decrease substance use. An evaluation of this program reported a 25% decrease in fatal car crashes, and a greater than 40% decrease in alcohol related accidents overall compared to a control community.

A third example comes from a five year protocol aimed at decreasing alcohol related problems in three communities. The components involved mobilizing community support groups, alcohol beverage server training, and enhancement of enforcement of DUI laws, along with changes in the density of alcohol outlets and enforcement of laws against sales to minors. The subsequent evaluation revealed significant decreases in underage alcohol sales and offered other evidence of achievement of goals.

1.10.3 A Brief Summary

Prevention of substance-related problems is something that we all do, although sometimes we don't realize it. Any type of healthcare promotion, educational efforts offered to our patients and clients, and the support that we give to school systems and to general population education programs help increase the level of awareness of potential problems related to substance. This section has offered a brief outline to help us to understand how our efforts contribute to prevention and to offer potential additional avenues we can choose to follow in our home communities.

1.11. ONWARD

You have now been introduced to my general philosophy regarding substances, problems, and their treatment. The next chapter offers a detailed discussion of the depressants and is followed by two chapters on alcohol and the treatment of alcohol related acute clinical problems. These three serve as a prototype for the remaining chapters. Each of the clinically relevant drug types is then discussed, and the final chapters emphasize emergency problems of substance misusers in general and an introduction to rehabilitation.

REFERENCES

1. White, F. J. The history of 'medicinal specifics' as addiction cures in the United States. *Addiction 98:*261–267, 2003.
2. Goldstein, A. *Addiction from Biology to Drug Policy* (2nd ed.). New York: Oxford University Press, Inc., 2001.
3. Corder, R., Douthwaite, J. A., Lees, D. M., Khan, N. Q., Viseu Dos Santos, A. C., Wood, E. G., & Carr, M. J. Endothelin-1 synthesis reduced by red wine. *Nature 414:*863–864, 2001.
4. Ruitenberg, A., van Swieten, J. C., Witteman, J. C. M., Mehta, K. M., van Duijn, C. M. M., Hofman, A., & Breteler, M. M. B. Alcohol consumption and risk of dementia: The Rotterdam Study. *Lancet 359:*281–286, 2002.
5. Zajicek, J., Fox, P., Sanders, H., Wright, D., Vickery, J., Nunn, A., & Thompson, A. Cannabinoids for treatment of spasticity and other symptoms related to multiple-sclerosis (CAMS study): Multicentre randomized placebo-controlled trial. *Lancet 362:*1517–1526, 2003.

6. Johnston, L. D., O'Malley, P. M., Bachman, J. G., & Schulenberg, J. E. *Monitoring the Future National Survey Results on Drug Use, 1975–2003, Vol. II: College Students and Adults Ages 19–40* (NIH Publication No. 04-5506). Bethesda, MD: National Institute on Drug Abuse, 2004.
7. Slutske, W. S. Alcohol use disorders among US college students and their non-college-attending peers. *Archives of General Psychiatry 62*:321-327, 2005.
8. Swartz, J. A., Hsieh, C.-M., & Baumohl, J. Disability payments, drug use and representative payees: An analysis of the relationships. *Addiction 98:*965–975, 2003.
9. Hardman, J. G., Limbird, L. E., & Goodman, A. G. (Eds.). *The Pharmacological Basis of Therapeutics* (10th ed.). New York: McGraw-Hill, 2001.
10. Miller, N. S., Sheppard, L. M., & Magen, J. Barriers to improving education and training in addiction medicine. *Psychiatric Annals 31:*649–656, 2001.
11. Kaner, E. F. S., Wutzke, S., Saunders, J. B., Powell, A., Morawski, J., & Bouix, J.-C. Impact of alcohol education and training on general practitioners' diagnostic and management skills: Findings from a World Health Organization Collaborative Study. *Journal of Studies on Alcohol 62:*621–627, 2001.
12. McClellan, A. T. Have we evaluated addiction treatment correctly? Implications from a chronic care perspective. *Addiction 97:*249–252, 2002
13. McLellan, A. T., Lewis, D. C., O'Brien, C. P., & Kleber, H. D. Drug dependence, a chronic medical illness: Implications for treatment, insurance, and outcomes evaluation. *JAMA 284:*1689–1695, 2000.
14. Fleming, M. F., Mundt, M. P., French, M. T., Manwell, L. B., Stauffacher, E. A., & Barry, K. L. Brief physician advice for problem drinkers: Long-term efficacy and benefit-cost analysis. *Alcoholism: Clinical & Experimental Research 26:*36–43, 2002.
15. Barrowclough, C., Haddock, G., Tarrier, N., Lewis, S. N., Moring, J., O'Brien, R., Schofield, N., & McGovern, J. Randomized controlled trial of motivational interviewing, cognitive behavior therapy and family intervention for patients with comorbid schizophrenia and substance use disorders. *American Journal of Psychiatry 158:*1706–1713, 2001.
16. Smith, T. L, Volpe, F. R., Hashima, J. N., & Schuckit, M. A. Impact of a stimulant-focused enhanced program on the outcome of alcohol- and/or stimulant-dependent men. *Alcoholism: Clinical & Experimental Research 23:*1772–1779, 1999.
17. Schuckit, M. A. *Educating Yourself About Alcohol and Drugs.* New York: Plenum Publishing Co., 1998.
18. Dowling, N., Smith, D., & Thomas, T. Electronic gaming machines: Are they the "crack-cocaine" of gambling? *Addiction 100:*33-45, 2005.
19. Kasper, D. L, Braunwald, E., Fauci, A. S., *et al.* (Eds.) *Harrison's Principles of Internal Medicine* (16th ed.). New York: McGraw-Hill, 2004.
20. Ma, O. J. & Cline, D. M. *Emergency Medicine Manual* (6th ed.). New York: McGraw-Hill, 2004.
21. Schuckit, M. A., Smith, T. L., Eng, M. Y., & Kunovac, J. Women who marry men with alcohol-use disorders. *Alcoholism: Clinical & Experimental Research 26:*1336–1343, 2002.
22. O'Brien, C. P. Drug addiction and drug abuse. In J. G. Hardman, L. E. Limbird, & A. G. Goodman (Eds.), *The Pharmacological Basis of Therapeutics* (10th ed.). New York: McGraw-Hill, 2001, pp. 621–642.
23. American Psychiatric Association. *Diagnostic and Statistical Manual of Mental Disorders*, Fourth Edition, Text Revision (DSM-IV-TR). Washington, DC: American Psychiatric Press, 2000.
24. Schuckit, M. A., Smith, T. L., Danko, G. P., Kramer, J., Godinez, J., Bucholz, K. K., Nurnberger, J. I., Jr., & Hesselbrock, V. A prospective evaluation of the four DSM-IV criteria for alcohol abuse in a large population. *American Journal of Psychiatry 162:*350–360, 2005.
25. Hasin, D. S., Schuckit, M. A., Martin, C. S., Grant, B. F., Bucholz, K. K., & Helzer, J. E. The validity of DSM-IV alcohol dependence: What do we know and what do we need to know? *Alcoholism: Clinical and Experimental Research 27:*244–252, 2003.

26. Schuckit, M. A., Danko, G. P., Smith, T. L., Hesselbrock, V., Kramer, J., & Bucholz, K. A 5-year prospective evaluation of DSM-IV alcohol dependence with and without a physiological component. *Alcoholism: Clinical and Experimental Research 27:*818–825, 2003.
27. Schuckit, M. A., Smith, T. L., Danko, G. P., Bucholz, K. K., Reich, T., & Bierut, L. Five-year clinical course associated with DSM-IV alcohol abuse or dependence in a large group of men and women. *American Journal of Psychiatry 158:*1084–1090, 2001.
28. World Health Organization. *The ICD-10 Classification of Mental and Behavioural Disorders.* Geneva: World Health Organization, 1992.
29. Hasin, D., & Paykin. A. Alcohol dependence and abuse diagnoses: Concurrent validity in a nationally representative sample. *Alcoholism: Clinical and Experimental Research 23:*144–150, 1999.
30. Schuckit, M. A., Daeppen, J. B., Danko, G. P., *et al.* Clinical implications for four drugs of the DSM-IV distinction between substance dependence with and without a physiological component. *American Journal of Psychiatry 156:*41–49, 1999.
31. Nestler, E. J. & Malenka, R. C. The addicted brain. *Scientific American 290:*78–85, 2004.
32. Koob, G. F., Le Moal, M. Drug addiction, dysregulation of reward, and allostasis. *Neuropsychopharmacology 24:*97–129, 2001.
33. Nestler, E. J., & Aghajanian, G. K. Molecular and cellular basis of addiction. *Science 278:*58–63, 1997.
34. Saal, D., Dong, Y, Bonci, A., & Malenka, R. C. Drugs of abuse and stress trigger a common synaptic adaptation in dopamine neurons. *Neuron 37:*577–582, 2003.
35. Gawin, F. H. The scientific exegesis of desire: Neuroimaging crack craving. *Archives of General Psychiatry 58:*342–344, 2001.
36. Kilts, C. D., Gross, R. E., Ely, T. D., & Drexler, K. P. G. The neural correlates of cue-induced craving in cocaine-dependent women. *American Journal of Psychiatry 161:*233–241, 2004.
37. Cole, J. C., Bailey, M., Sumnall, H. R., Wagstaff, G. F., & King, L. A. The content of ecstasy tablets. Implications for the study of their long-term effects. *Addiction 97:*1531–1536, 2002.
38. Substance Abuse and Mental Health Services Administration. *Overview of Findings from the 2002 National Survey on Drug Use and Health* (Office of Applied Studies, NHSDA Series H-21, DHHS Publication No. SMA 03-3774). Rockville, MD, 2003.
39. McIntosh, J., Gannon, M., McKeganey, M., & MacDonald, F. Exposure to drugs among pre-teenage schoolchildren. *Addiction 98:*1615–1623, 2003.
40. Wallace, J. M., Jr., Bachman, J. G., O'Malley, P. M., Johnston, L. D., Schulenberg, J. E., & Cooper, S. Tobacco, alcohol, and illicit drug use: Racial and ethnic differences among U.S. high school seniors, 1976–2000. *Public Health Report 117(Suppl.):*67–75, 2002.
41. Wagner, E. F., Lloyd, D. A., & Gil, A. G. Racial/ethnic and gender differences in the incidence and onset age of DSM-IV alcohol use disorder symptoms among adolescents. *Journal of Studies on Alcohol 63:*609–619, 2002.
42. Wallace, J. M., Jr., Bachman, J. G., O'Malley, P. M., Schulenberg, J. E., Cooper, S. M., & Johnston, L. D. Gender and ethnic differences in smoking, drinking and illicit drug use among American 8th, 10th, and 12th grade students, 1976–2000. *Addiction 98:*225–234, 2003.
43. Webb, E., Ashton, C. H., Kelly, P., & Kamali, F. Alcohol and drug use in UK university students. *Lancet 348:*922–925, 1996.
44. Wright, J. D., & Pearl, L. Knowledge and experience of young people regarding drug misuse. *British Medical Journal 310:*20–24, 1995.
45. Mora, M. E., Villatoro, J., & Rojas, E. Drug use among students in Mexico's northern border states. In The Department of Health and Human Services (Ed.), *Epidemiologic Trends in Drug Abuse.* Washington, DC: U.S. Government Printing Office, 1996, pp. 367–375.
46. Royo-Bordonada, M. A., Cid-Ruzafa, J., Martin-Moreno, J., *et al.* Drug and alcohol use in Spain: Consumption habits, attitudes and opinions. *Public Health 111:*277–284, 1997.

47. Knight, J. R., Wechsler, H., Kuo, M., Seibring, M., Weitzman, E. R., & Schuckit, M. A. Alcohol abuse and dependence among U.S. college students. *Journal of Studies on Alcohol 63:*263–270, 2002.
48. Grant, B. F., Stinson, F. S., Dawson, D. A., Chou, S. P., Ruan, J., & Pickering, R. P. Co-occurrence of 12-month alcohol and drug use disorders and personality disorders in the United States. *Archives of General Psychiatry 61:*361–368, 2004.
49. Westermeyer, J., & Thuras, P. Association of antisocial personality disorder and substance disorder morbidity in a clinical sample. The *American Journal of Drug and Alcohol Abuse 1:*93-110, 2005.
50. Brooke, D. Why do some doctors become addicted? *Addiction 91:*317–319, 1996.
51. Morrison, J., & Wickersham, P. Physicians disciplined by a state medical board. *Journal of the American Medical Association 279:*1889–1893, 1998.
52. Bloom, F. E. Neurotransmission and the central nervous system. In J. G. Hardman, L. E. Limbird, & A. G. Gilman (Eds.), *The Pharmacological Basis of Therapeutics* (10th ed.). New York: McGraw-Hill, 2001, pp. 293–320.
53. California Board of Pharmacy. *Pharmacy Law*. Sacramento, CA: LawTech Publishing Co., 1998.
54. Preuss, U. W., Schuckit, M. A., Smith, T. L., Danko, G. P., Dasher, A. C., Hesselbrock, M. N., Hesselbrock, V. M., & Nurnberger, J. I., Jr. A comparison of alcohol-induced and independent depression in alcoholics with histories of suicide attempts. *Journal of Studies on Alcohol 63:*498–502, 2002.
55. Preuss, U. W., Schuckit, M. A., Smith, T. L., Danko, G. P., Bucholz, K. K., Hesselbrock, M. N., Hesselbrock, V., & Kramer, J. R. Predictors and correlates of suicide attempts over 5 years in 1,237 alcohol-dependent men and women. *American Journal of Psychiatry 160:*56–63, 2003.
56. Schuckit, M. A., Tipp, J. E., Bergman, M., *et al.* Comparison of induced and independent major depressive disorders in 2,945 alcoholics. *American Journal of Psychiatry 154:*948–957, 1997.
57. Ries, R. K., Demirsoy, A., Russo, J. E., Barrett, J., & Roy-Byrne, P. P. Reliability and clinical utility of DSM-IV substance-induced psychiatric disorders in acute psychiatric inpatients. *The American Journal on Addictions 10:*308–318, 2001.
58. Welp, E. A. E., Bosman, I., Langendam, M. W., Totte, M., Maes, R. A. A., & van Ameijden, E. J. C. Amount of self-reported illict drug use compared to quantitative hair test results in community-recruited young drug users in Amsterdam. *Addiction 98:*987–994, 2003.
59. Dolan, K., Rouen, D., & Kimber, J. An overview of the use of urine, hair, sweat and saliva to detect drug use. *Drug and Alcohol Review 23:*213–217, 2004.
60. Liu, R., & Goldberg, B. (Eds.). *Handbook of Workplace Drug Testing.* Washington, DC: American Association of Clinical Chemists, 1995.
61. Darke, S., Hall, W., Kaye, S., Ross, J., & Duflou, J. Hair morphine concentrations of fatal heroin overdose cases and living heroin users. *Addiction 97:*977–984, 2002.
62. White, E. L. *The History of Addiction Treatment and Recovery in America. Slaying the Dragon*. Bloomington, IL: Chestnut Health Systems/Lighthouse Institute, 1998.
63. Springer, A. Heroin control: A historical overview. *European Addiction Research 2:*177–184, 1996.
64. Hoder, G., Flay, B., Howard, J., *et al.* Phases of alcohol problem prevention research. *Alcoholism: Clinical and Experimental Research 23:*183–194, 1999.
65. Heeb, J.-L., Gmel, G., Zurbrügg, C., Kuo, M., & Rehm, J. Changes in alcohol consumption following a reduction in the price of spirits: A natural experiment in Switzerland. *Addiction 98:*1433–1446, 2003.
66. Kuo, M., Heeb, J.-L., Gmel, G., & Rehm, J. Does price matter? The effect of decreased price on spirits consumption in Switzerland. *Alcoholism: Clinical and Experimental Research 27:*720–725, 2003.

67. Cunningham, J. K., & Liu, L.-M. Impacts of federal precursor chemical regulations on methamphetamine arrests. *Addiction 100:*479-488, 2005.
68. Norström, T., & Skog, O.-J. Saturday opening of alcohol retail shops in Sweden: An impact analysis. *Journal of Studies on Alcohol 64:*393–401, 2003.
69. Voas, R. B., Lange, J. E., & Johnson, M. B. Reducing high-risk drinking by young Americans south of the border: The impact of a partial ban on sales of alcohol. *Journal of Studies on Alcohol 63:*286–292, 2002.
70. Smithson, M., McFadden, M., Mwesigye, S.-E., & Casey, T. The impact of illicit drug supply reduction on health and social outcomes: The heroin shortage in the Australian Capital Territory. *Addiction 98:*340–348, 2004.
71. Wagenaar, A. C., Toomey, T. L., & Erickson, D. J. Preventing youth access to alcohol: Outcomes from a multi-community time-series trial. *Addiction 100:*335-345, 2005.
72. Furr-Holden, C. D. M., Ialongo, N. S., Anthony, J. C., Petras, H., & Kellam, S. G. Developmentally inspired drug prevention: Middle school outcomes in a school-based randomized prevention trial. *Drug and Alcohol Dependence 73:*149–158, 2004.
73. Spoth, R. L., Guyll, M., & Day, S. X. Universal family-focused interventions in alcohol-use disorder prevention: Cost-effectiveness and cost-benefit analyses of two interventions. *Journal of Studies on Alcohol 63:*219–228, 2002.
74. Larimer, M. E., Turner, A. P., Anderson, B. K., Fader, J. S., Kilmer, J. R., Palmer, R. S., & Cronce, J. M. Evaluating a brief alcohol intervention with fraternities. *Journal of Studies on Alcohol 62:*370–380, 2001.
75. Sobell, L. C., Sobell, M. B., Leo, G. I., Agrawall, S., Johnson-Young, L., & Cunningham, J. A. Promotion self-change with alcohol abusers: A community-level mail intervention based on natural recovery studies. *Alcoholism: Clinical and Experimental Research 26:*936–948, 2002.
76. Palmgreen, P., Donohew, L., Pugzles Lorch, E., Hoyle, R. H., & Stephenson, M. T. Television campaigns and adolescent marijuana use: tests of sensation seeking targeting. *American Journal of Public Health 91:*292–296, 2001.
77. Yanovitsky, I. Effect of news coverage on the prevalence of drunk-driving behavior: Evidence from a longitudinal study. *Journal of Studies on Alcohol 63:*342–351, 2002.
78. Johnsson, K. O., & Berglund, M. Education of key personnel in student pubs leads to a decrease in alcohol consumption among the patrons: A randomized controlled trial. *Addiction 98:*627–633, 2003.
79. Wallin, E., Gripenberg, J., & Andrèasson, S. Too drunk for a beer? A study of overserving in Stockholm. *Addiction 97:*901–907, 2002.
80. Trockel, M., Williams, S. S., & Reis, J. Considerations for more effective social norms based alcohol education on campus: An analysis of different theoretical conceptualizations in predicting drinking among fraternity men. *Journal of Studies on Alcohol 64:*50–59, 2003.
81. Clapp, J. D., Lange, J. E., Russell, C., Shillington, A., & Voas, R. B. A failed norms social marketing campaign. *Journal of Studies on Alcohol 64:*409–414, 2003.
82. Wechsler, H., Nelson, T. F., Lee, J. E., Seibring, M., Lewis, C., & Keeling, R. Perception and reality: A national evaluation of social norms marketing interventions to reduce college students' heavy alcohol use. *Journal of Studies on Alcohol 64:*484–494, 2003.
83. Wyllie, A., Zhang, J. F., & Casswell, S. Responses to televised alcohol advertisements associated with drinking behavior of 10–17 year-olds. *Addiction 93:*361–371, 1998.
84. Saffer, H. Studying the effects of alcohol advertising on consumption. *Alcohol Health & Research World 20:*266–272, 1996.
85. C'de Baca, J., Lapham, S. C., Liang, H. C., & Skipper, B. J. Victim impact panels: Do they impact drunk drivers? A follow-up of female and male, first-time and repeat offenders. *Journal of Studies on Alcohol 62:*615–620, 2001.
86. Polacsek, M., Rogers, E. M., Woodall, W. G., Delaney, H., Wheeler, D., & Rao, N. MADD victim impact panels and stages-of-change in drunk-driving prevention. *Journal of Studies on Alcohol 62:*344–350, 2001.

87. Rigotti, N. A., DiFranza, J. R., Chang, Y. C., *et al.* The effect of enforcing tobacco-sales laws on adolescents' access to tobacco and smoking behavior. *New England Journal of Medicine 337:*1044–1051, 1997.
88. Marques, P. R., Tippetts, A. S., & Voas, R. B. Comparative and joint prediction of DUI recidivism from alcohol ignition interlock and driver records. *Journal of Studies on Alcohol 64:*83–92, 2003.
89. Quaglio, G., Talamini, G., Lugoboni, F., Lechi, A., Venturini, L., Gruppo Intersert di Collaborazione Scientifica (GICS), Des Jarlais, D. C., & Mezzelani, P. Compliance with hepatitis B vaccination in 1175 heroin users and risk factors associated with lack of vaccine response. *Addiction 97:*985–992, 2002.
90. Zarkin, G. A., Bray, J. W., Karuntzos, G. T., & Demiralp, B. The effect of an enhanced employee assistance program (EAP) intervention on EAP utilization. *Journal of Studies on Alcohol 62:*351–358, 2001.
91. Winnick, C., & Larson, J. J. Prevention and education, community action programs. In J. H. Lowinson, P. Ruiz, R. B. Milman, & J. G. Langrod (Eds.), *Substance Abuse: A Comprehensive Textbook* (3rd ed.). Baltimore, MD: Williams & Wilkins, 1996, pp. 753–764.
92. Abel, E. L. Prevention of alcohol abuse-related birth effects. I. Public education efforts. *Alcohol & Alcoholism 33:*411–416, 1998.
93. Borland, R. Tobacco health warnings and smoking-related cognition and behaviors. *Addiction 92:*1427–1435, 1997.
94. Holder, H. D., Saltz, R. F., & Grube, J. W. Summing up: Lessons from a comprehensible community preventative trial. *Addiction 92(Suppl.):*5293–5301, 1997.
95. Hingson R., McGovern, T., Howland, J., *et al.* Reducing alcohol-impaired driving in Massachusetts. *American Journal of Public Health 86:*791–797, 1996.

CHAPTER 2

Depressants

2.1. INTRODUCTION

The classical depressants include hypnotics (sleeping pills), most antianxiety medications (e.g., diazepam or Valium), and alcohol.[1–5] This chapter focuses on the most commonly used drugs of this class (other than alcohol which is discussed in Chapters 3 and 4), including benzodiazepines, barbiturates, and barbiturate-like medications. Several related compounds, including kava and gamma-hydroxybutyric acid (GHB), are also briefly presented here, as their effects resemble those of the more classical depressants.[6–8] All depressants have the potential for being misused, and many prescription drugs of this class find their way into the street marketplace. The prototypical depressant is the barbiturate, which has been available in many forms since the 1860s and has been prescribed for a wide variety of problems. The generic names of all barbiturate medications in the United States end in *-al* and in Britain, in *-one*. These drugs differ in some ways from benzodiazepines and where appropriate, these two subgroups are discussed separately.

2.1.1. Pharmacology

2.1.1.1. Predominant Effects, Including Sedative, Hypnotic, or Anxiolytic Intoxication (304.10 in DSM-IV)

The depressants result in reversible depression of the activity of excitable neuronal tissues—especially those of the CNS—with the greatest effects on specific receptors and the synapse (the space between two nerve cells).[4,9,10] The resulting depression in activity can range from a slight lethargy or sleepiness, through levels of anesthesia, to death from breathing and heart depression.

2.1.1.2. Tolerance and Dependence

2.1.1.2.1. Tolerance

Tolerance to depressants occurs through both increased metabolism (*drug dispositional or metabolic tolerance*) and adaptation of the CNS to the presence of the drug (*pharmacodynamic tolerance*).[1,4,11] The metabolic tolerance can also produce an enhanced metabolism if some other substances, including the anticoagulant medications, result in lowered blood levels of these additional agents. The degree of tolerance can be huge, as case histories of 1000 mg per day of benzodiazepines have been reported in individuals still awake and talking. As is true of all medications, tolerance is not an all-or none phenomenon, and users can reach a point where tolerance stops and the next increment in the dose is lethal.

An important aspect of tolerance occurs with the concomitant administration of additional depressant drugs. If a second drug is consumed when the body is free of the first, cross-tolerance can be seen, as a reflection of both metabolic and pharmacodynamic mechanisms. However, if the second depressant drug is administered at the same time as the first, the opposite can be seen as the two drugs compete for metabolism and can potentiate the effects of each other in the brain. For example, a patient regularly using high doses of alcohol who undergoes surgery while in an alcohol-free state is likely to show significant cross-tolerance to some preanesthetic and anesthetic medications. If, however, the same patient uses a barbiturate or a benzodiazepine while intoxicated with alcohol, he is likely to experience a potentiation of drug effects with a resulting toxic reaction or overdose. Therefore, even an individual tolerant to one drug can have a fatal overdose with a concomitantly administered second depressant drug.

2.1.1.2.2. Dependence and Abuse (304.10 and 305.40 in DSM-IV)

All depressants including benzodiazepines such as chlordiazepoxide (Librium), diazepam (Valium), and alprazolam (Xanax), produce a withdrawal state when stopped abruptly after a relatively continuous administration of high doses.[12–15] The same may be true for benzodiazepine-like drugs such as zolpidem (Ambien), eszopiclone (Lunesta) and zaleplon (Sonata).[16,17] The withdrawal picture resembles a rebound hyperexcitability characterized by body changes in a direction opposite to that seen with the first administration of the drug.

Signs of withdrawal can be seen with abstinence after several weeks of frequent intoxication. In general, the severity of the abstinence syndrome increases with the strength of the drug, with higher doses, and with longer periods of administration. For a substance like pentobarbital, for example, stopping the drug after the administration of 400 mg a day for 3 months results in EEG changes in at least 30% of the individuals; 600 mg for 1–2 months results in a mild to moderate level of withdrawal in 50% of the individuals, including 10% with severe withdrawal symptoms including seizures;

and 900 mg for 2 months results in seizures in 75%, often accompanied by states of confusion. As a general rule, use of 500 mg of a barbiturate or an equivalent dose of other drugs will result in a risk of withdrawal seizures.

With the benzodiazepines, moderate withdrawal symptoms can be seen in individuals taking two or three times the usual clinical dose for several weeks, although most people for whom these drugs are prescribed do not use them for intoxication. Symptoms of withdrawal are likely to include headaches and anxiety (in about 80%), insomnia (in about 70%), and tremor and fatigue (each seen in about 60%), as well as perceptual changes, tinnitus, sweating, and a decreased ability to concentrate.[5,14,18] Similar to alcoholic withdrawal, abrupt abstinence after higher doses of benzodiazepines can precipitate delirium and seizures.[5,18,19] There is also compelling evidence that mild symptoms are likely to occur with abstinence following months of daily benzodiazepines in therapeutic doses after long-term use.

Another indication of the dependence-producing properties of the benzodiazepines comes from observations of the use of these drugs "on the street," where the value of diazepam and clonazepam (Klonopin) is estimated to be between $2.00 and $4.00 per pill.[2] Although many men and women who seek out these drugs for a "high" appear to move on to other agents relatively quickly, several groups of people have especially high risks for the continued misuse of benzodiazepines. First are heroin-dependent individuals and those on methadone maintenance, 75% or more of whom have admitted to taking benzodiazepines to enhance their intoxication or to deal with discomfort related to withdrawal symptoms from opioids.[20,21] At least theoretically, individuals who are alcohol dependent are also at increased risk for benzodiazepine dependence, perhaps in an effort to diminish anxiety, insomnia, or other withdrawal symptoms that might be observed in a context of their alcoholism. However, it is difficult to marshal definitive data regarding an enhanced prevalence of benzodiazepine or other brain depressant dependence in men and women who misuse alcohol.

In summary, all of the DSM-IV items for abuse or dependence, can develop these in people taking high doses of depressants.[22] Regarding dependence, these can include tolerance, withdrawal, use for longer periods than intended, interference with functioning, and so on. Regarding abuse, users can develop repetitive legal, occupational, and social problems, take these drugs in the context of hazardous activities, and continue their use despite these problems.

2.1.1.3. Specific Drugs

Tables 2.1 and 2.2 give examples of members of the different classes of hypnotic and antianxiety drugs. However, the actions of agents in the two major subclasses can overlap. For example, antianxiety drugs in high enough doses induce sleep, whereas some barbiturate hypnotics were labeled hypnosedatives and administered to treat anxiety.[4,5]

Table 2.1
Nonbenzodiazepine CNS Depressants

Drug type	Generic name	Trade name
Hypnotics/medical Uses		
Barbiturates		
Ultrashort-acting	Thiopental	Pentothal
	Methohexital	Brevital
Intermediate-acting	Pentobarbital	Nembutal
	Secobarbital	Seconal
	Amobarbital	Amytal
	Butabarbital	Butisol
Long-acting	Phenobarbital	Luminal
Others	Chloral hydrate	Noctec
	Paraldehyde	—
Antianxiety drugs		
Carbamates	Meprobamate	Miltown, Equanil

See Table 2.2 for the benzodiazepines.

2.1.1.3.1. Hypnotics

Although the most commonly used sleeping pills are the benzodiazepines or similar drugs, other hypnotics include the barbiturates and barbiturate-like drugs. These are presented in Tables 2.1 and 2.2.

The first subclass of *barbiturates* consists of the rarely misused *ultra-short*-acting drugs (used to induce anesthesia) with lengths of action of a few minutes (e.g., thiopental and methohexital). The *short* to *intermediate*-acting barbiturates exert their major effect for a period of approximately 4 h, so they help people get to sleep. These include the drugs prescribed and misused as hypnotics, such as pentobarbital (Nembutal) and secobarbital (Seconal). Finally, the *long-lasting* drugs, such as phenobarbital, are most often used to treat neurological conditions such as epilepsy. Abuse and dependence on phenobarbitol-like drugs are relatively uncommon.

Another group of hypnotics discussed here is exemplified by chloral hydrate (Noctec) and paraldehyde. These drugs share most of the dangers outlined for the barbiturate and barbiturate-like hypnotics.

Four other hypnotic drugs are the benzodiazepines flurazepam (Dalmane), nitrazepam (Mogodan), temazepam (Restoril), and triazolam (Halcion). Overall, these drugs do not produce completely normal sleep, but disturb the sleep EEG less than most other hypnotics, benefiting the patient by decreasing the sleep latency and the number of awakenings while increasing total amount of sleep. At the same time, the amount of sleep in Stage 2 increases while the sleep in Stages 3 and 4 tends to decrease, and moderate changes in REM sleep are likely to occur.

Table 2.2
Benzodiazepines

Generic name	Trade name	Half-life (h)	Usual adult daily dose (mg)[a]
Alprazolam	Xanax	11–15	0.75–4
Chlordiazepoxide	Librium	5–30	5–25
Clonazepam[b]	Klonopin	20–50	0.5–10+
Clorazepate	Tranxene	30–60	15–60
Diazepam	Valium; Dizac	20–50	2–15
Eszopiclone	Lunesta	6–9	1–3
Flurazepam[c]	Dalmane	50–100	15–30 HS
Lorazepam	Ativan	10–20	2–6
Nitrazepam[c]	Mogodan	24	5–10 HS
Oxazepam	Serax	5–20	10–60
Temazepam[c]	Restoril	4–8	15–30 HS
Triazolam	Halcion	3–5	0.25–0.5
Zaleplon[c,d]	Sonata	1	5–10
Zolpidem[c,d]	Ambien	2–3	10–20

[a]HS indicates use at bedtime (hour of sleep).
[b]Used mostly as an anticonvulsant.
[c]Used only as a hypnotic.
[d]Not a true Bz, but similar in action.

There are also several relatively new hypnotics, including Zolpidem (Ambien), technically not a benzodiazepine but an agent that carries most of the dangers of that group of drugs. This medication, an imidazopyridine, induces sleep, but has no antianxiety or muscle-relaxant properties. Zolpidem has a 2–3-h half-life, and is less disruptive of Stages 3 and 4 of sleep than the benzodiazepines. Acting primarily through its effects on omega 1 (or Bz_1) benzodiazepine receptors, it shares some of the problems associated with classical benzodiazepines. Thus, zolpidem will be self-administered by animals, tolerance can be observed, and a mild withdrawal or rebound syndrome can be expected when the drug is stopped. Zaleplon (Sonata) has a short half-life, and little effect on respiratory depression or morning cognitive functioning, but is only helpful in falling asleep, not staying asleep.[23,24]

Two other hypnotics are available outside the United States. Zopiclone (marketed in Europe as Zimovane and known on the street as “Zim Zims”) has been associated with a number of problems, including dependence.[16] The second medication, flunitrazepam (Rohypnol), is marketed in Central and South America and has become a problem in the United States, especially in locales close to the Mexican border. Known on the street as roSHAY, roofies, and Roche, and used to induce sleep at levels of 1–2 mg, it is misused for intoxication, and has also gained a reputation as a “date rape drug.”[25,26] Here, similar to the mixture of chloral hydrate and alcohol (known as a Mickey Finn), when dissolved in alcohol the mixture can produce somnolence, poor judgment, and amnesia for the episode. In recent years, the

United Nations Commission on Narcotic Drugs has moved this agent to the more restrictive Schedule III. Another new drug is eszopiclone (Lunesta).

In summary, most hypnotics have drawbacks. They disturb the natural sleep pattern, they can be dangerous if taken in an overdose, and all have a potential for misuse. It appears that *all* hypnotic medications lose some of their effectiveness if taken nightly for more than 2 weeks, or produce a rebound insomnia when stopped.[4,27,28] Therefore, considering their potential as agents for suicide and their limited time of efficacy if used daily, it is not wise to prescribe these medications for anything more than a short-term, acute crisis.

Safer approaches to treating insomnia are available, and are discussed in detail in other texts.[28] For instance, after carefully ruling out problems to which insomnia might be secondary (e.g., sleep apnea), I prescribe a schedule of going to bed and getting up at the same time each day, no caffeinated beverages, and no naps. Milk at bedtime can be a useful adjunct, perhaps because of its tryptophan content.

2.1.1.3.2. Antianxiety Drugs

The class of drugs most frequently prescribed for acute anxiety is the benzodiazepines [e.g., diazepam (Valium, Table 2.2)]. These medications are effective in the short-term treatment of *acute* anxiety, but few well-controlled studies have proved that they work for more than 1 month when taken daily.[2,4] Long-term use of these drugs is likely to produce rebound anxiety and insomnia when they are stopped; some patients find it very difficult to become drug free.[29]

Dangers associated with benzodiazepines and with other antianxiety agents include disturbances in sleep pattern and a possible change in affect (increased irritability, hostility, and lethargy). The carbamates (Table 2.1) can be especially lethal when taken in overdose, and these drugs accumulate in the body over time because they have a length of action that exceeds the usual time between the administration of doses. I never prescribe the carbamates (meprobamate) because they also appear to have a higher potential for producing dependence and a greater possibility of fatality following overdose than the benzodiazepines.

Another drug has been marketed for the treatment of long-standing general feelings of anxiety, or Generalized Anxiety Disorder in DSM-IV. Buspirone (Buspar) is briefly discussed in Section 2.1.1.3.4, but it is not a true depressant drug and does not share most of their dangers.

2.1.1.3.3. Benzodiazepines

Although the drugs in this antianxiety subclass are depressants, they are discussed separately because of the richness of understanding of their mode of action, their widespread use, their lower intensity of physiological changes, and the less intense toxic reactions on overdose. These drugs have peripheral body effects, but most actions discussed here occur in the brain. Benzodiazepines (Bzs) are used as muscle relaxants (e.g., after strains or in spinal disk disease), as anticonvulsants (usually for non-grand-mal seizures and/or for status epilepticus), and as antianxiety agents. Their usefulness in treating anxiety states is best limited to short-term help (2 or 3 weeks) for severe situational problems. The more long-term and chronic major anxiety disorders (e.g., agoraphobia or obsessive–compulsive disease) are not usual targets for their use, as these drugs are not effective over a long enough period of time, and there is a possible rebound increase in symptoms when the drugs are stopped.

Some specific drugs are listed in Table 2.2. Although there are variations among the medications (especially related to their half-lives), the drugs in this class have great clinical similarities. Compared with most other types of sedative/hypnotics such as the barbiturates and the carbamates, these drugs are relatively safe in overdose, induce less prominent metabolic tolerance, cause fewer changes in sleep stages, and appear to be less likely to produce physical dependence. All drugs of this class can be administered orally, and most are better absorbed by mouth than by intramuscular injection (diazepam can be given intravenously, and lorazepam is well absorbed intramuscularly). They usually reach peak blood levels in 2–4 h after oral administration, and most have active metabolites (except lorazepam and oxazepam). The recommended frequency of administration varies with the half-life, so lorazepam and oxazepam may need to be given four times a day to remain effective, whereas clorazepate and diazepam may be used once per day (usually at bedtime). With the exception of the Bzs that have shorter half-lives (which are the drugs without active metabolites), most of these substances accumulate in the body, reaching a steady state in 7–10 days. Therefore, clinicians must be certain that sedative side effects do not progressively interfere with life functioning, especially in the elderly.[30]

The pharmacological mechanisms of the benzodiazepines have been extensively studied. All these drugs enhance the effects of the more sedating amino acid brain neurotransmitter, gamma-aminobutyric acid (GABA).[31,32] Two types of GABA receptors are most relevant, including $GABA_A$ which is most sensitive to the effects of depressants such as benzodiazepines, whereas $GABA_B$ receptors have little relationship with the actions of brain depressants in the CNS. When a benzodiazepine or a related drug occupies a subcomponent of a GABA receptor, it facilitates the flow of chloride ions into the cell, thus, potentiating the effects of GABA.

In addition to GABA receptors, there are also three benzodiazepine receptors in the brain[4] that work in conjunction with $GABA_A$ activity. The Bz_1 (or omega 1) receptors contribute to the sleep-inducing effects of these drugs and are the site of the most prominent actions of most sleeping pills, such as zolpidem. The Bz_2 and Bz_3 receptors (also called omega 2 and omega 3) appear to be most active regarding the anticonvulsant, muscle-relaxant, and antianxiety actions.

The link between benzodiazepine receptors and the actions of other depressants has not been as well established. However, at relevant doses, at least one barbiturate, pentobarbital, increases binding at these receptors. As might be predicted from these data, recent studies have also identified benzodiazepines such as flumazenil (Romazicon) that act at the Bz/GABA sites to inhibit and *antagonize* the actions of other drugs of this class. These drugs are important in treating overdoses with medications that affect this receptor complex, but they produce symptoms of anxiety and can precipitate withdrawal in a Bz-dependent person.[9,33]

2.1.1.3.4. Some Nonbenzodiazepine Anxiolytics and Hypnotics

A number of nonbenzodiazepine anxiety-affecting agents have been evaluated. This development reflects the recognition that benzodiazepines are not perfect, having associated problems of misuse, physical dependence, cognitive impairment, and interactions with other brain depressants as described elsewhere in this chapter. Even though these agents are technically not depressants, they are discussed here because they can be used in a manner similar to the benzodiazepines.

These substances have a variety of structures and potential activities. They include nabilone, a tetrahydrocannabinol homologue distinguished by its relationship to the active ingredient in marijuana, and fenobam, a potentially effective anxiolytic with few muscle-relaxant or sedative/hypnotic properties and minimal potential for interaction with other depressants.[34]

The best known and most thoroughly studied of the nonbenzodiazepine anxiolytics is buspirone (Buspar), an unusual fat-soluble molecule of multiple rings with a structure unlike that of any other anxiolytic agent.[35,36] This drug has either weak or no actions on benzodiazepine receptors, and it does not replace benzodiazepines from their binding sites, nor does it directly affect GABA binding. Buspirone is known to affect serotonin, norepinephrine, and acetylcholine systems, with the most clinically relevant effect probably being on serotonin.

In controlled trials for the treatment of generalized anxiety disorder, its key clinical target, buspirone shows no hypnotic effects but demonstrates some anxiolytic properties, usually after 2 weeks of administration. At the same time, this agent appears to offer fewer safety concerns, as there is little evidence of cognitive impairment with clinically relevant doses, and little evidence that it interacts with brain depressants such as alcohol. Additionally, animal or clinical studies do not demonstrate a high potential for misuse of this agent. Thus, buspirone may be the first effective anxiolytic without a clinically significant dependence risk. However, the clinical indications for this medication are rather narrow.

2.1.1.3.5. Some Additional Drugs

Gamma-hydroxybutyric acid is a depressant-like drug that boosts the brain activity of GABA and perhaps of dopamine.[6] This substance, formerly available in health food stores, has for many years been used by athletes and bodybuilders, but a series of overdoses in the early 1990s resulted in its restriction from the legal markets. GHB still appears on the "streets" as a product of kitchen laboratories. Although not well studied, it appears that this drug is capable of producing the same pattern of problems seen with the other more typical brain depressants including dependence, withdrawal, and overdose.[37–39]

A second drug with a much longer and more culturally syntonic history has been used in Polynesia and Micronesia since at least the 1700s.[40] Kava is a complex mixture of substances extracted as a powder and consumed as a tea. It is made from the pepper plant (*Piper methysticum*) that grows in the South Pacific. The active ingredients, few of which have been isolated, produce a variety of effects including sedation and incoordination that can quickly progress to deep sleep. Intoxication is also associated with a decrease in cognitive functioning, and it is generally believed that Kava produces an alcohol-like effect. It has traditionally been used in a sundown ceremony for men on Fiji and on similar islands but is now also sold in different parts of the world as these populations have disbursed globally.

2.1.2. Epidemiology and Patterns of Use

The depressants are prescribed in great quantities. Supporting the high prevalence of use are studies demonstrating that more than one in three American adults had symptoms of insomnia during the preceding year, including 10% with chronic sleeping problems.[41] As a result, 3–4% had used a prescribed hypnotic of some type, an additional 2% have taken other prescription drugs to help them sleep, and approximately 3% took over-the-counter sleeping pills.[41] These figures include a total of 0.3% of the population (11% of users) who had taken the medication regularly over the last year. In addition, over 8% of the general population have used benzodiazepines to deal with anxiety.[41,42]

Among the depressants, the Bzs receive the widest use.[43] In one year, over 2 billion tablets of diazepam were prescribed in the United States. Although use is widespread, these figures do not necessarily indicate abuse or dependence, as these drugs are generally used as prescribed for sleep and for anxiety. However, up to 10% of general medical/surgical patients and 30% of individuals with serious psychiatric histories have, at some time, felt psychologically dependent on these antianxiety or hypnotic drugs, with an outright substance use disorder in between 5 and 10%.

Many people in the United States have used depressant drugs for a high. In 2003, 10.2% of high school seniors reported having ever used a "tranquilizer," a figure similar to the 10.3% in 2001.[44] For this age group, 6.7% had used in the prior year (6.9% in 2001) and 2.8% in the prior 30 days. Among college students, the ones who had ever used depressants for intoxication were 10.7% overall, 6.7% in the prior year, and 3.0% in the last 30 days.

It is more difficult to establish the lifetime prevalence of abuse or dependence on these agents. According to a 2002 survey, during the prior year, almost 200,000 Americans had received treatment for a condition related to depressant drugs, often in the context of additional drugs of misuse.[45] However, to place this into perspective, during that same period, 2.2 million Americans had received treatment for alcohol-related disorders, thus, while the rate of treatment for alcoholism was as high as about 1% of the population, the proportion in treatment for depressants was one in almost 1500 people.

Some subgroups of the population are more likely than others to engage in depressant abuse or dependence. Probably the best studied of these are individuals who are opioid dependent, especially those taking part in methadone maintenance programs.[20] Here, a substantial proportion (perhaps almost a majority) report having used a Bz or a barbiturate to help them cope with the opioid withdrawal syndrome or to enhance their levels of intoxication while taking methadone. In some locales, 65% or more of stimulant or intravenous (IV) opioid drug users also reported a history of imbibing or injecting depressants.[46]

Thus, misuse of depressant drugs should be considered in the evaluation of almost any patient seen in a usual medical setting, an emergency room, or in a crisis clinic. In light of the limited time that these medications stay effective when taken daily, there is rarely a valid clinical need to prescribe them for more than 2–4 weeks.

2.1.3. Establishing a Diagnosis

Identification of the individual misusing depressants requires a high index of suspicion, especially for patients with a delirium, a dementia, or with paranoid delusions, and for all men and women who insist on receiving prescriptions for any of these medications. It is imperative that special care be taken before these drugs are given to patients who are not known to the physician. Also, when they are prescribed, the script should be for only relatively small amounts, both to decrease the suicide overdose potential and to discourage misuse. No "repeats" should be allowed, bottles should be labeled as to the contents, and records should be evaluated to determine how long the patient has been on the medication.

2.2. EMERGENCY PROBLEMS

The following outline follows the general format presented in Table 1.5, reviewing the possible areas of difficulty seen in emergency rooms, in the outpatient office, and in crisis clinics. The most common problems seen with the CNS depressants are toxic overdose, temporary psychosis, and withdrawal.

2.2.1. Toxic Reactions

See Sections 4.2.1, 6.2.1, and 13.2.1

As this is the first chapter to discuss overdose, it is important to remind the reader that this text only gives very general guidelines. It is essential to also consult a textbook of medicine or a text on emergency medicine.[47,48]

2.2.1.1. Clinical Picture

2.2.1.1.1. History

The toxic reaction or overdose usually develops over a matter of minutes to hours, and the patient often presents in a confused or obtunded state with severe memory impairment.[49–51] This reaction is more likely to be seen when an individual mixes two or more depressants (usually alcohol and hypnotics), develops a confused state that results in inadvertent repeated administration of the drug, unintentionally takes too high a dose of a street drug, or makes a deliberate suicide attempt.

2.2.1.1.2. Physical Signs and Symptoms

Toxic reactions are characterized by various levels of anesthesia and decreased CNS, cardiac, and respiratory functioning. Additional signs include a decreased temperature, diminished reflexes, and decreased gut motility.[52] An overdose of a depressant drug can be very serious. The physical signs must be carefully evaluated in a manner similar to that suggested in Section 6.2.1 for opioids. Examination includes the following:

1. A careful evaluation of the vital signs and the reflexes, with the findings depending on the drug dose, the time elapsed since ingestion, and any complicating brain conditions, such as hypoxia.
2. A neurological exam to help establish the degree of coma. Important aspects include the following:
   a. *Pupillary reflexes:* Usually midpoint and slowly reactive, with which pupils tend to be enlarged.
   b. *Corneal reflexes:* Diminished or absent, except in mild coma.
   c. *Tendon reflexes and pain reflexes:* Tend to be depressed.
3. An evaluation of possible cardiac arrhythmias, especially with the short-acting barbiturates.
4. Oscultation of lungs for congestion from heart failure or from positional or infective pneumonia.

2.2.1.1.3. Psychological State

Because the patient often presents in a stupor or in a coma, there are usually few other distinctive psychological attributes.

2.2.1.1.4. Relevant Laboratory Tests

See Section 6.2.1.1.4.

As with any shock-like state or comparable medical emergency, it is important to carefully monitor the vital signs and the blood gases (arterial oxygen and CO_2) to evaluate the need for a respirator. A toxicological screen on either urine (50 ml) or on blood (10 cc) should also be carried out to determine the specific drug involved and the amount of the substance in the blood, and baseline blood chemistries and blood counts should be taken as outlined in Table 1.6. If the cause of the stupor or the coma is not obvious, a thorough neurological evaluation for additional medical problems (including an EEG, skull x-rays, a spinal tap, and so on) must be done. Routine tests should include an EKG, chest film, glucose, and electrolytes. Arterial blood gases should be evaluated if necessary.

2.2.1.2. Treatment

See Section 6.2.1.2.

Treatment begins with emergency procedures to guarantee an adequate airway, to make sure that the heart is functioning, and to deal with any concomitant bleeding; i.e., the ABCs of care.[53] The general goal is to support the vital signs until enough of the drug has been metabolized so the patient is stable, following the general approach presented in Table 2.3. The specific emergency maneuvers will depend on the patient's clinical status. These steps may range from simple observation for mild overdoses to starting an IV infusion, placing the patient on a respirator, and admitting him to an intensive care unit.

Although toxic reactions involving the Bzs should not be taken lightly, the clinical picture tends to be more mild, and fewer than 5% of patients require intensive-unit care for 48 h or more.[54] If treatment is initiated quickly, deaths are relatively rare (fewer than 1%), and especially rapid recovery is to be expected with the short-acting drugs such as lorazepam and oxazepam, even if the blood levels are initially high.[54,55]

A possible step for benzodiazepine overdose is to administer flumazenil (Romazicon). The usual dose is 0.2 mg IV every minute, up to 3 mg. If a Bz was involved, sedation should be quickly reversed, but there is a danger of precipitating seizures or increasing intracranial pressure.[52] Because of the short half-life of flumazenil, it may need to be repeated in 20–30 min.[9,33]

The additional steps for approaching the patient with a toxic reaction to depressants, not necessarily to be taken in the numbered order, include the following:

Table 2.3
Treatment of the Depressant Toxic Reaction

Diagnose	History, clinical signs
First steps	Airway, assist respiration
	Cardiac
	Check electrolytes
	Treat shock
	Lavage (use cuff if obtunded; activated charcoal; castor oil?)
Consider	Forced diuresis (limited value)
	Hemodialysis
Avoid	Stimulants

1. Establish a *clear airway*, *intubate* if needed (using an inflatable cuff in case you want to do a gastric lavage), and place on a *respirator* if necessary. The respirator should use compressed air (oxygen can decrease the respiratory drive) at a rate of 10–12 breaths per minute.
2. Evaluate the *cardiovascular status* and control *bleeding*; treat shock with plasma expanders, saline, dextran, or other relevant drugs.
3. Begin an IV (large-gauge needle), replacing all fluid loss (e.g., urine) plus 20 ml for insensible loss (from respiration and perspiration) each hour.
4. Establish a means of measuring *urinary output* (bladder catheter, if needed). Send 50 ml of urine for a toxicological screen.
5. Carry out *gastric lavage* with saline if oral medication was taken in the last 1–4 h. Continue lavage until you get a clear return. Consider giving 60 ml of *castor oil* via the stomach tube.
6. Repeated administration of activated charcoal or a similar agent (e.g., 1 g/kg or more of activated charcoal suspended in water and administered every 4 h or so, over the first 2 days) appears to help decrease absorption.
7. Because opioid overdoses can cause a similar clinical picture, and the patient may have ingested more than one type of medication, consider the possibility of a narcotic overdose. This is tested for through the administration of an opioid antagonist such as *naloxone* (Narcan) at a dose of 0.4–2 mg, given either intramuscularly (IM) or IV. If the patient has ingested opioids to the point of obtundation, a rapid reversal of the picture should be demonstrated. Doses of this short-acting opioid antagonist will need to be repeated as often as every 30 min, if initially effective.
8. Carry out a more thorough *physical* and *neurological exam*—which must include *pupils*, *corneal reflexes*, *tendon reflexes*, presence of *pathological reflexes* (e.g., snout reflex), *pain perception* (use Achilles tendon), and *awake/alert status* (see Sections 6.2.1.2 and 13.4.1).

9. Draw *bloods* for arterial blood gases if needed, general blood tests to evaluate liver and kidney functioning, blood counts, and a toxicological screen.
10. Gather a thorough *history* of
    a. Recent drugs (type, amount, time)
    b. Recent alcohol
    c. Chronic diseases
    d. Allergies
    e. Current treatments

    Obtain this information from the patient and/or from an available additional informant.
11. For the comatose patient, protect against *decubitus ulcers* (bedsores) by frequent turning, and *protect the eyes* by taping the lids closed if necessary.
12. Establish a *flow sheet* for
    a. Vital signs
    b. Level of reflexes
    c. Urinary output
    d. IV fluids

    These should be recorded up to every 30 min.
13. Consider *forced diuresis* especially for barbiturate overdose. This is not needed for patients with stable vital signs or for those where deep tendon reflexes are present (e.g., grade I or II coma), and rarely helps for chlordiazepoxide (Librium) or for diazepam (Valium). If either diuresis or dialysis is used, special care must be taken to maintain proper electrolyte levels and to avoid precipitating congestive failure. If diuresis is needed, you may use
    a. Furosemide (Lasix), 40–120 mg, as often as needed to maintain 250 ml or more per hour;
    b. IV fluids, with the general approach of giving enough saline and water with glucose to maintain urinary output in excess of 250 ml/h.
14. Alkalinization of the urine can be helpful with long-acting barbiturate overdose.[52] This can be accomplished with an IV bolus of 1–2 mEq/kg of sodium bicarbonate, followed by 50–100 mEq added to 500 ml of a 5% dextrose solution
15. Hemodialysis or peritoneal dialysis can be considered for the patient in a deep coma but is rarely needed. Hemoperfusion may be helpful for patients who have grade IV coma with associated apnea and hypotension, for patients who show deterioration despite supportive treatment, for those in prolonged coma with cardiorespiratory complications, or for individuals with very high plasma drug levels.
16. Evaluate the need for *antibiotics*. Do *not* use them prophylactically.
17. Do *not* use stimulants such as amphetamines.

18. For the unresponsive patient who requires admission to an intensive care unit, the prognosis is likely to relate to the levels and the degree of change in systolic pressure, the central venous pressure, and the acid–base balance (pH). A special word of warning is required regarding the ability of the depressant drugs to produce a temporary flat EEG, which can reverse within a matter of days.

2.2.2. The Depressant Withdrawal Syndrome (292.0 and 292.81 in DSM-IV)

See Sections 4.2.2 and 6.2.2.

The depressant withdrawal syndrome consists of a constellation of symptoms that might develop (during abstinence) in an individual taking any of these drugs daily in excessive doses. The clinical picture is usually a mixture of any or all of the possible symptoms, running a time course that tends to last 3–7 days for the acute syndrome related to short-acting drugs such as oxazepam or lorazepam that have half-lives similar to alcohol, but is longer for longer acting drugs like diazepam (Valium). Following the acute withdrawal period, less intense symptoms are likely to be observed for 3–6 months as part of a protracted withdrawal syndrome.

Although less likely to cause physical dependence than other depressants, all Bzs can do so.[4,15,56,57] As new Bz agents were introduced to the market, it was hoped that they might be less likely to be misused or associated with more mild abstinence syndromes, but this has usually not proven to be the case.

The Bzs are less popular as "street" drugs than other depressants, but they do have rewarding properties and are self-administered by animals. As is true of all depressants, the development of physical dependence relates to the drug dose and the period of time over which it was administered. Thus, physical withdrawal has been reported with diazepam in clinical dose ranges (e.g., 10–20 mg/day), as well as with alprazolam or with lorazepam (4 mg/day or less) when taken over a period of weeks to months.[27] When two to three times the normal maximal doses are ingested, physical dependence can probably be induced in a matter of days to weeks.

2.2.2.1. Clinical Picture

2.2.2.1.1. History

A depressant withdrawal syndrome must be considered in any individual who presents with signs of autonomic nervous system overactivity (e.g., a rapid pulse and elevated blood pressure) along with agitation, and who asks the physician for a depressant drug.[2,4] This syndrome can be seen in the person who fits DSM-IV dependence, as well as the middle class recent user who obtains the drug on prescription but takes more than recommended. The symptoms begin slowly over a period of hours and, similar to alcohol, may not peak until Day 2 or 3 for the short- to intermediate-half-life drugs.

The time course for the withdrawal from barbiturates, such as pentobarbital, or a drug like meprobamate (Miltown or Equanil) is outlined in Table 2.4. This table indicates the probable onset of symptoms within a half-day of stopping or decreasing the medications, a peak intensity at 24–72 hours, and diminished acute symptoms some time before Day 7. The time frame is a good deal longer for the longer acting barbiturates and the antianxiety drugs such as chlordiazepoxide (Librium), for which withdrawal seizures and delirium can begin as late as day 7 or 8. The acute stage of withdrawal is followed by the lingering symptoms of a protracted withdrawal condition that is likely to disappear by Months 3–6 following abstinence.[58]

2.2.2.1.2. Physical Signs and Symptoms

The withdrawal symptoms consist of a mixture of both psychological and physical problems. The patient usually develops a fine tremor, gastrointestinal (GI) upset, muscle aches, increased pulse and respiration rates, a fever, and a labile blood pressure.[2,43] Some atypical withdrawal syndromes can also be seen, especially with the Bzs, and may include headache, malaise, and abrupt weight loss. With any depressant, but especially the barbiturates, between 5 and 20% of individuals develop grand-mal convulsions—usually one or at the most two fits that only rarely progress to a state of repeated and continuous seizures known as status epilepticus.

2.2.2.1.3. Psychological State

The withdrawal symptoms include moderate to high levels of anxiety and a strong drive to obtain the drug.[12] In addition, between 5 and 20% of individuals develop a delirium, sometimes accompanied by hallucinations.

Table 2.4
Time Course of Acute Withdrawal from Short/Intermediate-Acting Barbiturates and Meprobamate

Time (after last dose)	Symptom	Severity
12–16 h	Intoxicated state	Mild
	Onset: Anxiety, tremors, anorexia, weakness, nausea/vomiting, cramps, hypotension, increased reflexes	
24 h	Weakness, tremors, increased reflexes, increased pleading for drug	Mild
	High risk for grand-mal seizures; delirium	Severe
24–72 h	Peak intensity	Greatest
3–7 days	Symptoms gradually disappear	Diminishing
1 week–6 months	Some anxiety, sleep disturbance, ANS irregularities	Mild

The state of confusion can include hallucinations or delusions similar to delirium tremens (DTs) described for alcohol in Chapter 4.

2.2.2.1.4. Relevant Laboratory Tests

Because the withdrawal syndrome is potentially more severe than most other drug withdrawals, it is essential that an adequate physical examination be carried out and that all baseline laboratory tests (including most of the chemistries and blood counts listed in Table 1.6) be evaluated. A toxicological screen (10 cc blood or 50 ml urine) may (or may not) reveal evidence of the drug, depending on the length of time since the last drug dose and the specific substance involved. It is imperative that the physical condition be carefully monitored throughout the acute withdrawal syndrome.

2.2.2.2. Treatment

See Sections 4.2.2.2 and 6.2.2.1.2.

An important aspect of treatment is prevention. Thus, patients should never be placed on a daily depressant for more than 2–3 weeks. Even with short-term use, the drug should be tapered off slowly rather than stopped abruptly.[27]

The treatment of depressant withdrawal follows a relatively simple paradigm. This includes a good physical evaluation, general supportive care, education and reassurance, and, if needed, medication.[2,13,59,60] The comments that follow apply to syndromes caused by withdrawal from depressants other than alcohol. Alcoholic withdrawal is discussed in Section 4.2.2.

1. To avoid delirium or convulsions, it is important to consider treatment of withdrawal in a *hospital setting*, although slow weaning off the drug as an outpatient is possible.
2. Each patient should receive an adequate *physical examination* and general *screening laboratory procedures*.
3. Assuming that the physical condition is stable and that the patient is being provided with good nutrition, rest, and multivitamins, treatment of the withdrawal itself can begin.
4. My preferred approach is to use the drug of abuse itself as a withdrawal agent, gradually tapering the doses over an approximate 4–8-week period (although this regimen does not result in a disappearance of all symptoms). There are few data to support the use of alpha adrenergic agonists (e.g., clonidine or Catapres) or beta blockers such as propranolol (Inderal) in the treatment of these syndromes. These agents run the risk of masking internal autonomic overactivity that can indicate impending seizures or delirium.
5. An alternate approach is to switch the patient to a long-acting depressant. This is listed for the sake of completeness, although I prefer

tapering the specific drug the patient is dependent upon. If a long-acting drug is chosen, you might consider phenobarbital (Luminal), which has a half-life of 12–24 h. This approach is based on the ease with which stable blood levels of this longer acting drug can be maintained, but suffers the drawback of some difficulty in determining the effective starting dose.

a. One begins by estimating the dose of the drug of dependence and giving approximately 32 mg of phenobarbital for each 100 mg of estimated barbiturate, for each 400 mg of meprobamate (Equanil), for each 5 mg of diazepam (Valium), or for each 25 mg of chlordiazepoxide (Librium). The total dose of phenobarbital is divided into portions to be given four times per day (QID), with extra medication given if the patient begins to demonstrate signs of withdrawal. Doses up to 500 mg of phenobarbital are sometimes needed.
b. One or two consecutive doses (or more) are withheld if the patient appears too sleepy or demonstrates some signs of intoxication, such as nystagmus or ataxia.
c. The required dose is then utilized for 2 days, given in divided doses at 6 A.M., noon, or 6 P.M., and midnight, with the largest dose (approximately 1.5 times the other dose) being given at midnight.
d. After this, the dose is decreased by approximately 30 mg per day—a 200 mg IM dose can be used if needed to control the emergence of serious withdrawal symptoms. If the patient looks sleepy or confused, the next dose should be withheld until he clears. It has not been shown that it is necessary to include phenytoin (Dilantin).
e. This is a rough outline and the individual dose must be titrated for the specific patient. The goal is to reach a drug level at 24 h that decreases withdrawal symptomatology without intoxicating the patient or making him too sleepy. As with any drug that has a half-life of more than a few hours, it is important to recognize that the drug could accumulate in the body over time. This danger is especially relevant in elderly patients, and those with chronic dementia or serious liver impairment—situations some might consider to be inappropriate for the phenobarbitol approach.

2.2.3. Delirium, Dementia, and Other Cognitive Disorders (292.81, 292.82, and 292.83 in DSM-IV)

See Section 1.7.3.

States of confusion can be seen with low doses of drugs in patients with an increased sensitivity to brain depressants (e.g., the elderly or people with brain damage) during severe intoxication, during an *overdose*, or in the context of depressant withdrawal.[9,30,61,62]

2.2.3.1. General Comments

Several special cases of a delirium or dementia need further discussion. Individuals with decreased brain functioning (e.g., older people and those who have had previous brain damage as a result of trauma, infections, or other causes) are probably more sensitive to the effects of all depressants, including the Bzs.[30,63] Thus, such individuals might be expected to show a clinically significant and relatively persistent, although rarely permanent, state of confusion when they take even moderate doses of hypnotics, alcohol, or most antianxiety drugs. Use or misuse of depressants should be considered as part of the differential diagnosis for all confused states of recent onset or for anyone demonstrating a rapid deterioration in his usual state of cognition.

A second important case involves the propensity of all of the brain depressants to interfere with the acquisition of new memories.[49,50] This condition of anterograde amnesia is similar to an alcoholic blackout (see Section 3.2.4), and is most likely to be observed when the drugs are taken in high doses or IV. In fact, minor medical procedures such as cardioversion and dental operations take advantage of this property. Although seen with all brain-depressant drugs, several agents, including triazolam, are especially likely to produce anterograde amnesia at clinically relevant doses.

Another important topic involves the possible development of more persistent neuropsychological deficits in heavy users of depressant drugs.[42,64] Significant memory problems have been reported in people who are depressant-dependent. These observations are corroborated by the demonstration of at least temporary psychological test deficits (e.g., on the Halstead–Reitan Battery) in a third or more of people with depressant dependence—deficits that can then remain during 3 weeks to 3 months of abstinence, or even longer.[64]

The treatment of a state of confusion induced by a depressant involves a series of common-sense steps. First, the patient should be evaluated for any life-threatening causes of the diminished level of cognition including trauma (e.g., a subdural hematoma), serious infections in the CNS or elsewhere, blood loss, electrolyte imbalances, hypoglycemia, and so on. Next, all depressants should be stopped, and the patient should be observed over the next several weeks to monitor improvement. As with alcohol, it is possible that some patients may demonstrate more permanent neuropsychological deficits.

The discussion now highlights two specific categories of delirium and dementia in greater detail.

2.2.3.2. Diminished Cognition Caused by Mild Overdose

2.2.3.2.1. Clinical Picture

A toxic syndrome short of a coma is characterized by abnormal vital signs and confusion, disorientation, decreased mentation, and impaired memory. This picture resembles the one seen during severe alcohol intoxication.

It may develop even at low doses in individuals at high risk for confusion, such as older people.

2.2.3.2.2. Treatment

This state is best treated with observation and general support, usually in an inpatient setting where the patient is protected from wandering or from harming himself. For younger individuals, the confusion usually clears within a matter of hours to days, but for older people, it might require an extended treatment period of 2 weeks or longer. In either instance, it is best to avoid the concomitant administration of any other drug.

2.2.3.3. States of Confusion Observed During Withdrawal

2.2.3.3.1. Clinical Picture

A rapidly evolving delirium can be seen during withdrawal from these drugs.[18] It is usually temporary, rarely lasting more than a few days even without treatment. When it develops, signs of withdrawal are usually prominent, but one must take care to rule out other potentially lethal causes of dementia, including trauma, occult bleeding, and brain damage.

2.2.3.3.2. Treatment

Treatment of a delirium during withdrawal is discussed in Section 2.2.2.2.

2.2.4. Psychosis (292.11 and 292.12 in DSM-IV)

See Sections 1.7.4, 4.2.4, and 5.2.4.

2.2.4.1. Clinical Picture

High repetitive doses of depressant drugs can produce a temporary psychosis, or a depressant-induced psychotic disorder, characterized by a relatively acute onset in a clear sensorium (the patient is alert and oriented), of auditory hallucinations, and/or paranoid delusions (e.g., thinking that someone is plotting against or trying to harm him). This picture has been more clearly established as it relates to alcohol, and thus is discussed in greater depth in Section 4.2.4. However, similar pictures can be expected with the misuse of any depressant.[65] It is probable that the generalizations presented for alcohol hold for the other depressants as well.

2.2.4.2. Treatment

With supportive care, the psychosis is likely to clear within 2 days to 4 weeks of abstinence. Antipsychotic medications do not have to be given unless the paranoia and/or hallucinations create a danger to the patient or to those around him. Then, such drugs—that is, haloperidol (Haldol), or risperidone (Risperdal), 1–3 mg twice a day can be used until the clinical picture clears.

2.2.5. Flashbacks

There are no recognized flashbacks with depressants.

2.2.6. Anxiety and Depression (292.89 and 292.84 in DSM-IV)

See Sections 1.7.6, 5.2.6, 7.2.6, and 8.2.6.

Withdrawal from depressant drugs can produce temporary symptoms similar to major anxiety disorders, which is discussed as sedative-, hypnotic, or anxiolytic-induced anxiety disorders in DSM-IV.[12,66] These can include symptoms of panic disorder, social phobia, agoraphobia, or generalized anxiety disorder. Intense *intoxication* with any brain depressant can mimic major depressive disorders, at least temporarily, although the syndrome is highly likely to disappear with continued abstinence.[67,68]

2.2.6.1. Clinical Picture

During intoxication, people can demonstrate pervasive sadness, hopelessness, the inability to concentrate, problems in sleeping, loss of appetite, and so on.[68] Withdrawal states are likely to include panic attacks that resemble panic disorder, high levels of anxiety regarding social situations that can be misdiagnosed as social phobia, along with high levels of feelings of anxiety that could be mislabeled as generalized anxiety disorder. Whereas independent major depressive and anxiety syndromes tend to be long-term, and for the latter, lifelong, the substance-induced pictures are time limited, with symptoms likely to improve markedly within a month or so of abstinence, and then to totally disappear over the next several months.

2.2.6.2. Treatment

When observed in any clinical condition, intense depressions, especially those with associated suicidal thoughts, must be taken seriously.[69] Thus, depressant-induced temporary mood disorders might require short-term hospitalizations with suicide precautions until the intensity of the depressive symptoms decreases over the subsequent days to weeks. In addition, in the context of these mood disturbances, it is important that patients be reassured that, although the symptoms are troubling, they are only temporary and will improve with continued abstinence. Of course, if the severe depressions interfering with life functioning remain at intense levels beyond the first month or so of abstinence, there may be a careful psychiatric evaluation for the possibility that an independent long-term major depressive disorder is present.

Anxiety conditions, whether representing independent lifelong anxiety disorders or as part of depressant withdrawal, usually do not require emergency intervention. Patients are likely to respond to education and to reassurance regarding the temporary nature of their symptoms. Active efforts to help individuals learn relaxation approaches, and more formal cognitive therapies to help them adjust to the acute and more protracted (but temporary) brain depressant-related syndromes can also be beneficial. However, because of the temporary nature of these substance-induced anxiety syndromes, medications are rarely, if ever, justified.

2.2.7. Medical Problems

Whereas few medical disorders are known to be unique to people who are depressant-dependent, daily use of hypnotics is associated with a slight, but significant, overall increased mortality rate (1.22–1.35 fold in women and in men), even after controlling for all other factors.[70] The conditions that develop depend on the specific drug taken and the route of administration. A few "special" problems are discussed in this section.

1. Anecdotal information indicates an ability of extended use of these drugs to *impair memory* over an extended period of time—perhaps even permanently. However, this phenomenon has not been definitely established.
2. IV users are vulnerable to all the complications that can result from contaminated needles.[71] These include hepatitis, tetanus, abscesses, acquired immunodeficiency syndrome (AIDS), and so on, as described for opioids in Section 6.2.7.
3. A special problem can result from the injection of these drugs into an artery. The resulting painful muscle and nervous tissue necrosis can necessitate amputation of a limb. Injection into veins can cause venous thrombosis.
4. A major difficulty with any depressant, including the Bzs, is the product of excessive *sedation*. This may cause impaired judgment and deterioration in work and motor performance, especially with longer acting drugs, which may accumulate in the body over time.[72] Although the actual number of cases is unknown, it is likely that depressants contribute to many motor vehicle accidents each year. Cognitive problems are exaggerated in the presence of liver disease or decreased albumin in the blood, but all patients should be warned to avoid activities demanding high levels of alertness and/or motor performance if they are experiencing sedation side effects. An additional problem, especially in the elderly who are more sensitive to the effects of brain depressants, is the possibility of falls with a subsequent heightened risk for hip fractures.[42,63]

5. At the usual doses, these drugs are not likely to induce serious *cardiac* symptoms in the average healthy individual. However, all depressants can suppress respirations, and thus, might precipitate respiratory failure in individuals with chronic obstructive lung disease.
6. All of these drugs can decrease inhibitions and have been reported to increase angry outbursts. Some patients with depression can react to depressants with an intensification of their sadness and irritability.
7. *Drug interactions* are a potential problem with all medications. The depressants are likely to potentiate the side effects of tricyclic-type antidepressants and anticonvulsants, and (through possible interference with liver metabolism) may increase blood levels of digoxin.[73] The actions of L-dopa may be inhibited by this class of drugs, and cimetidine may interfere with benzodiazepine metabolism and excretion. Of course, the interaction between two or more depressants can be severe, and an enhancement of Bz actions are likely to be noted after an individual drinks ethanol. Long-term oral contraceptive use can interfere with benzodiazepine metabolism, and antacids can interfere with their absorption.
8. No drug can be considered safe during *pregnancy*. Although there is some controversy, and other depressants such as thalidomide are highly toxic to the fetus, there is no strong evidence of specific teratogenicity for most of the currently used depressants.[74] Because this class of drugs is rarely necessary for sustaining life functioning, pregnant women should be told to avoid these medications, especially during the first trimester. This caveat probably extends to the neonatal period for women who are breast-feeding, as there is evidence that Bzs pass through the mother's milk to the baby and may be responsible for an accumulation of bilirubin.[75,76]

REFERENCES

1. Ballenger, J. C. Benzodiazepine receptor agonists and antagonists. In B. J. Sadock, & V. A. Sadock (Eds.), *Kaplan & Sadock's Comprehensive Textbook of Psychiatry* (7th ed.). Baltimore, MD: Lippincott, Williams & Wilkins, 2000, pp. 2317–2323.
2. Wesson, D. R., Smith, D. E., Ling, W., & Seymour, R. B. Sedative-hypnotics. In J. H. Lowinson, P. Ruiz, R. B. Millman, & J. G. Langrod (Eds.), *Substance Abuse: A Comprehensive Textbook* (4th ed.). Baltimore, MD: Lippincott, Williams & Wilkins, 2004, pp. 302–312.
3. Evers, A. S., & Crowder, C. M. General anesthetics. In J. G. Hardman, L. E. Limbird, & A. G. Goodman (Eds.), *The Pharmacological Basis of Therapeutics* (10th ed.). New York: McGraw-Hill, 2001, pp. 337–366.
4. Charney, D. S., Mihic, J., & Harris, R. A. Hypnotics and sedatives. In J. G. Hardman, L. E. Limbird, & A. G. Goodman (Eds.), *The Pharmacological Basis of Therapeutics* (10th ed.). New York: McGraw-Hill, 2001, pp. 399–427.
5. O'Brien, C. P. Drug addiction and drug abuse, In J. G. Hardman, L. E. Limbird, & A. G. Goodman (Eds.), *The Pharmacological Basis of Therapeutics* (10th ed.). New York: McGraw-Hill, 2001, pp. 621–642.

6. Brancucci, A., Berretta, N., Mercuri, N. B., & Francesconi, W. Presynaptic modulation of spontaneous inhibitory postsynaptic currents by gamma-hydroxyburyrate in the substantia nigra pars compacta. *Neuropsychopharmacology 29:*537–543, 2004.
7. Stoops, W. W., & Rush, C. R. Differential effects in humans after repeated administrations of zolpidem and triazolam. *The American Journal of Drug and Alcohol Abuse. 29:*281–299, 2003.
8. Szabo, S. T., Gold, M. S., Goldberg, B. A., & Blier, P. Effects of sustained gamma-hydroxybutyrate treatments on spontaneous and evoked firing activity of locus coeruleus norepinephrine neurons. *Biological Psychiatry 55:*934–939, 2004.
9. Girdler, N. M., Lyne, J. P., Wallace, R., Neave, N., Scholey, A., Wesnes, K. A., & Herman, C. A randomized controlled trial of cognitive and psychomotor recovery from midazolam sedation following reversal with oral flumazenil. *Anaesthesia 57:*868–876, 2002.
10. Bloom, F. E. Neurotransmission and the central nervous system. In J. G. Hardman, L. E. Limbird, & A. G. Goodman (Eds.), *The Pharmacological Basis of Therapeutics* (10th ed.). New York: McGraw-Hill, 2001, pp. 293–320.
11. Flaishon, R., Weinbroum, A. A., Veenman, L., Leschiner, S., Ruddick, V., & Gavish, M. Flumazenil attenuates development of tolerance to diazepam after chronic treatment of mice with either isoflurane or diazepam. *Anesthesia & Analgesia 97:*1046–1052, 2003.
12. Allison, C., Claase, L. A., & Pratt, J. A. Diazepam withdrawal-induced anxiety and place aversion in the rat: Differential effects of two chronic diazepam treatment regimes. *Behavioral Pharmacology 13:*417–425, 2002.
13. Gerra, G., Zaimovic, A., Giusti, F., Moi, G., & Brewer, C. Intravenous flumazenil versus oxazepam tapering in the treatment of benzodiazepine withdrawal: A randomized, placebo-controlled study. *Addictive Biology 7:*385–395, 2002.
14. McGregor, C., Machin, A., & White, J. M. In-patient benzodiazepine withdrawal: Comparison of fixed and symptom-triggered taper methods. *Drug and Alcohol Review 22:*175–180, 2003.
15. Chand, P. K., & Murthy, P. Megadose lorazepam dependence. *Addiction 98:*1633–1636, 2003.
16. Hajak, G., Müller, W. E., Wittchen, H. U., Pittrow, D., & Kirch, W. Abuse and dependence potential for the non-benzodiazepine hypnotics zolpidem and zopiclone: A review of case reports and epidemiological data. *Addiction 98:*1371–1378, 2003.
17. Rosenberg, R., Caron, J., Roth, T., & Amato, D. An assessment of the efficacy and safety of eszopiclone in the treatment of transient insomnia in healthy adults. *Sleep Medicine 6*:15-22, 2005.
18. Cammarano, W. B., Pittet, J. F., Weitz, S., Schlobohm, R. M., & Marks, J. D. Acute withdrawal syndrome related to the administration of analgesic and sedative medications in adult intensive care unit patients. *Critical Care Medicine 26:*676–684, 1998.
19. Gatzonis, S. D., Angelopoulos, E. K., Daskalopoulou, E. G., *et al.* Convulsive status epilepticus following abrupt high-dose benzodiazepine discontinuation. *Drug and Alcohol Dependence 59:*95–97, 2000.
20. Darke, S., Topp, L., & Ross, J. The injection of methadone and benzodiazepines among Sydney injecting drug users 1996–2000: 5-year monitoring of trends from the illicit drug reporting system. *Drug and Alcohol Review 21:*27–32, 2002.
21. Ross, J., & Darke, S. The nature of benzodiazepine dependence among heroin users in Sydney, Australia. *Addiction 95:*1785–1793, 2000.
22. American Psychiatric Association. *The Diagnostic and Statistical Manual of Mental Disorders* (4th ed. revised text) Washington, DC: American Psychiatric Press, 2000.
23. Beaumont, M., Batejat, D., Coste, O., van Beers, P., Colas, A., Clere, J.-M., & Pierard, C. Effects of zolpidem and zaleplon on sleep, respiratory patterns and performance at a simulated altitude of 4,000 m. *Neuropsychobiology 49:*154–162, 2004.
24. Drover, D. R. Comparative pharmacokinetics and pharmacodynamics of short-acting hypnosedatives: Zaleplon, zolpidem, and zopiclone. *Clinical Pharmacokinetics 43:*227–238, 2004.

25. Berthelon, C., Bocca, M. L., Denise, P., & Pottier, A. Do zopiclone, zolpidem and flunitrazepam have residual effects on stimulated task of collision anticipation? *Journal of Psychopharmacology 17:*324–331, 2003.
26. Gahlinger, P. M. Club drugs: MDMA, gamma-hydroxybutyrate (GHB), rophynol and ketamine. *American Family Physician 69:*2619–2626, 2004.
27. Lader, M. Iatrogenic sedative dependence and abuse—Have doctors learnt caution? *Addiction 93:*1133–1135, 1998.
28. Ancoli-Israel, S. *All I Want is a Good Night's Sleep.* St. Louis, MO: Mosby Publishing Co., 1996.
29. Rickels, K., DeMartinis, N., Garcia-Espana, F., Greenblatt, D. J., *et al.* Imipramine and buspirone in treatment of patients with generalized anxiety disorder who are discontinuing long-term benzodiazepine therapy. *American Journal of Psychiatry 57:*1973–1979, 2000.
30. Wang, P. S., Bohn, R. L., Glynn, R. J., Mogun, H., & Avorn, J. Hazardous benzodiazepine regimens in the elderly: Effects of half-life, dosage, and duration on risk of hip fracture. *American Journal of Psychiatry 158:*892–898, 2001.
31. Buck, K. J., & Finn, D. A. Genetic factors in addiction: QTL mapping and candidate gene studies implicate GABAergic genes in alcohol. *Addiction 96:*139–149, 2000.
32. McKernan, R. M., Rosahl, T. W., Reynolds, D. S., Sur, C., Wafford, K. A., *et al.* Sedative but not anxiolytic properties of benzodiazepines are mediated by the GABAa receptor a! subtype. *Nature Neuroscience 3:*587–592, 2000.
33. Olshaker, J. S., & Flanigan, J. Flumazenil reversal of lorazepam-induced acute delirium. *Journal of Emergency Medicine 24:*181–183, 2003.
34. Sanders-Bush, E., & Mayer, S. E. 5-Hydroxytryptamine (Serotonin): Receptor Agonists and Antagonists. In J. G. Hardman, L. E. Limbird, & A. G. Goodman (Eds.), *The Pharmacological Basis of Therapeutics* (10th ed.). New York: McGraw-Hill, 2001, pp. 205–222.
35. Liu, Y. P., Wilkinson, L. S., & Robbins, T. W. Effects of acute and chronic buspirone on impulsive choice and efflux of 5-HT and dopamine in hippocampus, nucleus accumbens, and prefrontal cortex. *Psychopharmcology 173:*175–185, 2004.
36. Rynn, M., Garcia-Espana, F., Greenblatt, D. J., Mandos, L. A., Schweizer, E, & Rickels K. Imipramine and buspirone in patients with panic disorder who are discontinuing long-term benzodiazepine therapy. *Journal of Clinical Psychopharmacology 25:*505–508, 2003.
37. Carter, L. P., Chen, W., Wu, H., Mehta, A. K., Hernandez, R. J., Ticku, M. K., Coop, A., Koek, W., & France, C. P. Comparison of the behavioral effects of gamma-hydroxybutyric acid (GHB) and its 4-methyl-substituted analog, gamma-hydroxyvaleric acid (GVB). *Drug and Alcohol Dependence 78:*91–99, 2005.
38. Reeves, J., & Duda, R. GHB/GBL intoxication and withdrawal: A review and case presentation. *Addictive Disorders & Their Treatment 2:*25–28, 2003.
39. Rosenberg, M. H., Deerfield, L. J., & Baruch, E. M. Two cases of severe gamma-hydroxbutyrate withdrawal delirium on a psychiatric unit: Recommendations for management. *The American Journal of Drug and Alcohol Abuse 29:*487–496, 2003.
40. Cairney, S., Clough, A. R., Maruff, P., Collie, A., Currie, B. J., & Currie, J. Saccade and cognitive function in chronic kava users. *Neuropsychopharmacology 28:*389–396, 2003.
41. Nowell, P. D., Mazumdar, S., Buysse, D. J., *et al.* Benzodiazepines and zolpidem for chronic insomnia: A meta-analysis of treatment efficacy. *Journal of the American Medical Association 278:*2170–2177, 1997.
42. McCabe, S. E. Correlates of nonmedical use of prescription benzodiazepine anxiolytics: Results from a national survey of U.S. college students. *Drug and Alcohol Dependence 79:*53-62, 2005.
43. Boixet, M., Batlle, E., & Bolibar, I. Benzodiazepines in primary health care: A survey of general practitioners prescribing patterns. *Addiction 91:*549–556, 1996.
44. Johnston, L. D., O'Malley, P. M., & Bachman, J. G. *Monitoring the Future National Survey Results on Drug Use, 1975–2003. Vol. II: College Students and Adults Ages 19–40.* (NIH Publication No. 04-5506). Bethesda, MD: National Institute on Drug Abuse, 2004.

45. Substance Abuse and Mental Health Services Administration. *Overview of Findings from the 2002 National Survey on Drug Use and Health* (Office of Applied Studies, NHSDA Series H-21, DHHS Publication No. SMA 03–3774). Rockville, MD, 2003.
46. Ross, J., Darke, S., & Hall, W. Transitions between routes of benzodiazepine administration among heroin users in Sydney. *Addiction 92:*697–705, 1995.
47. Kasper, D. L., Braunwald, E., Fauci, A. S., *et al.* (Eds.), *Harrison's Principles of Internal Medicine* (16th ed.). New York: McGraw-Hill, 2005.
48. Ma, O. J., & Cline, D. M. (Eds.), *Emergency Medicine Manual* (6th ed.). New York: McGraw-Hill, 2004.
49. Pomara, N., Willoughby, L., Wesnes, K., Greenblatt, D. J., & Sidtis, J. J. Apoliprotein E ∊4 allele and lorazepam effects on memory in high-functioning older adults. *Archives of General Psychiatry 62*:209–216, 2005.
50. Verster, J. C., Volkerts, E. R., & Verbaten, M. N. Effects of alprazolam on driving ability, memory functioning and psychomotor performance: A randomized, placebo-controlled study. *Neuropsychopharmacology 27:*260–269, 2002.
51. Sperling, R., Greve, D., Dale, A., Killiany, R., *et al.* Functional MRI detection of pharmacologically induced memory impairment. *PNAS 99:*455–460, 2002.
52. Mausner, K. L. Sedatives and hypnotics. In O. J. Ma, & D. M. Cline (Eds.), *Emergency Medicine Manual* (6th ed.). New York: McGraw-Hill, 2004, pp. 489–493.
53. Najarian, S. L. General management of the poisoned patient. In O. J. Ma, & D. M. Cline (Eds.), *Emergency Medicine Manual* (6th ed.). New York: McGraw-Hill, 2004, pp. 467–475.
54. Chang, G., & Kosten, T. R. Detoxification. In J. H. Lowinson, P. Ruiz, R. B. Millman, & J. G. Langrod (Eds.), *Substance Abuse: A Comprehensive Textbook* (4th ed.). Baltimore, MA: Lippincott, Williams & Wilkins, 2004, pp. 579–586.
55. Weinbroum, A. A., Flaishon, R., Sorkine, P., *et al.* A risk-benefit assessment of flumazenil in the management of benzodiazepine overdose. *Drug Safety 17:*181–196, 1997.
56. Salzman, C. The APA task force report on benzodiazepine dependence, toxicity, and abuse. *American Journal of Psychiatry 148:*151–152, 1991.
57. Kaminski, B. J., Sannerud, C. A., Weerts, E. M., Lamb, R. J., & Griffiths, R. R. Physical dependence in baboons chronically treated with low and high doses of diazepam. *Behavioral Pharmacology 14:*331–342, 2003.
58. Satel, S. L., Kosten, T. R., Schuckit, M. A., & Fischman, M. W. Should protracted withdrawal from drugs be included in DSM-IV? *American Journal of Psychiatry 150:*695–704, 1993.
59. Vorma, H., Naukkarinen, H., Sarna, S., & Kuoppasalmi, K. Treatment of out-patients with complicated benzodiazepine dependence: Comparison of two approaches. *Addiction 97:*851–859, 2002.
60. Morin, C. M., Bastien, C., Guay, B., Radouco-Thomas, M., Leblanc, J., & Vallières, A. Randomized clinical trial of supervised tapering and cognitive behavior therapy to facilitate benzodiazepine discontinuation in older adults with chronic insomnia. *American Journal of Psychiatry 161:*332–342, 2004.
61. Koski, A., Ojanperä, I., & Vuori, E. Alcohol and benzodiazepines in fatal poisonings. *Alcoholism: Clinical and Experimental Research 26:*956–959, 2002.
62. Anthenelli, R. M., Klein, J. L., Smith, T. L., & Schuckit, M. A. Comparison of the subjective and amnestic effects of diazepam and amobarbital in healthy young men. *The American Journal of Addictions 2:*131–140, 1993.
63. Cummings, S. R., Nevitt, M. C., Browner, W. S., *et al.* Risk factors for hip fracture in white women. *New England Journal of Medicine 332:*767–773, 1995.
64. Tönne, U., Hiltunen, A. J., Vikander, B., *et al.* Neuropsychological changes during steady-state drug use, withdrawal and abstinence in primary benzodiazepine-dependent patients. *Acta Psychiatrica Scandinavica 91:*299–304, 1995.
65. Fraser, A. A., & Ingram, I. M. Lorazepam dependence and chronic psychosis. *British Journal of Psychiatry 147:*211, 1985.

66. Martínez-Cano, H., de Iceta Ibáñez de Gauna, M., Vela-Bueno, A., & Wittchen, H. U. DSM–III–R co-morbidity in benzodiazepine dependence. *Addiction 94:*97–107, 1999.
67. Schuckit, M. A., Tipp, J. E., Bucholz, K. K., *et al.* The life time rates of three major mood disorders and four major anxiety disorders in alcoholics and controls. *Addiction 92:*1289–1304, 1997.
68. Schuckit, M. A., Tipp, J. E., Bergman, M., *et al.* Comparison of induced and independent major depressive disorders in 2,945 alcoholics. *American Journal of Psychiatry 154:*948–957, 1997.
69. Preuss, U. W., Schuckit, M. A., Smith, T. L., Danko, G. P., Dasher, A. C., Hesselbrock, M. N., Hesselbrock, V. M., & Nurnberger, J. I., Jr. A comparison of alcohol-induced and independent depression in alcoholics with histories of suicide attempt. *Journal of Studies on Alcohol 63:*498–502, 2002.
70. Kripke, D. F., Klauber, M. R., Wingard, D. L., *et al.* Mortality hazard associated with prescription hypnotics. *Biological Psychiatry 43:*687–693, 1998.
71. Dobbin, M., Martyres, R. F., Clode, D., & Champion de Crespigny, F. E. Association of benzodiazepine injection with the prescription of temazepam capsules. *Drug and Alcohol Review 22:*153–157, 2003.
72. Barbone, F., McMahon, A. D., Davey, P. G., *et al.* Association of road-traffic accidents with benzodiazepine use. *Lancet 352:*1331–1336, 1998.
73. Schuckit, M. A. A clinical review of interactions among medications. *Developmental Disabilities: Clinical Insights 11*, San Diego Regional Center for the Developmentally Disabled, 1998.
74. Bergman, U., Rosa, F. W., Baum, C., Wilhom, B. E., & Faich, G. A. Effects of exposure to benzodiazepine during fetal life. *Lancet 340:*694–696, 1992.
75. Steingart, R. A., Abu-Roumi, M., Newman, M. E., Silverman, W. F., Slotkin, T. A., & Yanai, J. Neurobehavioral damage to cholinergic systems caused by prenatal exposure to heroin or phenobarbital: Cellular mechanisms and the reversal of deficits by neural grafts. *Developmental Brain Research 122:*125–133, 2000.
76. Burt, V. K., Suri, R., Altshuler, L., Stowe, Z., *et al.* The use of psychotropic medications during breast-feeding. *American Journal of Psychiatry 158:*1101–1109, 2001.

CHAPTER 3

Alcoholism: An Introduction

3.1. INTRODUCTION

3.1.1. General Comments

Alcohol, nicotine, and caffeine are the most widely used drugs in Western civilizations, and alcohol is the most acutely destructive of the three. Thus, alcohol is used in this text as a prototype for the discussion of other pharmacological agents, with information presented in Chapters 3, 4, and 14. This chapter covers some definitions, pharmacology and effects on body systems, epidemiology, the natural history of alcoholism, and some data on etiology. Chapter 4 is an overview of treatment of acute problems, and Chapter 14 offers information on rehabilitation of the alcoholic.

3.1.2. Some Definitions

3.1.2.1. Alcohol Abuse and Dependence (305.00 and 303.90 in DSM-IV)

As a clinician, I diagnose a patient in order to know about prognosis and to help me select the best treatment. The criteria I use must be clear and relatively precise so that they can be utilized by different clinicians in different settings. Over the last 20 years, progress has been made to meet these demands for both alcohol abuse and dependence, as presented in Table 1.1.[1–7] Dependence requires a positive response to three of seven items, indicating repetitive problems that interfere with functioning and that cluster together, so that three or more items have occurred during the same 12-month period. Thus, the age of onset of dependence can be considered as the age at which three or more items get clustered together, not the age of the first problem. DSM-IV also advises clinicians to place special emphasis on the diagnosis of dependence with a physiological component (i.e., tolerance and/or withdrawal have been reported at some time in the course of alcoholism).[8,9] Several papers have reported that this diagnostic subtype is associated with more concurrent problems and a worse prognosis.[10,11]

Abuse, a diagnosis only relevant if the person is not dependent on that substance, centers on four items separate from those used for dependence, including social, interpersonal, and legal problems, or continued use despite such difficulties. For abuse, the problems must have occurred repeatedly over a 12-month period and caused clinically significant impairment or distress. Several studies have documented that, among adults, the diagnosis of alcohol abuse is likely to remain stable over time, with only about 10% going into alcohol dependence.[5,6,12–14]

The clinical validity of the diagnosis of DSM-IV dependence has been established through several approaches.[4,15] Individuals with this diagnosis have very high levels of alcohol intake, and at least 70–80% continue to show repetitive alcohol problems over follow-ups from 1– to 5 years and beyond.[5,12,16–19] The diagnosis tends to run in families, is strongly genetically influenced, and the criteria overall appear to work when applied to special populations including adolescents, older individuals, and the homeless.[20–24] The four criteria for abuse may be a bit less reliable than dependence, but still identify individuals with a relatively predictable clinical course.[25,26] Regardless of the socioeconomic status, at least 50–60% of those with abuse continue to show alcohol-related difficulties over the next 5 years.[7,12,26]

A diagnostic system that relies upon two clinical entities defined by separate criteria (i.e., abuse and dependence) does create some potential problems.[27,28] One difficulty is that it is possible for an individual to have one or two of the dependence criteria, but not the criteria for abuse. These "diagnostic orphans" (demonstrating problems but not meeting criteria for either major diagnosis) appear to have a clinical course midway between the problems over time expected for individuals with dependence and those relevant to the diagnosis of abuse.[27] Subsequent diagnostic manuals, such as DSM-V, will need to take this important group into consideration.

Although the majority of clinicians in the United States use DSM-IV criteria for the substance-use disorders, in some other parts of the world ICD-10 is preferred. Fortunately, the criteria for dependence are similar in the two major diagnostic approaches. ICD-10 lists six items for dependence, most of which are roughly the same as those offered in DSM-IV. The threshold for a diagnosis requires three or more of the items to have occurred during the previous year (remember that DSM-IV asks for clustering during any 12-month period).[2] The criteria for harmful use (the rough parallel of abuse) are, unfortunately, quite different from those outlined for abuse in DSM-IV, with evidence that the syndromes do not greatly overlap. In ICD-10, harmful use is diagnosed only in the presence of actual damage to health, which can be physical (as in the cases of hepatitis from alcohol) or mental (e.g., episodes of depressive disorders secondary to heavy drinking). Of course, harmful use is not diagnosed if dependence on that same substance is present.

3.1.2.2. Some Additional Diagnostic Considerations

To be clinically useful, diagnostic criteria must be stated in relatively objective terms, avoiding such judgments as "He drinks too much" or "I *feel* that he is becoming too psychologically dependent".[29] Several additional approaches and concepts have been proposed for consideration for substance-use disorders, but each has potential problems.

1. The *quantity–frequency–variability* (QFV) approach attempts to gather accurate information on drinking patterns, and then to place an individual in a "deviant" category when the alcohol intake differs statistically from the average. Although this scheme is relevant to studies of drinking patterns, its usefulness is limited by the difficulty of obtaining good information about alcohol intake because of the reticence of the individual to admit his pattern, and because of his decreased memory at rapidly rising blood-alcohol levels.
2. A second rubric, *psychological dependence*, is based on the occurrence of a series of subjective experiences relating drinking to such problems as stockpiling liquor, taking drinks before going to a party, and otherwise demonstrating that the individual is psychologically uncomfortable unless there is alcohol around. It is difficult to objectively quantify this approach.
3. A third diagnostic scheme, widely used by physicians in the past, centers on the occurrence of *withdrawal* or *abstinence* symptoms when an individual stops drinking alcohol.[9] However, most people experiencing withdrawal have relatively mild symptoms[30] that can be difficult to distinguish from a hangover or a case of flu. In any event, limiting the definition of dependence to those who have evidenced withdrawal is restrictive, as many individuals who have serious life-impairment and medical problems and who may die of an alcohol-related complication have never demonstrated obvious signs of physical withdrawal.
4. Before leaving the topic of diagnostic approaches, it is important to recognize that an alternative scheme could involve a dimensional, as opposed to categorical, approach.[31,32] Here, for example, the seven DSM-IV dependence criteria might be used to generate a scale score from zero to seven, depending upon the number of criteria endorsed in the appropriate time period. This approach is attractive for research endeavors, but has some drawbacks in clinical settings. Diagnostic criteria are often used as guidelines by healthcare provider organizations and insurance companies to determine the level of intensity of care appropriate for an individual.[31] In this instance, the relevant agency is likely to choose a cutoff point (perhaps three or more items endorsed in a relevant time period), which, in effect, reverts to a categorical system. As both a researcher and

> clinician, I favor a continuation of the categorical diagnosis because it is more useful in clinical situations, but recognize the potential relevance of using a dimensional approach as an additional scheme in research projects.

As is true of any clinical diagnosis, the criteria must be "bent" for an individual who comes close but does not quite fit the research definition and is thus labeled a "probable" alcoholic. For instance, someone who is self-employed, whose spouse appears to be "long-suffering and uncomplaining," and who appears to be at low risk for arrest (possibly because he either is in a powerful position or lives in a small community where he knows the police), may have many alcohol-related life problems, but may not fulfill the diagnostic criteria. In this instance, the patient would be labeled as having probable alcoholism or alcohol dependence, and would receive the same general treatment as a person with definite alcoholism. However, one should constantly recheck the diagnosis and recognize the lowered level of certainty in predicting the future course.

Understanding the effects of alcohol on the body can facilitate proper diagnosis. As described in Section 3.2.3, there are patterns of laboratory results and physical signs and symptoms that, although not diagnostic, can raise the clinician's suspicion regarding the presence of alcoholism. Similarly, there are a variety of simple paper-and-pencil tests asking about alcohol-related life problems that can help in establishing the diagnosis. The most widely used are the 25-item Michigan Alcohol Screening Test (MAST), its shorter 10-question counterpart, and the 10-item Alcohol Use Disorders Identification Test (AUDIT).[32,33] Although screening tests like this can be helpful, they do not in themselves diagnose alcoholism and cannot take the place of a clinical history carefully obtained from the patient and from a relevant resource person. More details on these tests are offered in Chapter 4, Section 4.1.1.

3.1.2.3. Issues of Dual Diagnosis or Comorbidity (see also Section 3.2.4)

Two out of every three alcohol-dependent individuals meet criteria for an additional psychiatric disorder.[34–37] This subset of alcoholics is heterogeneous, with about half of them (i.e., a third of the total) meeting criteria for another substance-use disorder or a major preexisting personality disorder, especially antisocial personality disorder. This means that about 35% or so of alcohol-dependent men and women appear to have a DSM-IV-like psychiatric condition, especially major depressive episodes, major anxiety conditions, manic depressive disease, and schizophrenia.

There is important heterogeneity of these conditions when observed in alcoholics. It is of key importance to remember that alcohol has a major effect on the brain, and, thus, severe intoxication and withdrawal states are capable of mimicking several major psychiatric disorders. When a psychiatric picture is observed only in the context of heavy drinking or during the abstinence syndrome, this can closely resemble a major psychiatric disorder, except for one major difference. The substance-induced conditions are highly likely to improve within several days or weeks of abstinence, with a great probability that the symptoms will fall below the severity appropriate for the diagnosis of an independent psychiatric disorder within several weeks to at the most one month. The result is that the prognoses and the optimal treatments for alcohol-induced psychiatric pictures are quite different than the approaches most appropriate for independent disorders.

Intoxication with alcohol, a typical depressant drug, is likely to mimic major depressive episodes. The higher the dose of alcohol and the longer the period of heavy drinking, the greater the likelihood that such depressions will occur, with an estimate that between 40% or more alcohol-dependent individuals will have one or more such alcohol-induced episodes. However, the rate of independent major depressions (i.e., severe depressions lasting weeks on end, all day, every day, and interfering with functioning) that are observed outside of the context of heavy drinking may be no more prevalent in alcoholics than in the general population.[36,38,39] Independent major depressions are likely to require many months of treatment with cognitive therapy and/or antidepressant medications, while alcohol-induced mood disorders are likely to benefit from short-term (several weeks) cognitive behavioral approaches, and there are no data to date indicating that they routinely respond to antidepressants.

Withdrawal states from depressants such as alcohol are likely to include high levels of anxiety and insomnia. During the first several weeks to a month following abstinence in alcohol-dependent individuals, these symptoms can be severe enough to resemble major anxiety disorders such as generalized anxiety disorder, panic disorder, and social phobia, as described in DSM-IV.[38,40] It is also likely that the withdrawal states intensify symptoms of posttraumatic stress disorder (PTSD), and, theoretically, might be capable of inducing temporary PTSD-like syndromes in individuals who would otherwise be much less symptomatic. Independent (i.e., not alcohol related) severe anxiety conditions are likely to require long-term (sometimes over many years) cognitive behavioral approaches, as well as some long-term medications, with the specific pharmacological agent differing among the disorders. Alcohol-related anxiety conditions, however, are likely to improve a great deal during the first week or two of abstinence, with continued improvement over the subsequent weeks. The result is that at the end of one month of abstinence, the alcohol-induced anxiety disorders are no longer likely to meet the diagnostic criteria for DSM-IV major anxiety conditions.

In the context of severe repeated intoxication, an estimated 3% or so of alcoholics develop severe paranoid delusions (suspiciousness) and/or auditory hallucinations (hearing voices), while otherwise appearing alert and oriented to time, place, and person. This condition resembles schizophrenia, a disorder that usually requires lifelong prescription of antipsychotic medications, such as risperidone (Risperdal). While alcohol-induced psychotic syndromes may benefit from antipsychotic medications for several days to several weeks, the hallucinations and delusions usually clear fairly rapidly with abstinence, and are almost always gone by one month after the cessation of drinking. Thus, antipsychotic medications for these alcohol-related psychoses are not justified beyond 2 to at most 4 weeks of treatment.

The clinician can distinguish between substance-induced versus independent psychiatric conditions in two ways. The first is to take advantage of the fact that the past behavior is the best predictor of future problems. Therefore, it is worth investing the 5 to 10 min required for a time line-based longitudinal history to determine whether the major psychiatric condition (e.g., a major depression or panic disorder) existed before the onset of dependence.[1,38,39] Note here that it is not a question of whether the major depression, for example, can be documented before the first drink, nor even before the first alcohol-related problem. Rather, the emphasis is on regular and repeated impairment from alcohol (e.g., three or more of the dependence criteria) as might be observed in dependence. It is also worthwhile to evaluate whether the full psychiatric syndrome can be documented as having ever occurred during periods of abstinence of 1 or 2 months or more since the onset of dependence. If the psychiatric condition was noted to be independent in the past (i.e., either antedated the alcoholism or occurred during a 1+ month abstinence), the probability is much higher than for the average alcoholic that the current episode is also independent of the heavy drinking and may require antidepressant medications.

The second and essential step in establishing an independent versus alcohol-induced psychiatric disorder is to work with the patient and the family to encourage at least a 1-month period of abstinence during which the patients' symptoms can be observed. Even for an individual with no evidence of prior independent episodes of the psychiatric condition, maintenance of symptoms severe and debilitating enough to justify a DSM-IV diagnosis after a month of abstinence should cause the clinician to consider revising the label from a probable substance-induced condition to a probable independent psychiatric disorder.

It may be worthwhile to describe this time line-based approach in a little more detail:

1. The *first* key step in attempting to differentiate independent and alcohol-induced syndromes is to determine whether an individual fits actual criteria for an additional psychiatric disorder. For instance, it is important to differentiate sadness (a temporary mood change) and major depressive disorder, to recognize the difference between

someone who "drinks" and a person who fulfills criteria for actual alcohol abuse or dependence.

2. The *second* key step is to gather the best information possible to determine the approximate *age* at which the individual first met the criteria for each disorder. In doing this, it can be useful to help the patients place events in a chronological order by having them establish some important markers in their lives. Thus, a line can be drawn on paper and the ages of high school graduation, marriages, birth of children, longest jobs, etc., noted. Then, the onset of a disorder (e.g., major depression) is based on the full syndrome, not a symptom. Similarly, regarding alcohol dependence, it is not the first alcohol use or isolated problem that is the focus, but the age at which substance-related difficulties clustered together for a diagnosis. Thus, a man could have experienced sadness at age 12, started drinking at age 13, actually fulfilled criteria for alcohol dependence at age 31, and developed an alcohol-induced major depressive disorder at age 35. In this instance, the patient is likely to run the course of alcohol dependence, and the depressive episode is likely to clear within days to weeks of abstinence.
3. A *third* step is to see if the patient had any periods of abstinence since the onset of dependence, and to look for evidence of an independent psychiatric disorder during that period.
4. *Finally*, the patient should be closely observed over time to see if the psychiatric symptoms diminish with continued abstinence over the next month or so.

Although the majority of cases where psychiatric symptoms are observed in the course of alcohol dependence represent alcohol-induced syndromes, the clinician must be careful not to overlook independent disorders when they occur. There are several psychiatric conditions which have relatively close ties to alcohol dependence and, therefore, where independent diagnoses are seen in the course of alcoholism more often than expected by chance alone. These include the antisocial personality disorder, bipolar or manic depressive disease, schizophrenia, and, to a lesser extent, panic disorder and perhaps social phobia. When these independent disorders are identified, they often require long-term treatment in addition to the steps used to address the substance-use disorder. These are discussed in the following section.

3.1.2.3.1. Independent Manic Depressive Disease, Schizophrenia, and Panic Disorders

A variety of hypotheses have been put forth to explain why several independent psychiatric conditions might have higher risks for *both* alcohol and drug use disorders. Some researchers have theorized that both substance-related and psychiatric conditions might be affected by overlapping groups of genes, others have hypothesized that the substance-related problems might occur through impaired judgment inherent in the Axis I (i.e., not personality disorder) psychiatric conditions, and yet others proposed that substances might be used to diminish either the psychiatric symptoms or the side effects of medications used for the Axis I disorders.[41,42] There is probably some truth to each of these explanations, although few studies have supported the last named "self-medication" hypotheses.

An important point here is to note that while manic depressive disease and schizophrenia, for example, are relatively rare conditions (seen in less than 1% of the population), the two to fourfold higher risk for substance-use disorders in these syndromes contributes to the difficulty involved in treating such complicated patients.[43,44] Once a diagnosis of an independent psychiatric condition is established, it is important that either a clinician, knowledgeable in both types of disorders, occupy a key role in treatment, or that clinical groups expert in each, work together as a team to come up with a treatment plan. For independent schizophrenia and manic depressive disease, it is essential to first stabilize the psychiatric condition, while paying attention to any acute need for treatment of an alcohol withdrawal syndrome. Once the mania or psychotic episode, for example, has improved sufficiently, additional treatment aimed at enhancing motivation for abstinence from alcohol and other drugs must be implemented. It is important that clinicians providing long-term treatment recognize the need to continue to address both types of problems.

Independent moderate depressive episodes (lacking acute suicidal ideation) and independent anxiety conditions can often be initially handled in alcohol treatment settings. Here, cognitive treatment can be used to initially treat the independent disorder, with decisions made on a case-by-case basis regarding the advisability of instituting additional medications relevant to the Axis I disorder, and the timing of such interventions.

3.1.2.3.2. Some Thoughts on Axis II Personality Disorders

Alcohol-dependent individuals are likely to present to the clinician with a wide variety of problems in interpersonal functioning, and in handling life stresses. These often contribute to the decision to seek treatment, and occur as a consequence of the impact that alcohol has on brain neurochemistry and overall functioning. It is easy to mislabel these substance-related impairments as lifelong personality disorders. In DSM-IV, a personality disorder is a lifelong condition that regularly and significantly impairs life functioning.[1] It is usually first apparent during childhood or adolescence, and must be observed in diverse situations, as it is not appropriate to apply this label for patterns of problems that only appear in the context of relatively unique circumstances.

Several of the DSM-IV personality disorders have adequate data to document their reliability and ability to predict long-term problems including the schizotypal personality disorder, the antisocial personality disorder (ASPD), and, perhaps, the borderline personality disorder.[45,46] None of these conditions, nor any other personality disorder, should be diagnosed in an alcohol-dependent individual unless it is clear that the symptoms were observable before the onset of the substance-use disorder and remained clinically relevant during extended periods of abstinence.

The Axis II condition with the closest and most thoroughly documented relationship to alcoholism (as well as substance-related disorders) is ASPD.[45–48] This condition is characterized by severe impulsivity, problems in learning from mistakes, and a general lack of empathy. Establishing the diagnosis requires that such characteristics have been observed in childhood, in a condition known as conduct disorder as related to difficulties with peers, school, police, and family. The symptoms are obvious before the onset of substance use, and well established before repetitive enough problems with substances develops to justify a diagnosis of dependence. The fact that as many as 80% of individuals with ASPD have dependence on alcohol or other drugs helps to explain why about 20% of alcohol-dependent men and perhaps 5% of alcohol-dependent women fulfill criteria for this disorder that is only seen in 1–3% of the general population. It seems likely that in these instances representing a minority of alcoholics, the heavy drinking and alcohol-related problems may have occurred, as a consequence of the easy availability of alcohol, in an individual who is impulsive and has difficulty learning from prior errors and punishment.

Some clinicians and researchers have also documented a relationship between borderline personality disorder and alcoholism.[46] The borderline condition is characterized by an onset, early in life, of chaotic and inconsistent interpersonal relationships in an individual who frequently demonstrates depressive and anxiety syndromes, especially in the context of life stress. Perhaps reflecting the greater reliability of the ASPD criteria, as well as the more recent inclusion of borderline personality disorder in the diagnostic manual, few data are available regarding the degree of relationship between this condition and a variety of substance-use disorders, including alcoholism.

The importance of discussing these personality conditions is twofold. First, reflecting the fact that the true personality disorders tend to be lifelong conditions and do not disappear with abstinence, it is important to avoid assigning these Axis II DSM-IV labels when observations are based solely on problems that developed in the context of alcoholism or other substance-use disorders. Second, while the treatment of individuals with both alcoholism and a personality disorder is generally similar to that for the usual alcoholic, the personality characteristics and subsequent manner in which the individuals relate to others around them must be kept in mind when interpreting how the person is responding to treatment and functioning in life, in general. It is also important to remember that the maximal level of life functioning likely to be observed after successful treatment for alcoholism will probably be, in effect, what one would expect from a sober individual carrying these additional conditions.

3.1.2.3.3. Placing These Issues of Comorbidity into a Clinical Perspective

It might be good to pull together some of the major conclusions relevant to the information presented in this section. First, men and women who are alcohol dependent are more likely, than people in the general population, to present with psychiatric symptoms. When these syndromes are potentially life-threatening, they must be immediately addressed, regardless of whether they represent substance-induced or independent disorders. For example, men and women who are alcohol dependent have perhaps an 8–10% lifetime risk for death by suicide.[37] Thus, suicidal plans must be taken seriously in alcoholics. This means that immediate psychiatric hospitalization must be considered, and suicide precautions should be implemented. Only after these steps are taken will a careful time line-based history be important in identifying the probability that the depressive and suicidal symptoms are likely to rapidly improve on their own without antidepressant medication (i.e., are alcohol induced) versus the need for the institution of antidepressants over a 9–12-month period as a reflection of an independent psychiatric disorder.

A similar situation exists regarding potentially dangerous hallucinations and/or delusions in a substance-dependent individual. The first step is to protect the patients and those around them from harm as a consequence of the psychotic thinking. This often requires immediate psychiatric hospitalization (sometimes involuntary), and it can necessitate the prescription of antipsychotic drugs. At this point, the distinction between an independent and a substance-induced psychotic disorder is an essential step for determining whether long-term versus short periods of medication or close observation will be required. The appropriate diagnosis is also necessary for an estimation of the highest level of function likely to be observed in this individual in the future and to determine the potential need for long-term antipsychotic medications.

Another general conclusion related to the material presented here is the need to always supplement the time line review with the close observation of the clinical syndrome over the subsequent 4 weeks or so. Abstinence during this period should be monitored through information gathered from others, seeing (or at least talking on the phone with) the patient multiple times per week to document possible intoxication, and supplementing information with urine toxicology screens or state markers of heavy drinking when possible. The clinician can expect that the anxiety, depressive, and psychotic symptoms, for example, will improve during that period of observation, usually falling below a diagnostic threshold by week 4. On the other hand, the observation that a person with a provisional diagnosis of a substance-induced condition does not show this pattern of improvement despite apparent continued abstinence, means that the clinician should consider revising the diagnosis and perhaps, initiating treatment with the most appropriate longer term medication.

The next general implication is the need to remember, that independent psychiatric disorders should be as aggressively treated among individuals who are alcohol or other drug-dependent, as they are in any other patient or client. It appears as if the response to treatment of independent major depressive disorders or manic depressive disorders, for example, among people with alcoholism is comparable to the outcome likely to be observed in individuals who are non-alcohol dependent.

3.2. PHARMACOLOGY AND EFFECTS OF ALCOHOL SEE ALSO SECTION 3.2.5

3.2.1. CNS Actions

A great deal is known about the actions of alcohol in the brain. Unfortunately, that is both good and bad news, because the effects on different neurochemical systems are so complex, seen in such diverse areas of the CNS, and so likely to be altered by various conditions, that it is difficult to identify any one alteration as relating to any specific effect.[49–51] Changes in brain chemistry are different for acute than for chronic administration of alcohol, vary with the dose, are impacted by the specific situations, and appear to relate to a series of genetic susceptibilities. These complexities make it wise to focus on the cascade of events related to the administration of alcohol, impacting on a variety of neurochemical actions rather than to study a specific "one drug–one effect" phenomenon.

In prior years, one theory of alcohol actions was based on the observation that alcohol alters the properties of lipids (fats) in the membranes of neurons. There is a direct relationship between the anesthetic properties of alcohol and the amount of changes in the lipid solubility of these membranes, with the final result that alcohol increases the permeability or fluidity of these structures. Although this general property of alcohol might contribute to some of the clinical effects of this drug, it is likely that other major effects are even more important.

An example relates to the theory that most pleasurable effects of drugs are mediated through changes in the brain neurochemical dopamine, especially in a section of the brain called the ventral tegmental area.[50,52] Alcohol does, indeed, cause increases in the metabolites of dopamine; chronic alcohol administration results in an increase in the number of receptors in the brain that are sensitive to dopamine; and it is likely that changes in this neurochemical system are important in the effects observed with alcohol. Changes in a relative of dopamine, norepinephrine, also relate to the effects of alcohol, and at least in animals, the amount of norepinephrine in the brain might have an impact on the preference for alcohol.

Closely related to the interaction between alcohol and norepinephrine or dopamine are the effects of alcohol on serotonin, another important brain chemical. Alcohol, given acutely, increases the release of serotonin within the brain, but chronic administration of this drug tends to decrease the amount of serotonin stored in the CNS. The levels of serotonin (and its metabolites) in the brain or cerebrospinal fluid (CSF) appear to be related to whether an organism will voluntarily seek out higher or lower amounts of alcohol, and it has been hypothesized that a specific area of the brain, the dorsal raphe nucleus, is especially important in this phenomenon. More recent data have also highlighted the potential importance of several specific serotonin receptors including the 2_A, 2_C, and 1_B varieties.[53,54] Interesting data also relate the alcoholism risk, to the protein that transports serotonin from the synaptic space back into the cell (the serotonin transporter).[55–57] As one might predict, treating animals or humans with drugs that affect serotonin or specific transmitters has a modest effect on alcohol intake.

Another neurochemical mechanism thought to have a major impact on the effects of alcohol relates to the inhibitory transmitter system involving gamma-aminobutyric acid (GABA).[55,58,59] It is this system that is most responsive to the effects of the benzodiazepine medications (e.g., diazepam or Valium). Through a mechanism that might be distinct from the actions of benzodiazepines, acute doses of alcohol appear to increase the actions of this inhibitory system. Interestingly, animals that are more likely to self-administer alcohol appear to have a GABA receptor system that is less sensitive to the effects of alcohol. In addition, some subunits of GABA receptor subtypes have been reported to relate to the level of reaction to alcohol and to the alcoholism risk.

In recent years, a fourth important neurochemical system has been linked to the effects of alcohol. Receptors sensitive to the actions of the stimulatory neurochemical glutamate, as part of the *N*-methyl-D-aspartate (NMDA) system also appear to be important.[60,61] Acutely administered alcohol has inhibitory effects on the actions of NMDA receptors, with a potentially enhanced sensitivity of the same receptors following chronic use of alcohol and during withdrawal.

In this brief review of some of the neurochemical effects of alcohol, there are also possible interactions between alcohol and the brain's opioid receptor system (see Chapter 6).[50,62,63] For example, at least theoretically, some important metabolites of alcohol, including acetaldehyde, can combine or condense with any of the several neurochemicals to produce opiate-like substances, the tetrahydroisoquinolines (THIQs) and the beta carbolines. Alcohol is also felt to have an effect on some of the body's own opioids, with a possibility that the severity of the alcohol withdrawal syndrome might be related to body levels of beta-endorphin.

Finally, it should be remembered that this very superficial overview hardly does justice to the complexity of the issues. Readers must be aware of the fact that other neurochemical systems, including the ones rich in acetylcholine, might also play direct and indirect roles in the final results of alcohol intake.[64] Recent studies have also documented the effects of alcohol on cannabinoid receptors.[65,66] Other key elements in alcohol's CNS effects include adenosine receptors, potassium channels, and elements of the intracellular second messenger systems.[67,68] Thus, even a review as brief as this can highlight how many different neurochemical systems are likely to be involved in the effects of alcohol and the complexities of the interactions that are observed.

If the story relating to the effects of alcohol itself was not complicated enough, there are additional considerations. The alcoholic beverages consumed by individuals contain a great deal more than just the ethanol, and these can have a major impact on intoxication and on some of the possible beneficial effects of some beverages such as red wine.[69,70] The procedures for manufacturing beer, wine, whiskey, gin, and so on, all add ingredients to the alcoholic beverages, substances referred to as *congeners*. These constituents affect the rate of absorption and distribution of alcohol, contain diverse substances with a variety of direct body effects including alterations in sex hormones, and can themselves have an impact on the brain.

3.2.2. Behavioral Changes (Intoxication 303.00)

The final level of behavioral impairment depends on the person's age, weight, gender, consumption with food, and prior experience with alcohol as well as on his level of tolerance.[71] Table 3.1 gives a rough outline of what can be expected in a non-tolerant individual, with results ranging from minor impairment of motor coordination, sensation, and mood at low doses, to amnesia and Stage 1 anesthesia for blood levels exceeding 300 mg alcohol/100 ml blood (30 mg%). The cognitive and motor functioning problems observed at even relatively low alcohol concentrations can be considerable. Levels of 400–700 mg% can cause coma, respiratory failure, and death, although tolerant individuals may be awake and able to talk at blood levels exceeding 780 mg%. For each of these values, the level of impairment at falling blood-alcohol concentrations (BACs) is usually less than the effects observed at rising BACs.[71] Note that 100 mg% is equivalent to 0.1 g/100 ml. The usual drink contains about 10–12 g of absolute alcohol and (for those watching their weight) a minimum of 70 calories, and raises the BAC about 15–20 mg/dl, the same amount that is metabolized in 1 h.

An additional topic worthy of brief mention is the age-old search for amethystic (sobering) agents. Probably the most useful data come from the

Table 3.1
Rough Correlation between Blood-Alcohol Level and Behavioral/Motor Impairment

Rising blood-alcohol level[a]	Expected effect
20–99	Impaired coordination, euphoria
100–199	Ataxia, decreased mentation, poor judgment, labile mood
200–299	Marked ataxia and slurred speech, poor judgment, labile mood, nausea and vomiting
300–399	Stage I anesthesia, memory lapse, labile mood
400 and above	Respiratory failure, coma, death

[a]mg/100 ml blood (mg% or mg/dl).

demonstration that fruit sugar (fructose) increases the rate of disappearance of ethanol from the body by 10% or more, thus helping the individual sober up more rapidly. Clinical application of this finding is limited because of the possibility of resulting overhydration and changes in the body acid–base balance. Caffeine also appears to have some mild abilities to counteract some of the effects of ethanol, especially at low BACs.[72] Data from animal research suggests that Vitamin C might have some benefit in decreasing some of the toxic effects of alcohol.[73] Additional preliminary data indicate fairly unimpressive results on the use of stimulants, precursors of brain neurochemicals such as L-dopa, and prostaglandin synthetase inhibitors such as ibuprofen (Nuprin) as potential sobering agents.

3.2.3. Effects on the Body

Alcohol is a very attractive drug, as its immediate effects at moderate doses are perceived by most users as pleasant. In addition, for individuals who are not alcoholic, not taking medications, and are in good physical condition, alcohol in amounts up to two drinks per day has the beneficial effects of increasing socialization, stimulating the appetite, and decreasing the risk for macular degeneration and gallstones.[74–76] Modest doses of alcohol in any form are also thought to decrease the risk of cardiovascular disease through an increase in high-density lipoproteins (HDLs), a decrease in platelet adhesion, and the effects of different chemicals, some of which may be specific for red wines.[77,78] Additional data suggest possible protective effects of moderate drinking on some forms of dementia.[79] However, as consumption increases to more than two to three drinks daily, or when some individuals who have preexisting medical disorders drink, damage to various body systems can be serious, and early signs of some of these changes may give the clinician reason to increase his level of suspicion that the patient being seen may be alcoholic.[80] Because the toxicity of alcohol has been presented in depth in other texts, only a brief review is given here.

The average person with alcoholism is likely to appear in the clinical setting sober, well groomed, and with no obvious aura of alcohol problems. He or she may complain of any of a variety of medical and emotional problems. These must be properly diagnosed as alcohol-related if the clinician hopes to avoid unexpected calls in the middle of the night and nonresponse to ill-advised treatments that should never have been given in the first place (e.g., sleeping pills). Thus, it is in the clinician's best interest to identify the person with alcoholism to be certain of offering maximal care at minimal risk.

Changes in body systems that can be expected in the course of alcoholism include those discussed in the following sections. These can help identify the person with alcoholism and outline important information to be shared with men and women who are alcohol dependent and their families and friends.

3.2.3.1. Effects on Blood Cells

Alcohol affects the production of all types of blood cells, with resulting large-red-blood-cell anemia (a macrocytosis), decreased production and efficiency of white cells (probably leading to an increased predisposition toward infection), and decreased production of clotting factors and platelets (probably causing increased bruising and gastrointestinal bleeding).[81–84] There is also a decrease in T-cells and in thymus-derived lymphocytes, which might contribute to the increased rates of cancers seen in people with alcoholism. The combination of impairments in the immune system along with poor judgment that can be seen during intoxication might increase the chances of developing AIDS or impair a person's response to treatment.[85,86] In addition, the decreased functioning of aspects of the immune system may contribute to an increased vulnerability to tuberculosis, viral and bacterial infections, and cancers (see Section 3.2.3.4).

3.2.3.2. Digestive System

In the digestive system, alcohol is associated with high rates of ulcer disease as well as elevated rates of inflammation of the stomach (gastritis). The stomach problems reflect alcohol stimulation of gastric acid, especially prominent with beer and wine, as well as the promotion of colonization of a bacterium associated with the development of ulcer disease.[87]

Inflammation of the pancreas probably reflects blockage of pancreatic ducts along with concomitant stimulation of the production of digestive enzymes.[88,89] The latter relates to a probable fragility of enzyme storage structures in the cells, and the combination leads to both acute and chronic pancreatitis.[89] Related to pancreatic functioning and insulin, even at low doses, alcohol disturbs the liver's sugar-producing function (gluconeogenesis) and shunts building blocks for sugars into the production of fats. Thus, reflecting this and other mechanisms, glucose and insulin abnormalities are relatively common in heavy drinkers and may revert to normal with abstinence.[90]

Major problems in the liver may be secondary to the use of alcohol by liver cells as a "preferred fuel," with resultant scarcity of nicotinamide adenine dinucleotide (NAD) as a hydrogen receptor. The liver problems can progress from fatty liver (probably seen with repeated blood-alcohol levels of 80 mg/dl or more), to alcoholic hepatitis (probably not directly related to the fatty liver), and to subsequent cirrhosis. The latter may begin with early fiber deposition around the central hepatic veins, that is, a process of central hyaline sclerosis.[91–93] Some adverse liver changes can be seen with consumption of as little as 20 g of alcohol per day in women and 40 g per day in men, although higher doses over longer periods of time are usually required for cirrhosis. In reviewing this material, however, the clinician must remember that less than one in five people with alcoholism present with clinically significant cirrhosis. A special case of potentially fatal liver deterioration occurs with the coadministration of as little as 2.5 g or more per day of acetaminophen (e.g., Tylenol) in the context of heavy drinking (even as few as six drinks per day), a condition often heralded by extremely high levels of aspartate aminotransferase (AST).[92]

3.2.3.3. Alcohol and Cancer

Through a number of mechanisms, people with alcoholism also have significantly elevated rates of a wide range of cancers, including in the digestive tract (especially the esophagus and stomach), the head and neck, and the lungs.[94,95] This high risk might relate to problems from local irritation of lung or digestive tract linings, a decrease in the protective actions of mucous coverings of these regions, or a decrease in immune system components that identify and destroy cancer cells. The data on the increased prevalence of cancer in people with alcoholism remain robust even when the effects of dietary changes, smoking habits, and other factors are considered. Although most of the increase in cancerous lesions is associated with high levels of alcohol intake, recent data indicate that for one type of cancer, carcinoma of the breast, intake of even as little as one or two drinks per day might be associated with a moderately increased risk.[96,97] In the final analysis, people with alcoholism or those who are heavy drinkers must be carefully evaluated for the possibility of cancer, and alcoholism must be considered as a possible additional diagnosis in patients with cancerous lesions, especially those of the head and neck, the digestive tract, and the lung.

3.2.3.4. Nervous System Adverse Effects

See also Section 3.2.4.

As recognized by DSM-IV, the most prevalent form of alcohol-related confusion occurs with intoxication. Although most individuals show a clearing of clouded consciousness over a matter of hours as they sober up, those with preexisting brain damage (e.g., some older people and those with prior brain trauma) may evidence confusion lasting for days or weeks. Thus, alcohol must be considered a part of the differential diagnosis of all fairly rapid-onset states of confusion.

The association between alcoholism and more permanent dementias is less clear.[98,99] The majority of people with alcoholism who present for detoxification show some signs of intellectual impairment, and 40–70% may show increased brain ventricular size (possibly indicating decreased brain tissue).[100] Although some investigators feel that there is a correlation between increased size of brain ventricles and decreased functioning on psychological testing, not all agree, and it is probable that most people with alcoholism will recover in both parameters after months of abstinence.[101,102] The etiology of these changes is not known, but it probably represents the combination of trauma, vitamin deficiencies, and a direct neurotoxic effect of alcohol on the brain.

One rare condition (seen in less than 1% of alcoholics) carries with it a mortality of greater than 15%, and a probability that only approximately one third of patients will demonstrate clinically relevant levels of recovery. Wernicke–Korsakoff syndrome is a consequence of a thiamine deficit in predisposed individuals, especially those who have a deficiency in transketolase, one of the three types of enzymes for which thiamine is a cofactor.[103,104] Brain imaging and autopsy material of such patients reveal changes (including microhemorrhages) in the mammillary bodies, in the dorsomedial nucleus of the thalamus, and in the periventricular gray matter of the brain. The Wernicke aspect of this condition involves neurological abnormalities including those affecting the sixth cranial nerve, whereas the Korsakoff syndrome is characterized by an intense anterograde amnesia that is much more intense than the general level of dementia. Treatment of the Wernicke–Korsakoff syndrome involves the administration of thiamine (usually orally), with partial or full recovery seen in perhaps one to two thirds of these patients, a process that often requires several months.

The chronic intake of alcohol can also result in deterioration of the peripheral nerves to both the hands and the feet (a peripheral neuropathy seen in 5–15% of people with alcoholism).[105] Additional potential problems associated with the CNS involve a rapidly developing permanent incoordination (cerebellar degeneration), which is seen in fewer than 1% of people with alcoholism, and other more dramatic but even rarer neurological disorders that can result in rapid death including Marchiafava-Bymani and Central Pontine-related problems.[106,107] Although modest drinking might decrease the risk for ischemic stroke, higher levels of drinking are related to an elevated risk for hemorrhagic stroke, even when other factors such as blood pressure are controlled.

3.2.3.5. Cardiovascular System

It has been estimated that one quarter of people with alcoholism develop an early onset of diseases of the heart or the cardiovascular system.

This occurs in part, because alcohol is a striated muscle toxin that produces a heart inflammation, or myocardiopathy, with resulting preclinical left ventricular abnormalities.[108] Heart problems also develop as a consequence of alcohol-induced hypertension and elevations in blood fats, including cholesterol.[108–112] Thus, coronary diseases occur at as high as a sixfold increased rate in individuals who are alcohol dependent, contributing to at least 20% of the excess mortality.[113] Such heart-related problems, along with electrocardiographic abnormalities, can be especially prominent during withdrawal but are also observed in the context of persistent heavy drinking. In addition, alcohol in doses as low as one drink can temporarily decrease the cardiac output of blood and cardiac contractility in nonalcoholics with heart disease, and can diminish the warning signs of pain while increasing the potential heart damage or ischemia in patients with angina. Alcoholism must also be considered in all individuals who demonstrate mild elevations in blood pressure (e.g., 145/95), especially if the pressure appears to fluctuate with time (e.g., higher early in the week), and as little as 1 g/kg body weight per day of ethanol over 5 days can result in a significant pressure increase, especially among individuals with prior hypertension.

3.2.3.6. Body Muscle

Body muscle is also sensitive to alcohol, and an alcoholic binge can result in muscle inflammation or, with chronic heavy use, muscle wasting, primarily in the shoulders and the hips.[114] The rapid destruction of muscle tissue can produce a condition known as rhabdomyolysis with acute muscle pain and kidney failure.

3.2.3.7. Hormonal Changes and Problems in Sexual Functioning

Acute doses of alcohol can produce numerous transitory alterations in important hormones, including prolactin, growth hormone, adrenocorticotropin hormone (ACTH), and cortisol.[98,115] Alcohol consumption can also produce a decrease in parathyroid hormone functioning with associated decreased blood levels of calcium and magnesium. Continued administration of alcohol at relatively high doses results in tolerance to some of these effects, but problems can develop.

Consequences of some of these changes, as well as the direct effects of alcohol, include menstrual irregularities, altered feelings of sexuality, and possible effects on a developing fetus as described in Section 4.2.7.2.[116–118] Men can develop decreased sperm production and motility through the direct effects of ethanol on the testes; decreased ejaculate volume, sperm count, and sperm motility (all of which tend to improve with 3 months of abstinence); changes in testosterone including decreased production of this hormone in the presence of elevated leutenizing hormone; and impotence (through psychological mechanisms, peripheral neuropathy involving the perineal nerves, and/or the direct destruction of the testes).[119,120]

3.2.3.8. Changes in Bones

Data also support significant changes in bone strength or density in people with alcoholism.[121,122] There is an increased risk for bone fractures among men and women who are alcohol dependent, along with x-ray evidence that bone density is decreased. The specific mechanisms involved are not fully understood, but it may reflect chronic changes in parathyroid hormone with high doses of alcohol (as opposed to low doses of alcohol as alluded to previously), coupled with the possible consequences of high levels of cortisol associated with chronic heavy drinking, and anti-proliferative effects of alcohol on osteoblasts.

3.2.3.9. Alcohol, Nutrition, and Vitamins

As discussed briefly above, alcohol has a profound effect on the body's metabolism of fats and carbohydrates.[123] Acute doses are likely to impair the ability of cells to respond appropriately to insulin, with a decreased sensitivity to this hormone during alcohol withdrawal. Carbohydrate-regulation abnormalities can contribute to a difficulty in maintaining normal acid–base balance, which can subsequently help produce a condition known as alcoholic lactic acidosis or ketacidosis.[124] In this condition, the patient can present with a life-threatening emergency, complaining of nausea and abdominal pain, with vomiting. The blood sugar and other mechanisms can contribute to decreased blood levels of a variety of electrolytes including sodium, potassium, magnesium, calcium, and phosphorus.[125,126]

Alcohol interferes with the absorption, storage, or distribution of a number of essential vitamins including B_1, B_6, D, and E.[127] Through additional alcohol-related pathology, it is also possible to find deficient levels in Vitamin B_2, A, and K in people with alcoholism. On the other hand, most people who are alcohol dependent do not present for treatment with significantly altered blood levels of these vitamins, and thus, most potential deficiencies are likely to be mild and easily corrected through abstinence, appropriate nutrition, and oral administration of multivitamins.

3.2.3.10. Other Abnormalities

Through a variety of mechanisms, a number of other alcohol-related problems can develop. These include dental changes such as gum disease, enlargement of the parotid gland, and potential increased risks for tooth decay, as well as increased rates of cancer of the mouth.[128,129] Changes in the eyes can include cataracts and keratitis.[130]

Alcohol not only impairs the normal kidney regulation of substances such as uric acid, but it also appears to interfere with the rapidity of recovery of the kidney following damage.[131] The kidney appears to be especially vulnerable to damage in the context of concomitant liver disease or evidence of ischemia. Most of the alcohol-induced changes in the kidney produce alterations in the acid–base balance of the body, the regulation of fluids, and the appropriate maintenance of sodium, potassium, and other electrolytes. Fortunately, most of these changes are associated with intoxication and tend to reverse with abstinence.

Through direct effects as well as interference with immune functioning, heavy doses of alcohol appear to increase the risk for infections of the skin and the development of eczema.[132] There is a particularly close relationship between drinking and either the precipitation or the intensification of psoriasis.[133] Additional problems include the potential intensification of some aspects of AIDs.[134]

3.2.3.11. Accidents and Driving Impairment

Any discussion of the effects of alcohol on the body would be incomplete without mentioning the one, that probably has the most dramatic impact on morbidity and mortality.[135,136] Perhaps 40% or more of Americans have ever driven after drinking enough to cause impairment, including 7% of young men in the prior month. There is evidence that even at a BAC as low as 15 mg/dl (i.e., approximately one drink), the ability to operate a motor vehicle is significantly impaired.[137] Alcohol is also an important contributor to bicycle accidents.[138] Similar dramatic levels of impairment have even been observed with experienced pilots operating flying simulators, and studies have shown impairment of piloting skills lasting 14 h or more after BACs reached 100 mg/dl.[139] Thus, the likelihood of accidents (in the home and in the workplace as well as on the highways or in the skies) is significantly increased after even moderate doses of alcohol.

It is not surprising that almost 55% of individuals treated for severe traumatic injury have been diagnosed of a substance-use disorder at some time in their lives. In 60% of these, the disorder was observed within the prior 6 months.[140] Serious injuries that occur in the context of alcohol intoxication appear to be more closely associated with rapid death than other similar injuries in sober patients.[141]

3.2.4. Effects on Mental Processes

See also Sections 3.1.2.3 and 3.2.3.4.

In addition to the physiological changes that occur with alcohol, there are a number of important emotional consequences. With modest intake, at decreasing BACs most people experience sadness, anxiety, irritability, and a host of resulting interpersonal problems.[42] At persistent higher doses, alcohol can cause almost any psychiatric symptom, including temporary pictures of intense sadness, auditory hallucinations and/or paranoia in the presence of clear thought processes (a clear sensorium), and intense anxiety. These symptoms are discussed in Sections 4.2.3 and 4.2.4. This section reviews some additional aspects of the effects of alcohol in brain functioning.

Insomnia can occur as a consequence of simple alcohol intoxication, as this drug tends to fragment the sleep, with the result of both a decrease in deep sleep stages and frequent awakenings.[142–144] These problems can be expected to persist in alcoholics for up to 3–6 months as part of a "protracted" abstinence phase and might enhance the risk for relapse.[145]

Another consequence of alcohol that impacts both physical and mental functioning is the *hangover*.[146,147] This syndrome consists of a mixture of symptoms that can include headache, nausea and vomiting, thirst, decreased appetite, dizziness, fatigue, and tremor. This is a highly prevalent phenomenon that contributes to lost time and efficiency at work and at school. At least one hangover is likely to be reported in 40% or more of men age 18 or older and in 27% of women of similar age, including 5 and 1% of the two genders, respectively, who have had an average of one or more hangovers a month during the preceding year. A number of hypothesized mechanisms for this phenomenon have been presented, including consequences of changes in vasopressin or in dopamine levels in the hypothalamus, changes in prostaglandins or in beta-adrenergic activity, as well as the possibility that these symptoms represent a mild degree of alcohol withdrawal. Other than prevention by limiting the ethanol intake, no effective treatment approaches to this prevalent phenomenon have yet been developed.

A third phenomenon related to the use of any brain depressant, including alcohol, is an anterograde amnesia or *blackout*.[148,149] This label applies to individuals who have consumed enough of a depressant, rapidly enough, to experience the drug's ability to interfere with the acquisition and storage of new memories. Perhaps one third of drinkers report at least one alcoholic blackout, with the same being true of two thirds or more of individuals who fulfill criteria for alcohol dependence. The problem appears to involve an inability to acquire new memories while intensively intoxicated, with the information being unretrievable from the memory within minutes of its occurrence. By itself the history of a blackout is a useful indication that a person has, on at least one occasion, rapidly consumed an excessive amount of alcohol. However, in the absence of additional alcohol-related problems, a blackout, on its own, is not a highly specific predictor of the development of alcohol dependence.

3.2.5. Alcohol Metabolism

See also Section 3.2

Alcohol is fully absorbed from the lining or membranes of the digestive tract, especially in the stomach and the proximal portion of the small intestine. Only 5–15% is excreted directly through the lungs, sweat, and urine, the remainder being metabolized in the liver at a rate of approximately one drink per hour, the equivalent of 7 g or more of ethanol per hour, with 1 g equaling 1 mg of 100% alcohol.[150] The usual route of metabolism is via the enzyme alcohol dehydrogenase (ADH), although some additional alcohol is metabolized in the liver microsomal system, as shown in Fig. 3.1, as well as by catalase, (especially in the brain).[151] Thus, the major product of alcohol metabolism is acetaldehyde, a toxic substance that, fortunately, is quickly metabolized to carbon dioxide and water through a variety of mechanisms, the most prominent of which is via aldehyde dehydrogenase (ALDH).[152]

ADH and ALDH perform a variety of tasks in addition to the metabolism of ethanol. Both enzymes are under genetic control, and ADH has eight or more isoenzymes in humans, each with different metabolic properties and with different patterns in various national groups.[153] Women appear to have less ADH in their gastric mucosa (stomach lining) and are subsequently likely to have higher BACs when they drink because less alcohol is being metabolized before it is distributed throughout the body.[154,155] Factors that increase the BAC are likely to be associated with a lower risk for heavy drinking.[21] There are at least four clinically significant ALDH isoenzymes in humans, and the most physiologically active regarding acetaldehyde, the mitochondrial form, is deficient in perhaps as many as 50% of Asian (e.g., Japanese, Chinese, or Korean) men and women.[156,157]

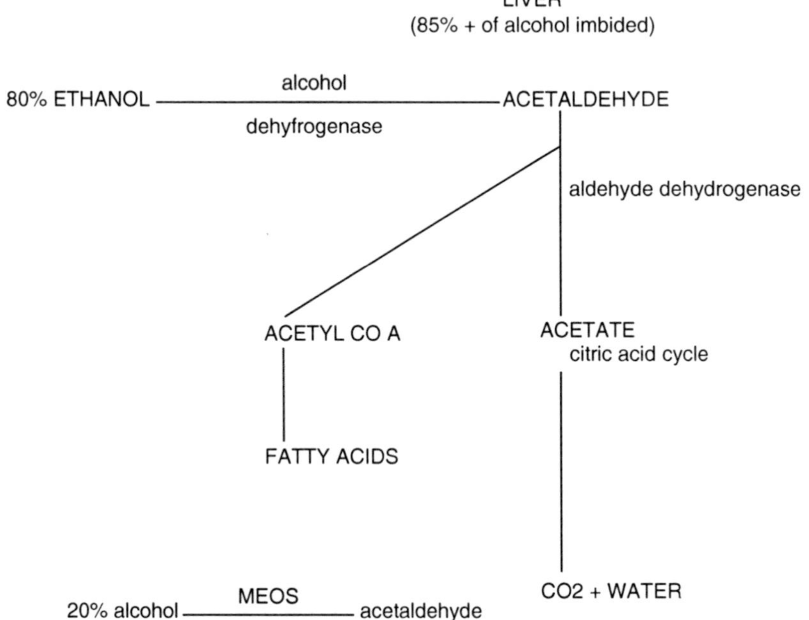

Figure 3-1. Metabolism of alcohol. Abbreviations: ACETYL CO A, acetyl-coenzyme A; MEOS, microsomal ethanol-oxidizing system

This is responsible for the higher rate of facial flushing (probably acetaldehyde-mediated) when some Asian people drink, a factor that is linked with the lower level of alcoholism in Asians. Ethnic groups also differ in their pattern of forms of ADH, which may contribute to the faster production of acetaldehyde, a more intense response to alcohol, and, perhaps, to the lower prevalence of alcohol-use disorders in African-Americans and Jews.[21,156]

3.2.6. Tolerance and Physical Dependence

See also Section 3.1.2.1

Toleration of higher doses of ethanol can develop rapidly and it parallels the toleration of the depressants discussed in Section 2.1.1.3. Part of this phenomenon is metabolic, primarily through a slight increase in both ADH activity and in the liver microsomal ethanol-oxidizing system (MEOS); part is pharmacodynamic, the apparent result of a direct adaptation of CNS tissues to alcohol and finally; part is behavioral.[158,159] Cross tolerance to other depressing drugs occurs, but it must be remembered that the concomitant administration of two or more depressants may potentiate the effects of both. Alcohol also produces a level of physical dependence that results in a withdrawal syndrome almost identical to that described for the other depressants. The alcohol withdrawal syndrome is discussed in Section 4.2.2.

3.3. EPIDEMIOLOGY OF DRINKING AND ALCOHOLISM

A great many people drink, and many have minor problems, but fewer demonstrate a persistent lifestyle centered on alcohol despite alcohol-related problems (i.e., alcoholism).[160,161]

3.3.1. Drinking Patterns and Problems

The per capita consumption of alcohol in the United States increased progressively between 1961 and 1980. Since that time, there has been a slow, but steady, decrease of about 1% per year in the amount of absolute alcohol consumed per adult, so that in more recent years, the average American drank about 2.2 gallons of absolute alcohol yearly, down from 2.4 gallons. The decreases have been seen for all types of alcoholic beverages, although they are most prominent for spirits and least for wine.

The 2002 National Survey on Drug Use and Health[162] reported that about 80% of men and women have ever consumed alcoholic beverages. About 5% used in the prior month, with the highest figure (71%) for subjects age 21. About 45% in this age group had consumed five or more drinks in an evening over the prior month, and about 15% had done so on five or more different times. Almost 15% of Americans age 12+ drove under the influence of alcohol in the prior year.

Among men, the proportion who have ever used alcohol differs a bit across ethnic groups. In general, drinking and heavy drinking is higher in men than women, and higher among Native Americans and Latino men, with lower figures for African-Americans.[163–165]

Regarding teenagers, the 2003 Monitoring the Future Study reported that 77% of teenagers had ever used alcohol by Grade 12, including 48% in the prior month and 62% who had ever been intoxicated (30% in the recent 3 days). Among college students, 86% ever used alcohol and 86% had ever been intoxicated.

3.3.2. Alcohol Abuse and Dependence

It has been estimated that at least 15% of men and about 10% of women in the US ever met the criteria for alcohol dependence. Current (e.g., prior year) overall are about 10% with dependence and 7% with abuse.[166] A 2002 national survey estimated prior year rates of abuse or dependence of about 8% overall, including 18% in 18–25-year olds.[162] Among college students, the 12-month prevalence of dependence was 6%, with more than twice that figure for abuse.[166]

The armed services have a reputation for high rates of alcohol problems, an observation that implies possible high rates of alcoholism.[167] These findings must be considered from the perspective that the military has a high percentage of young males (i.e., those at the highest risk for alcohol-related difficulties). Indeed, once one controls for age, gender, and socioeconomic stratum, the rate of probable alcoholism might not be greatly different from those of the population in general. It has also been reported that there are differences in alcoholism rates across occupations, with higher figures for less well paid unskilled and semiskilled jobs.[168,169]

Regarding ethnic groups, as briefly reviewed above, lower rates of alcoholism are seen among Asians and in Jews, and high rates in most groups of North American Indians and Eskimos.[170,171] It is not known whether these differences are related to social factors, either protecting from heavy drinking or encouraging drunkenness (for lower or higher rates, respectively) and/or genetic influences.

3.4. NATURAL HISTORY OF ALCOHOLISM

Once the diagnosis of alcohol dependence has been established, it is possible to estimate the likely prognosis or the natural course of the disorder (see Table 3.2).[5–7,10,19] The average person with alcoholism first demonstrates the clustering of major alcohol-related life problems in the mid-20s to early 30s, and most people with alcoholism present for treatment in their early 40s—after more than a decade of difficulties. Consistent with these findings, it is likely that by age 31, approximately half of those who will fulfill the criteria for alcoholism have already done so. However, an earlier onset of regular drinking and associated problems may be related to a higher prevalence and more severe causes of alcoholism.[172,173]

Table 3.2
Natural History of Alcohol Dependence

1. Age at which first drink is taken[a]		12–14
2. Age at first intoxication[a]		14–18
3. Age at which minor alcohol problem is experienced[a]		18–25
4. Usual age of onset (3+ DSM-IV problems)		23–33
5. Usual age on entering treatment		40
6. Usual age of death		55–60
Leading cause:	Heart disease	
	Cancer	
	Accidents	
	Suicide	
7. In any year, abstinence alternates with active drinking.		1/4 to 1/3

[a]These ages are about the same in the general population.

If alcohol problems continue, the person with alcoholism is likely to die 15 years earlier than the average expected age for the general population, with the leading causes of death (in approximately decreasing order of frequency) being heart disease, cancer, accidents, and suicide.[37,174–177] Alcohol is estimated to contribute to 11% to almost 25% of premature deaths, with a sixfold increase in the number of expected deaths in follow-up evaluations.[178] The figures for suicide, a 3–10% lifetime risk, probably reflect, what would otherwise be temporary but intense alcohol-induced mood disorders that develop in the context of heavy drinking.[37] Other disorders, such as cirrhosis, are seen much more frequently in people with alcoholism than in the general population, but do not contribute to the majority of deaths. As discussed in Section 3.2.2, these findings reflect the diverse organ systems affected by ethanol. Thus, it is estimated that over 90% of people with alcoholism coming in for treatment had important medical problems, including hypertension, ulcer disease, or chronic obstructive lung disease, gastritis, or peripheral neuropathy, and, to a lesser extent, with cardiomyopathy. For most of these forms of physical pathology, extended periods of abstinence are associated with a return toward normal levels of risk.

The course of alcoholism is a fluctuating one, with very few, if any, people with alcoholism staying persistently drunk until they die.[19,179] The usual alcoholic is a blue-collar or a white-collar worker who alternates periods of abstinence (and times when he is drinking very little) with periods of serious alcohol misuse.[180] In any given month, one half of people with alcoholism will be abstinent, with a mean of 4 months of being dry in any 1–2-year period. Thus, the average person with alcoholism has spontaneous periods of abstinence and marked decreases in drinking that alternate with times of heavy drinking. An additional aspect of the course of alcoholism is the high associated risk for heavy smoking.

Reflecting overall differences between the genders in the general population, most studies agree that women have a higher proportion of abstainers (thus contributing to their lower risk for developing alcohol problems). Women with alcoholism (as with women in general) are less likely than men to commit acts of violence, have fewer alcohol-related driving accidents, and develop fewer major problems from work, related to drinking when compared to males with alcoholism.[165,181] The age of onset of drinking in women with alcoholism is several years later than that of male alcoholics, but men and women who are alcohol dependent are likely to come for treatment at similar ages. This foreshortening of the period between the onset of drinking and seeking out of treatment has been reported as "telescoping" of the course of alcohol dependence. Although probably a real phenomenon, in most studies it only represents a several year differential between the genders. Some studies have reported a higher risk for alcohol-related liver and perhaps brain damage in women with alcoholism compared to men, but not all agree. In the final analysis, the general attributes of the natural history of alcoholism are more similar than different in men and women.

A second important subgroup of individuals who are alcohol dependent are those in older age groups.[19,182,183] Similar to the comparison of men and women who are alcohol dependent, the course of alcoholism in older individuals resembles that of younger people, with some notable exceptions. First, perhaps a third to half of men and women who are alcohol dependent in their 50s and 60s did not develop their dependence until after the age of 40. Second, it is probable that the older age people with alcoholism are less likely to have a close family member with alcoholism. Third, as might be expected from older people in the general population, compared to younger people with alcoholism, the older individual is more likely to have alcohol-related physical problems but is less likely to demonstrate alcohol-related police difficulties, violence, or job problems.

The question of a person with alcoholism returning to "controlled" or nonproblem drinking has been hotly debated.[17,19] The lack of agreement reflects, in part, the definition of *controlled drinking*, with some reports including individuals drinking as many as eight drinks per day and accepting self-reports of a lack of problems without thorough record checks or interviewing of additional relatives. However, both anecdotal information and follow-ups have indicated that only 1–5% of individuals who are alcohol dependent ever achieve a persistent state of drinking low amounts of ethanol without associated problems for years on end. These people are likely to have had less severe and pervasive alcohol-related problems in the past. Therefore, it is best to advise people with alcoholism that abstinence is the only appropriate goal of treatment because 95% or more of people with alcoholism are unlikely to achieve any long period of controlled drinking; short periods of drinking without problems are part of the natural course of most people with alcoholism but usually give way to serious problems and there are difficulties in identifying those who will be able to do this successfully.

It is also important to remember that alcoholism is not a hopeless disorder. Not only can one expect improvement with treatment, but 10–30% of people with alcoholism learn to abstain or to seriously limit their drinking without any exposure to a formal treatment regimen.[184,185] The chance of demonstrating spontaneous remission probably increases with the same factors that indicate a good prognosis for those entering treatment (e.g., having a job, living with a family, and having no police record). Anecdotally, men and women with spontaneous remission tend to name alcohol-related physical problems, changes in lifestyle, or spiritual experiences as having contributed to their decision to maintain abstinence. The process seems to be aided by a general cognitive reappraisal, especially if supported by a spouse.

3.5. ETIOLOGY OF ALCOHOLISM

The process of developing a substance-use disorder is very complex. Individuals go through stages of experimentation with a drug, periods where they choose to continue to use despite early problems, and the experience of severe repetitive difficulties that might fulfill criteria for abuse or dependence. This progression develops in the context of the person's genetic makeup, the family in which he or she lives, pressures from peers, strengths or weaknesses in schooling, and so on. Every external influence has a potential impact on the progression from experimentation to persistent problems. Therefore, a thorough description of the causes of alcoholism and drug dependence is the focus of many texts.

Lacking space for an in depth discussion of these issues, this section briefly presents some thoughts on genetic and environmental factors that contribute to substance-use disorders overall, using alcoholism as an example. Reflecting the fact that my own research is on genetics, the greatest emphasis is placed in that domain. However, it is important to remember the larger picture, and we must pay equal attention to both environment and genetics.

3.5.1. Some Useful Models

A variety of models recognize the importance of social learning processes and reinforcement as they relate to genetic predispositions to produce heavier substance-use and related problems. Some approaches place an emphasis on both protective and detrimental domains that include *cultural/societal elements*, interpersonal factors, psycho-behavioral aspects, as well as genetic influences, especially regarding their importance during the teenage years.

Other models tie together biological predispositions, diminished cognitive controls (i.e., executive functioning), and *disinhibition*, visualizing acting out (externalizing) disorders, as central elements of repetitive substance exposure and subsequent problems.[186] Here, the externalizing behaviors and associated cognitive problems are felt to interact with lack of stability in the home and the selection of heavy-drinking peers to increase the risk for substance-related problems.

A third model proposes that a central element of a predisposition towards substance-related difficulties rests with *mood and anxiety symptoms*, especially during adolescence.[187,188] In this context, a family history of both mood and substance-related problems, along with difficulties in the home are felt to contribute to relatively ineffective strategies for coping with stress. These all result in a greater vulnerability to the problematic use of substances.

In reality, however, no one model is likely to fully explain the risk for substance-related difficulties in any individual. Rather, the models are learning tools, with elements that are likely to combine in contributing to an individual's problem related to alcohol and drugs.

3.5.2. Some Elements of the Models Hypothesized to Contribute to Heavy Substance Use

As seen in several recent publications,[189,190] it is likely that the optimal understanding of substance-related patterns and problems rests with visualizing a system of interrelating components. Key elements of the models described above are briefly outlined in this section.

3.5.2.1. Peer Drinking

Peer characteristics, including their level of substance use and the amounts of social support they offer, are likely to be important in alcohol and drug use.[191] An overlapping phenomenon is a person's perception of the social norms of drinking behaviors, as these may impact on what the person believes are acceptable drinking and drug use patterns for themselves.[192] The intensity of drinking among peers and perceptions regarding their substance-use patterns are projected to amplify the impact of the absence of a stable family environment, externalizing symptoms, as well as anxiety and mood problems, combining together to produce an enhanced risk for substance-related difficulties.

3.5.2.2. The Impact of the Home Environment

Different attributes of the home environment are often cited as facilitating acting out behavior or helping an individual resist repetitive substance use and associated problems.[193] Relevant elements might include whether a parent engages in heavy drinking or drug use, if the family is intact or headed by a single parent, the levels of warmth or conflict between parents, the consistency of parenting styles, the level of bonding with the offspring, and types and consistency of discipline used.[194] Additional components include the absence of a parent's commitment to monitor homework and school performance, lower expectations regarding the child's achievements, and a lack of participation in family traditions or rituals.[195]

3.5.2.3. Stress

Alcohol and substance use can contribute to higher levels of stress, and the use of substances has been reported to be elevated in adults and adolescents during or following some periods of stress, although findings are likely to vary depending upon the specific stress involved.[196] The amount of stress experienced might also relate to the family environment, problems with peers, and so on, and thus, stress must be viewed as a component of a model of risk, rather than a unique cause of substance-related difficulties.

3.5.2.4. Social Support and Levels of Nurturance in the Environment

The feeling of social connectedness, the number of persons an individual feels can be depended upon, and the level of support they offer have been shown to relate to alcohol and other substance problems.[197,198] Higher levels of social support are associated with lower psychological problems and substance use in both adults and adolescents. The context of the support may be important with, for example, the perception by an adolescent of a close and confiding relationship with a parent, likely to be associated with lower levels of substance use, and presumably, fewer substance-related problems. A supportive peer group might be especially important in dampening or magnifying problems inherent in either an individual's psychological makeup and/or the family environment. The impact of these sources of support, however, might actually enhance substance problem risks if the key persons are heavy substance users themselves.

3.5.2.5. Alcohol and Drug Expectancies

A rich literature has evaluated the relationship between a person's expectations of the effects of a drug such as alcohol and their use behaviors.[199] For example, most studies report that the more positive an individual's expectations of the effects of alcohol, and the fewer negative effects that they foresee with alcohol and drug use, the higher the likelihood of heavy drinking.[200] Prospective studies have demonstrated the importance of aspects of alcohol expectancies to the subsequent onset, progression, and levels of alcohol consumption and problems in both teenagers and adults.[201]

3.5.2.6. Styles of Coping with Stress

Problems with substances have been reported in individuals who use alcohol or other drugs to cope with difficulties.[202] More problematical coping (e.g., avoidance-like distancing, and refusal to accept responsibility for one's own actions), has also been reported to characterize several groups at high risk for alcohol problems, and to relate to problematic drinking.

3.5.2.7. Self-Esteem and Self-Efficacy

A person's positive feelings of self-worth, or self-esteem, might buffer sadness or anxiety, while low values could enhance an association with deviant peers and contribute to higher rates of drinking and other substance use.[203] High levels of self-efficacy (or the ability of an individual to make his or her own decisions) also impacts on alcohol use and patterns of consumption, and relates to the probability of more severe substance-related difficulties.

3.5.2.8. A Brief Presentation of Some Other Possible External Influences

Religiosity or spirituality may relate to lower levels of social deviance and the pattern of substance use, sometimes through mitigating the effect of deviant peers or externalizing symptoms.[204] *Levels of school performance* and extracurricular activities may also reflect underlying cognitive problems, the impact of peers, and the home environment, and, in turn, have a major impact on a person's self-esteem and the ability to make decisions on one's own.[191] *The socioeconomic status* and levels of poverty also have a major impact on alcohol and other substance use and problems through stresses, availability of drugs, and peer influences.[205,206]

3.5.2.9. A Brief Summary

In summary, an understanding of factors that predispose an individual toward higher levels of alcohol intake and subsequent alcohol-related problems is probably best approached through considering many elements simultaneously. This might be best viewed as a series of models of risk. The purpose of the brief thoughts given above is to present examples of how these factors might operate.

3.5.3. Genetic Factors

All of the environmental and sociocultural factors discussed earlier in this section combine to explain an estimated 40–50% of the risk for alcohol-use disorders.[21,207] The remaining 50% or so of the risk is explained by genetic influences. In fact, alcoholism is typical of complex genetically influenced disorders, with many similarities to the ways that genetic influences add to the risk for adult onset diabetes, many forms of cancer, high blood pressure, and most major psychiatric disorders.

For any of these conditions, the first step was to determine whether genetic factors appear to contribute to the disorder overall. In the field of alcoholism, these studies began with the documentation that this disease runs strongly in families, with a fourfold increased risk for these disorders among close relatives of alcoholics compared to relatives of controls. Two types of investigations then established the fact that the familial nature of this disorder is, largely reflected by genetic influences. In the first approach, almost all relevant investigations have documented that the fourfold increased risk for alcoholism in children of alcoholics is still observed, even when those children were adopted out and raised by nonalcoholics. The second approach documented that even though pairs of twins (both identical and fraternal) share major childhood events together, the risk for alcoholism is at least twice as high in identical twins of alcoholics as it is in fraternal twins. Finally regarding establishing the importance of genes for the development of alcoholism, animal studies have documented the importance of genes in the probability that a strain of rodents, for example, will choose to drink alcohol, as well as the amount of alcohol they are likely to consume.[208,209] The twin and the family studies are able to compare the relative importance of genes and environment, and indicate that 40–60% of the risk for alcoholism rests with genetic factors.

The influence of environment is an important reminder that genes do not cause alcoholism, but only contribute to the risk. As a result, no one gene is likely to be able to explain whether someone will become an alcoholic. An additional important factor relates to heterogeneity, where it is likely that each of the multiple genetically influenced characteristics affect the risk. To use another complex disorder as an example, the risk for early onset heart attacks is likely to be genetically influenced, but some families might be carrying a variety of genes that enhance the variety of risk for high blood pressure, others might carry the genetically influenced risk through genes related to high blood fats, while yet others might carry a predisposition toward deterioration of heart muscle (i.e., a cardiomyopathy). Similar heterogeneity is seen for alcoholism.

For alcoholism, one set of genes relate to the alcohol-metabolizing enzymes. Higher blood levels of the first metabolite, acetaldehyde, will result from a variation in the alcohol-metabolizing enzymes that more rapidly produce the psychoactive breakdown product or any variation that diminishes the rate of metabolism of this substance.[208] A moderate increase in acetaldehyde contributes to a more intense (but not necessarily more aversive) reaction to alcohol, while very high levels produce vomiting, a rapid rise and drop in blood pressure, a rapid heart rate, diarrhea, and additional unpleasant symptoms. Ten percent of Japanese, Chinese, and Korean individuals cannot produce an active form of ALDH, have the severe aversive reaction to alcohol, and have virtually no risk for alcoholism. Forty percent produce some of the relevant ALDH form, but not enough to be fully effective, with a resulting more intense response to alcohol (including flushed skin and a modest increase in heart rate), which is associated with a lower than average alcoholism risk.[157,208,210]

A second genetically influenced characteristic, one that enhances the alcoholism risk, is higher levels of impulsivity or disinhibition.[21,211] In its extreme form, this presents as conduct disorder in childhood and antisocial personality disorder in adults, and is associated with high rates of dependence for most drugs, along with a predisposition toward criminal behavior and violence.[146,170] A third group of genetically influenced characteristics appears to operate indirectly through several major independent psychiatric disorders, most notably schizophrenia and manic depressive disease.[42] In these instances, it is not clear whether the substance-use disorders (including alcoholism) develop as a consequence of the underlying preexisting behaviors, develop in the context of poor judgment inherent in the disorders themselves, or share some specific genes which interact with other genes in the environment to determine which disorder is more likely to appear.

My own research has centered on a fourth genetically influenced characteristic, one that is unrelated to metabolism, disinhibition, or independent psychiatric disorders. About 40% of the children of alcoholics, when tested at a relatively young age, demonstrate less intense effects of alcohol at a given blood-alcohol level.[21,189,190] The diminished response to alcohol can be seen in subjective reports of intoxication, as well as by observing physiological and motor performance-related reactions to alcohol. Several studies have shown similar low responses to alcohol in some other groups at high risk for alcoholism including Native Americans and Koreans, along with at least one report that the opposite (a greater response to alcohol) is seen in Jewish subjects, a group at low overall alcoholism risk. We are now searching for genes that contribute to the low level of response to alcohol, while also prospectively following populations with low and high responses in order to identify additional characteristics and environmental events that might interact with the low response, to further enhance the alcoholism risk. It is hoped that the identification of specific genes contributing to this and other characteristics associated with alcoholism, will lead to the identification of more focused and effective prevention approaches, as well as to the development of additional more focused treatments.

REFERENCES

1. American Psychiatric Association. *The Diagnostic and Statistical Manual of Mental Disorders* (4th ed., Text Revision). Washington, DC: American Psychiatric Press, 2000.
2. World Health Organization. *The International Classification of Mental and Behavioural Disorders* (10th ed.). Geneva: World Health Organization, 1992.
3. Pollock, N. K., Martin, C. S., & Langenbucher, J. W. Diagnostic concordance of DSM-III, DSM-III-R, DSM-IV and ICD-10 alcohol diagnoses in adolescents. *Journal of Studies on Alcohol 61:*439–446, 2000.
4. Schuckit, M. A., & Smith, T. L. A comparison of correlates of DSM-IV alcohol abuse or dependence among more than 400 sons of alcoholics and controls. *Alcoholism: Clinical and Experimental Research 25:*1–8, 2001.
5. Schuckit, M. A., Smith, T. L., Danko, G. P., Bucholz, K. K., Reich, T., & Bierut, L. Five-year clinical course associated with DSM-IV alcohol abuse or dependence in a large group of men and women. *American Journal of Psychiatry 158:*1084–1090, 2001.
6. Schuckit, M. A., Danko, G. P., Smith, T. L., & Buckman, K. R. The five-year predictive validity of each of the seven DSM-IV items for alcohol dependence among alcoholics. *Alcoholism: Clinical and Experimental Research 26:*980–987, 2002.

7. Schuckit, M. A., Smith, T. L., Danko, G. P., Reich, T., Bucholz, K. K., & Bierut, L. J. Similarities in the clinical characteristics related to alcohol dependence in two populations. *American Journal of Addiction 11:*1–9, 2002.
8. Hasin, D., Paykin, A., Meydan, J., & Grant, B. Withdrawal and tolerance: Prognostic significance in DSM-IV alcohol dependence. *Journal of Studies on Alcohol 61:*431–438, 2000.
9. Langenbucher, J., Martin, C., Labouvie, E., Sanjuan, P., Bavly, L., & Pollock, N. Toward the DSM-V: The withdrawal-gate model vs. DSM-IV in the diagnosis of alcohol abuse and dependence. *Journal of Consulting and Clinical Psychology 68:*799–809, 2000.
10. Schuckit, M. A., Danko, G. P., Smith, T. L., Hesselbrock, V., Kramer, J., & Bucholz, K. A 5-year prospective evaluation of DSM-IV alcohol dependence with and without a physiological component. *Alcoholism: Clinical and Experimental Research 27:*818–825, 2003.
11. Schuckit, M. A., Smith, T. L., Daeppen, J.-B., Eng, M., Li, T.-K., Hesselbrock, V. M., Nurnberger, J. I., Jr., & Bucholz, K. K. Clinical relevance of the distinction between alcohol dependence with and without a physiological component. *American Journal of Psychiatry 155:*733–740, 1998.
12. Schuckit, M. A., Smith, T. L., & Landi, N. A. The 5-year clinical course of high-functioning men with DSM-IV alcohol abuse or dependence. *American Journal of Psychiatry 157:*2028–2035, 2000.
13. Hasin, D., & Paykin, A. DSM-IV alcohol abuse: Investigation in a sample of at-risk drinkers in the community. *Journal of Studies on Alcohol 60:*181–187, 1999.
14. Ridenour, T. A., Cottler, L. B., Compton, W. M., Spitznagel, E. L., & Cunningham-Williams, R. M. Is there a progression from abuse disorders to dependence disorders? *Addiction 98:*635–644, 2003.
15. Hasin, D. S., Schuckit, M. A., Martin, C. S., Grant, B. F., Bucholz, K. K., & Helzer, J. E. The validity of DSM-IV alcohol dependence: What do we know and what do we need to know? *Alcoholism: Clinical and Experimental Research 27:*244–252, 2003.
16. Dawson, D. Drinking patterns among individuals with and without DSM-IV alcohol use disorders. *Journal of Studies on Alcohol 61:*111–120, 2000.
17. Hasin, D., Liu, X., & Paykin, A. DSM-IV alcohol dependence and sustained reduction in drinking: Investigation in a community sample. *Journal of Studies on Alcohol 62:*509–517, 2001.
18. Hasin, D., Paykin, A., & Endicott, J. Course of DSM-IV alcohol dependence in a community sample: Effects of parental history and binge drinking. *Alcoholism: Clinical and Experimental Research 25:*411–414, 2001.
19. Vaillant, G. E. A 60-year follow-up of alcoholic men. *Addiction 98:*1043–1051, 2003.
20. Hilsenroth, M. J., Ackerman, S. J., Blagys, M. D., Baumann, B. D., Baity, M. R., Smith, S. R., Price, J. L., Smith, C. L., Heindselman, T. L., Mount, M. K., & Holdwick, D. J., Jr. Reliability and validity of DSM-IV axis I. *American Journal of Psychiatry 157:*1858–1863, 2000.
21. Schuckit, M. A. Vulnerability factors for alcoholism. In K. Davis (Ed.), *Neuropsychopharmacology: The Fifth Generation of Progress*. Baltimore: Lippincott, Williams & Wilkins, 2002, pp.1399–1411.
22. Baer, J. S., Sampson, P. D., Barr, H. M., Connor, P. D., & Streissguth, A. P. A 21-year longitudinal analysis of the effects of prenatal alcohol exposure on young adult drinking. *Archives of General Psychiatry 60:*377–385, 2003.
23. O'Neill, S. E., Sher, K. J., Jackson, K. M., & Wood, P. K. Dimensionality of alcohol dependence in young adulthood: current versus lifetime symptomatology. *Journal of Studies on Alcohol 64:*495–499, 2003.
24. Wagner, E. F., Lloyd, D. A., & Gil, A. G. Racial/ethnic and gender differences in the incidence and onset age of DSM-IV alcohol use disorder symptoms among adolescents. *Journal of Studies on Alcohol 63:*609–619, 2002.
25. Harford, T. C., & Muthen, B. O. The dimensionality of alcohol abuse and dependence: A multivariate analysis of DSM-IV symptom items in the National Longitudinal Survey of Youth. *Journal of Studies on Alcohol 62:*150–157, 2001.

26. Schuckit, M. A., Smith, T. L., Danko, G. P., Kramer, J., Godinez, J., Bucholz, K. K., Nurnberger, J. I., Jr., & Hesselbrock, V. A prospective evaluation of the four DSM-IV criteria for alcohol abuse in a large population. *American Journal of Psychiatry 162:*350–360, 2005.
27. Eng, M. Y., Schuckit, M. A., & Smith, T. L. A five-year prospective study of diagnostic orphans for alcohol use disorders. *Journal of Studies on Alcohol 64:*227–234, 2003.
28. Sarr, M., Bucholz, K. K., & Phelps, D. L. Using cluster analysis of alcohol use disorders to investigate 'diagnostic orphans': Subjects with alcohol dependence symptoms but no diagnosis. *Drug and Alcohol Dependence 60:*295–302, 2000.
29. Kendall, R., & Jablensky, A. Distinguishing between the validity and utility of psychiatric diagnoses. *American Journal of Psychiatry 1:*4–12, 2003.
30. Schuckit, M. A., Tipp, J. E., Reich, T., Hesselbrock, V. M., & Bucholz, K. K. The histories of withdrawal convulsions and delirium tremens in 1648 alcohol dependent subjects. *Addiction 90:*1335–1347, 1995.
31. Magura, S., Staines, G., Kosanke, N., Rosenblum, A., Foote, J., DeLuca, A., & Bali, P. Predictive validity of the ASAM patient placement criteria for naturalistically matched vs. mismatched alcoholism patients. *The American Journal on Addictions 12:*386–397, 2003.
32. Gomez, A., Conde, A., Santana, J. M., & Jorrin, A. Diagnostic usefulness of brief versions of Alcohol Use Disorders Identification Test (AUDIT) for detecting hazardous drinkers in primary care settings. *Journal of Studies on Alcohol 66:*305-308, 2005.
33. Reinert, D. F., & Allen, J. P. The alcohol use disorders identification test (AUDIT): A review of recent research. *Alcoholism: Clinical and Experimental Research 26:*272–279, 2002.
34. Kessler, R. C., Crum, R. M., Warner, L. A., Nelson, C. B., Schulenberg, J., & Anthony, J. C. Lifetime co-occurrence of *DSM–III–R* alcohol abuse and dependence with other psychiatric disorders in the National Comorbidity Survey. *Archives of General Psychiatry 54:*313–321, 1997.
35. Hasin, D. S., & Grant, B. F. Major depression in 6050 former drinkers: Association with past alcohol dependence. *Archives of General Psychiatry 59:*794–800, 2002.
36. Preuss, U. W., Schuckit, M. A., Mith, T. L., Danko, G. P., Dasher, A. C., Hesselbrock, M. N., Hesselbrock, V. M., & Nurnberger, J. I., Jr. A comparison of alcohol-induced and independent depression in alcoholics with histories of suicide attempts. *Journal of Studies on Alcohol 63:*498–502, 2002.
37. Preuss, U. S., Schuckit, M. A., Smith, T. L., Danko, G. P., Bucholz, K. K., Hesselbrock, M. N., Hesselbrock, V., & Kramer, J. R. Predictors and correlates of suicide attempts over 5 years in 1,237 alcohol-dependent men and women. *American Journal of Psychiatry 160:*56–63, 2003.
38. Schuckit, M. A., Tipp, J. E., Bucholz, K. K., Nurnberger, J. I., Jr., Hesselbrock, V. M., Crowe, R. R., & Kramer, J. The life-time rates of three major mood disorders and four major anxiety disorders in alcoholics and controls. *Addiction 92:*1289–1304, 1997.
39. Schuckit, M. A., Tipp, J. E., Bergman, M., Reich, W., Hesselbrock, V. M., & Smith, T. L. Comparison of induced and independent major depressive disorders in 2,945 alcoholics. *American Journal of Psychiatry 154:*948–957, 1997.
40. Brady, K. T., Sonne, S., Anton, R. F., Randall, C. F., Back, S. E., & Simpson, K. Sertraline in the treatment of co-occurring alcohol dependence and posttraumatic stress disorder. *Alcoholism: Clinical and Experimental Research 29:*395-401, 2005.
41. Schuckit, M. A., Kelsoe, J. R., Braff, D. L., & Wilhelmsen, K. C. Some possible genetic parallels across alcoholism, bipolar disorder and schizophrenia. *Journal of Studies on Alcohol 64:*157–159, 2003.
42. Raimo, E. R., & Schuckit, M. A. Alcohol dependence and mood disorders. *Addictive Behaviors 23:*933–946, 1998.
43. Wu, L.-T., Kouzis, A. C., & Leaf, P. J. Influence of comorbid alcohol and psychiatric disorders on utilization of mental health services in the National Comorbidity Survey. *American Journal of Psychiatry 156:*1230–1236, 1999.

44. Barrowclough, C., Haddock, G., Tarrier, N., Lewis, S. W., Moring, J., O'Brien, R., Schofield, N., & McGovern, J. Randomized controlled trial of motivational interviewing, cognitive behavior therapy, and family intervention for patients with comorbid schizophrenia and substance use disorders. *American Journal of Psychiatry 158:*1706–1713, 2001.
45. Kuperman, S., Schlosser, S. S., Kramer, J. R., Bucholz, K., Hesselbrock, V., Reich, T., & Reich, W. Risk domains associated with an adolescent alcohol dependence diagnosis. *Addiction 96:*629–636, 2001.
46. Zanarini, M. C., Frankenburg, F. R., Hennen, J., & Silk, K. R. The longitudinal course of borderline psychopathology: 6-year prospective follow-up of the phenomenology of borderline personality disorder. *American Journal of Psychiatry 160:*274–283, 2003.
47. Petry, N. M., Kirby, K. N., & Kranzler, H. R. Effects of gender and family history of alcohol dependence on a behavioral task of impulsivity in healthy subjects. *Journal of Studies on Alcohol 63:*83–90, 2002.
48. Verheul, R., Kranzler, H. R., Poling, J., Tennen, H., Ball, S., & Rounsaville, B. J. Axis I and Axis II disorders in alcoholics and drug addicts: Faco or artifact. *Journal of Studies on Alcohol 61:*101–110, 2000.
49. Boehm, S. L., III, Valenzuela, C. F., & Harris, R. A. Alcohol: Neurobiology. In J. H. Lowinson, P. Ruiz, R. B. Millman, & J. G. Langrod (Eds.), *Substance Abuse: A Comprehensive Textbook* (4th ed.). Baltimore, MD: Lippincott, Williams & Wilkins, 2004, pp. 121–150.
50. Robinson, D. L., Volz, T. J., Schenk, J. O., & Wrightman, R. M. Acute ethanol decreases dopamine transporter velocity in rat striatum: In vivo and in vitro electrochemical measurements. *Alcoholism: Clinical and Experimental Research 29*:746–755, 2005.
51. Krystal, J. H., & Tabakoff, B. Ethanol abuse, dependence, and withdrawal. Neurobiology and clinical implication. In K. L. Davis (Ed.), *Neurpsychopharmacology: The Fifth Generation of Progress*. Baltimore, MD: Lippincott, Williams & Wilkins, 2002, pp. 1423–1444.
52. Koob, G. F., & Le Moal, M. Drug addiction, dysregulation of reward, and allostasis. *Neuropsychopharmacology 24:*97–129, 2001.
53. Schuckit, M. A., Mazzanti, C., Smith, T. L., Ahmed, U., Radel, M., Iwata, N., & Goldman, D. Selective genotyping for the role of 5-HT2A, 5-HT2C and GABAa6 receptors and the serotonin transporter in the level of response to alcohol: A pilot study. *Biological Psychiatry 45:*647–651, 1999.
54. Hu, X., Oroszi, G., Chun, J., Smith, T. L., Goldman, D., & Schuckit, M. A. An expanded evaluation of the relationship of four alleles to the LR to alcohol and the alcoholism risk. *Alcoholism: Clinical and Experimental Research 29:*8–16, 2005.
55. Schuckit, M. A., Smith, T. L., & Kalmijn, J. The search for genes contributing to the low level of response to alcohol: Patterns of findings across studies. *Alcoholism: Clinical and Experimental Research, 28:*1449–1458, 2004.
56. Harrison, A. A., Liem, Y. T. B., & Markou, A. Fluoxetine combined with a serotonin-1A receptor antagonist reversed reward deficits observed during nicotine and amphetamine withdrawal in rats. *Neuropsychopharmacology 25:*55–71, 2001.
57. Twitchell, G. R., Hanna, G. L., Cook, E. H., Fitzgerald, H. E., & Zucker, R. A. Serotonergic function, behavioral disinhibition and negative affect in children of alcoholics: The moderating effects of puberty. *Alcoholism: Clinical and Experimental Research 24:*972–979, 2000.
58. Pierucci-Lagha, A., Covault, J., Feinn, R., Nellissery, M., Hernandez-Avila, C., Oncken, C., Morrow, A. L., & Kranzler, H. R. GABRA2 alleles moderate the subjective effects of alcohol, which are attenuated by finasteride. *Neuropsychopharmacology 30*:1193-1213, 2005.
59. Papadeas, S., Grobin, A. C., & Morrow, A. L. Chronic ethanol consumption differentially alters GABAa receptor a1 and a4 subunit peptide. *Alcoholism: Clinical and Experimental Research 25:*1270–1275, 2001.
60. Krystal, J. H., Petrakis, I. L., Limoncelli, D., Webb, E., Gueorgueva, R., D'Souza, D. C., Boutros, N. N., Trevisan, L., & Charney, D. S. Altered NMDA glutamate receptor antago-

nist response in recovering ethanol-dependent patients. *Neuropsychopharmacology 28:*2020–2028, 2003.

61. Camarini, R., Frussa-Filho, R., Monteiro, M. G., & Calil, H. M. MK-801 blocks the development of behavioral sensitization to ethanol. *Alcoholism: Clinical and Experimental Research 24:*285–290, 2000.
62. Bart, G., Kreek, M. J., Ott, J., LaForge, K. S., Proudnikov, D., Pollak, L., & Heilig, M. Increased attributable risk related to a functional μ-opioid receptor gene polymorphism in association with alcohol dependence in central Sweden. *Neuropsychopharmacology 30:*417–422, 2005.
63. Mascia, M. P., Maiya, R., Borghese, C. M., Lobo, I. A., Hara, K., Yamakura, T., Gong, & Beckstead, M. J. Does acetaldehyde mediate ethanol action in the central nervous system? *Alcoholism: Clinical and Experimental Research 25:*1570–1575, 2001.
64. Le, A. D., Corrigall, W. A., Harding, J. W. S., Juzytsch, W., & Li, T.-K. Involvement of nicotinic receptors in alcohol self-administration. *Alcoholism: Clinical and Experimental Research 24:*155–163, 2000.
65. Hungund, B. L., Szakall, I., Adam, A., Basavarajappa, B. S., & Vadasz, C. Cannabinoid CB1 receptor knockout mice exhibit markedly reduced voluntary alcohol consumption and lack alcohol-induced dopamine release in the nucleus accumbens. *Journal of Neurochemistry 84:*698–704, 2003.
66. Vinod, K. Y., Arango, V., Xie, S., Kassir, S. A., Mann, J. J., Cooper, T. B., & Hungund, B. L. Elevated levels of endocannabinoids and CB_1 receptor-mediated G-protein signaling in the prefrontal cortex of alcoholic suicide victims. *Biological Psychiatry 57:*480-486, 2005.
67. Choi, D.-S., Cascini, M.-G., Mailliard, W., Young, H., Paredes, P., McMahon, T., Diamond, I., Bonci, A., & Messing, R. O. The type 1 equilibrative nucleoside transporter regulates ethanol intoxication and preference. *Nature Neurscience 7:*855–861, 2004.
68. Davies, A. G., Pierce-Shimomura, J. T., Kim, H., VanHoven, M. K., Thiele, T. R., Bonci, A., Bargmann, C. I., & McIntire, S. L. A central role of the BK potassium channel in behavioral responses to ethanol in *C. elegans*. *Cell 225:*655–666, 2003.
69. Hidestrand, M., Shankar, K., Ronis, M. J. J., & Badger, T. M. Effects of light and dark beer on hepatic cytochrome P-450 expression in male rats receiving alcoholic beverages as part of total enteral nutrition. Alcoholism: *Clinical and Experimental Research 29:*888-895, 2005.
70. Romero, I., Paez, A., Ferruelo, A., Lujan, M., & Berenguer, A. Polyphenols in red wine inhibit the proliferation and induce apoptosis of LNCap cells. *BJU International 89:*950–954, 2002.
71. Pihl, R. O., Paylan, S. S., Gentes-Hawn, A., & Hoaken, P. N. S. Alcohol affects executive cognitive functioning differentially on the ascending versus descending limb of the blood alcohol concentration curve. *Alcoholism: Clinical and Experimental Research 27:*773–779, 2003.
72. Mackay, M., Tiplady, B., & Scholey, A. B. Interactions between alcohol and caffeine in relation to psychomotor sped and accuracy. *Human Psychopharmacology 17:*151–156, 2002.
73. Wickramasinghe, S. N., Hasan, R. & Zhalpey, Z. Differences in the serum levels of acetaldehyde and cytotoxic acetaldehyde-albumin complexes after the consumption of red and white wine: In vitro effects of flavonoids, vitamin E, and other dietary antioxidants on cytotoxic complexes. *Alcoholism: Clinical and Experimental Research 23:*835–841, 1999.
74. Hetherington, M. M., Cameron, F., Wallis, D. J., & Pirie, L. M. Stimulation of appetite by alcohol. *Physiological Behavior 74:*283–289, 2001.
75. Perreira, K. M., & Sloan, F. A. Excess alcohol consumption and health outcomes: A 6-year follow-up of men over age 50 from the health and retirement study. *Addiction 97:*301–310, 2002.
76. Leitzmann, M. F., Giovannucci, E. L., Stampfer, M. J., Spiegelman, D., Colditz, G. A., Willett, W. C., & Rimm, E. B. Prospective study of alcohol consumption patterns in relation to symptomatic gallstone disease in men. *Alcoholism: Clinical and Experimental Research 23:*835–841, 1999.
77. Cordova, A. C., Jackson, L. S. M., Berke-Schlessel, D. W., & Sumpio, B. E. The cardiovascular protective effect of red wine. *Journal of the American College of Surgeons 200:*428-439, 2005.

78. Mukamal, K. J., Conigrave, K. M., Mittleman, M. A., Camargo, C. A., Jr., Stampfer, M. J., Willett, W. C., & Rimm, E. B. Roles of drinking pattern and type of alcohol consumed in coronary heart disease in men. *New England Journal of Medicine 348:*109–118, 2003.
79. Ruitenberg, A., van Swieten, J. C., Witteman, J. C. M., Mehta, K. M., van Duijn, C. M., Hofman, M., & Breteler, M. M. Alcohol consumption and risk of dementia: The Rotterdam study. *The Lancet 359:*281–286, 2002.
80. Tolstrup, J. S., Jensen, M. K., Tjonneland, A., Overvad, K., & Gronbaek, M. Drinking pattern and mortality in middle-aged men and women. *Addiction 99:*323–330, 2004.
81. Sun, L., Konig, I. R., Jacobs, A., Seitz, H. K., Junghanns, K., Wagner, T., Ludwig, D., Jacrobs, A., & Homann, N. Mean corpuscular volume and ADH1C genotype in white patients with alcohol-associated diseases. *Alcoholism: Clinical and Experimental Research 29:*788-793, 2005.
82. Boyadjieva, N. I., Dokur, M., Advis, J. P., Meadows, G. G., & Sarkar, D. K. Beta-endorphin modulation of lymphocyte proliferation: effects of ethanol. *Alcoholism: Clinical and Experimental Research 26:*1719–1727, 2002.
83. Whitfield, J. B., Zhu, G., Heath, A. C., Powell, L. S., & Martin, N. G. Effects of alcohol consumption on indices of iron stores and of iron stores on alcohol intake markers. *Alcoholism: Clinical and Experimental Research 25:*1037–1045, 2001.
84. Volpato, S., Pahor, M., Ferrucci, L., Simonsick, E. M., Guralnik, J. M., Kritchevsky, S. B., Fellin, R., & Harris, T. B. Relationship of alcohol intake with inflammatory markers and plasminogen activator inhibitior-1 in well-functioning older adults: The health, aging, and body composition study. *Circulation 109:*607–612, 2004.
85. Samet, J. H., Horton, N. J., Traphagen, E. T., Lyon, S. M., & Freedberg, K. A. Alcohol consumption and HIV disease progression: Are they related? *Alcoholism: Clinical and Experimental Research 27:*862–867, 2003.
86. Kalichman, S. E., Cain, D., Zweben, A., & Swain, G. Sensation seeking, alcohol use and sexual risk behaviors among men receiving services at a clinic for sexually transmitted infections. *Journal of Studies on Alcohol 64:*564–569, 2003.
87. Lieber, C. S. Gastric ethanol metabolism and gastritis: Interactions with other drugs, *Helicobacter pylori*, and antibiotic therapy (1957–1997)—A review. *Alcoholism: Clinical and Experimental Research 21:*1360–1366, 1997.
88. Verlaan, M., Te Morsche, R. H. M., Roelofs, H. M. J., Laheij, R. J. F., Jansen, J. B. M. J., Peters, W. H. M., & Drenth, J. P. H. Genetic polymorphisms in alcohol-metabolizing enzymes and chronic pancreatitis. *Alcohol & Alcoholism 39:*20–24, 2004.
89. Maruyama, K., Takahashi, H., Matsushita, S., Nakano, M., Harada, H., Otsuki, M., Ogawa, M., Suda, K., Baba, T., Honma, T., Moroboshi, T., & Matsuno, M. Genotypes of alcohol-metabolising enzymes in relation to alcoholic chronic pancreatitis in Japan. *Alcoholism: Clinical and Experimental Research 23(Suppl.):*85S–91S, 1999.
90. Wannamethee, S. G., Camargo, C. A., Jr., Manson, J. E., Willett, W. C., & Rimm, E. B. Alcohol drinking patterns and risk of Type 2 diabetes mellitus among younger women. *Archives of Internal Medicine 163:*1329–1336, 2003.
91. Stinson, F. S., Grant, B. F., & Dufour, M. C. The critical dimension of ethnicity in liver cirrhosis mortality statistics. *Alcoholism: Clinical and Experimental Research. 25:*1181–1187, 2001.
92. Zimmerman, H. J., & Maddrey, W. C. Acetaminophen (paracetamol) hepatotoxicity with regular intake of alcohol: Analysis of instances of therapeutic misadventure. *Hepatology 22:*767–779, 1995.
93. Marsano, L. S. Hepatitis. Primary Care. *Clinics in Office Practice 30:*81–107, 2003.
94. Polednak, A. P. Recent trends in incidence rates for selected alcohol-related cancers in the *United States. Alcohol and Alcoholism 40:*234-238, 2005.
95. Albertsen, K., & Gronbaek, M. Does amount or type of alcohol influence the risk of prostate cancer? *Prostate 52:*297–301, 2002.
96. Zhang, Y., Kreger, B. E., Dorgan, J. F., Splansky, G. L., Cupples, L. A., & Ellison, R. C. Alcohol consumption and risk of breast cancer: The Framington Study revisted. *The American Journal of Epidemiology 149:*93–101, 1999.

97. Vachon, C. M., Cerhan, J. R., Vierkant, L. R. A., & Sellers, T. A. Investigation of an interaction of alcohol intake and family history on breast cancer risk in the Minnesota Breast Cancer Family Study. *Cancer 92:*240–248, 2001.
98. Stampfer, M. J., Kang, J. H., Chen, J., Cherry, R., & Grodstein, F. Effects of moderate alcohol consumption on cognitive functioning in women. *New England Journal of Medicine 352:*245-253, 2005.
99. Harris, C. R., Albaugh, B., Goldman, D., & Enoch, M. A. Neurocognitive impairment due to chronic alcohol consumption in an American Indian community. *Journal of Studies on Alcohol 64:*458–466, 2003.
100. Bjork, J. M., Grant, S. J., & Hommer, D. W. Cross-sectional volumetric analysis of brain atrophy in alcohol dependence: Effects of drinking history and comorbid substance use disorder. *American Journal of Psychiatry 160:*2038–2045, 2003.
101. Anttila, T., Helkala, E.-L., Viitanen, M., Kareholt, I., Fratiglioni, L., Winblad, B., Soininen, H., Tuomilehto, J., Nissinen, A., & Kivipelto, M. Alcohol drinking in middle age and subsequent risk of mild cognitive impairment and dementia in old age: A prospective population based study. *British Medical Journal 129:*539–542, 2004.
102. Mukamal, K. J., Longstreth, W. T., Jr., Mittleman, M. A., Crum, R. M., & Siscovick, D. S. Alcohol consumption and subclinical findings on magnetic resonance imaging of the brain in older adults: *The Cardiovascular Health Study. Stroke 32:*1939–1946, 2001.
103. Oscar-Berman, M., Kirkley, S. M., Gansler, D. A., & Couture, A. Comparisons of Korsakoff and Non-Korsakoff alcoholics on neuropsychological tests of prefrontal brain functioning. *Alcoholism: Clinical and Experimental Research 28:*667–675, 2004.
104. Wang, J. J. L., Martin, P. R., & Singleton, C. K. A transketolase assembly defect in a Wernicke–Korsakoff syndrome patient. *Alcoholism: Clinical and Experimental Research 21:*576–580, 1997.
105. Ammendola, A., Gemini, D., Iannaccone, S., Argenzio, F., Ciccone, G., Ammendola, K. E., Serio, L., Ugolini, G., & Bravaccio, F. Gender and peripheral neuropathy in chronic alcoholism: A clinical-electroneurographic study. *Medical Council on Alcoholism 35:*368–371, 2000.
106. Sullivan, E. V., & Pfefferbaum, A. Magnetic resonance relaxometry reveals central pontine abnormalities in clinically asymptomatic alcoholic men. *Alcoholism: Clinical and Experimental Research 25:*1206–1212, 2001.
107. Helenius, J., Tatlisumak, T., Soinne, L., Valanne, L., & Kaste, M. Marchiafava-Bignami disease: Two cases with favourable outcome. *European Journal of Neurology 8:*269–272, 2001.
108. Kajander, O. A., Kupari, M., Perola, M., Pajarinen, J., Savolainen, V., Penttilä, A., & Karhunen, P. J. Testing genetic susceptibility loci for alcoholic heart muscle disease. *Alcoholism: Clinical and Experimental Research 25:*1409–1413, 2001.
109. Minami, J., Yoshii, M., Todoroka, M., Nishikimi, T., Ishimitsu, T., Fukanaga, T., & Matsuoka, H. Effects of alcohol restriction on ambulatory blood pressure, heart rate, and heart rate variability in Japanese men. *American Journal of Hypertension 15:*125–129, 2002.
110. Rouillier, P., Boutron-Ruault, M.-C., Bertrais, S., Arnault, N., Daudin, J.-J., Bacro, J.-N., & Hercberg, S. Alcohol and atherosclerotic vascular disease risk factors in French men: Relationships are linear, J-shaped, and U-shaped. *Alcoholism: Clinical and Experimental Research 29:*84-88, 2005.
111. Foppa, M., Fuchs, F. D., Preissler, L., Andrighetto, A., Rosito, G. A., & Duncan, B. B. Red wine with the noon meal lowers post-meal blood pressure: A randomized trial in centrally obese, hypertensive patients. *Journal of Studies on Alcohol 63:*247–251, 2002.
112. Trevisan, M., Dorn, J., Falkner, K., Russell, M., Ram, M., Muti, P., Freudenheim, J. L., Nochajaski, T., & Hovey, K. Drinking pattern and risk of non-fatal myocardial infarction: A population-based case–control study. *Addiction 99:*313–322, 2003.
113. Romelsjö, A., Branting, M., Hallqvist, J., Alfredsson, L., Hammar, N., Leifman, A., & Ahlbom, A. Abstention, alcohol use and risk of myocardial infarction in men and women

taking account of social support and working conditions: the SHEEP case–control study. *Addiction 98:*1453–1462, 2003.

114. Estruch, R., Sacanella, E., Fernandez-Sola, J., Nicolas, J. M., Rubin, E., & Urbano-Marquez, A. Natural history of alcoholic myopathy: A 5-year study. *Alcoholism: Clinical and Experimental Research 22:*2023–2028, 1998.
115. Ginsburg, E. S., Mello, N. K., & Mendelson, J. H. Alcohol abuse: Endocrine concomitants, In *Hormones, Brain and Behavior* (Vol. 5). Elsevier Science, 2002, pp. 747–780.
116. Mumenthaler, M. S., O'Hara, R., Taylor, J. L., Friedman, L., & Yesavage, J. A. Influence of the menstrual cycle on flight simulator performance after alcohol ingestion. *Journal of Studies on Alcohol 62:*422–433, 2001.
117. Sarkola, T. Effect of alcohol on steroids in women. *Alcohol Research 7:*51–53, 2002.
118. Lindman, R. E., Koskelainen, B. M., & Eriksson, C. J. P. Drinking, menstrual cycle, and female sexuality: A diary study. *Alcoholism: Clinical and Experimental Research 23:*169–173, 1999.
119. Sarkola, T., & Eriksson, C. J. P. Testosterone increases in men after a low dose of alcohol. *Alcoholism: Clinical and Experimental Research 27:*682–685, 2003.
120. Yamauchi, M., Takeda, K., Sakamoto, K., Searashi, Y., Uetake, S., Kenichi, H., & Toda, G. Association of polymorphism in the alcohol dehydrogenase 2 gene with alcohol-induced testicular atrophy. *Alcoholism: Clinical and Experimental Research 25:*16S–18S, 2001.
121. Callaci, J. J., Juknelis, D., Patwardhan, A., Sartori, M., Frost, N., & Wezeman, F. H. The effects of binge alcohol exposure on bone resorption and biomechanical and structural properties are offset by concurrent bisphosphonate treatment. *Alcoholism: Clinical and Experimental Research 28:*182–191, 2004.
122. Elmali, N., Ertern, K., Ozen, S., Knan, M., Baysal, T., Güner, G., & Bora, A. Fracture healing and bone mass in rats fed on liquid diet containing ethanol. *Alcoholism: Clinical and Experimental Research 26:*509–513, 2002.
123. Risinger, F. O. Genetic analyses of ethanol-induced hyperglycemia. *Alcoholism: Clinical and Experimental Research 27:*756–764, 2003.
124. Ishii, K., Kumashiro, R., Koga, Y., Tanikawa, K., Furudera, S., Mitsuoka, M., Sakamoto, T., & Kaku, N. Two survival cases of alcoholic lactic acidosis complicated with diabetes mellitus and alcoholic liver disease. *Alcoholism: Clinical and Experimental Research 20:*387A–390A, 1996.
125. Elisaf, M., Liberopoulos, E., Bairaktari, E., & Siamopoulos, K. Hypokalaemia in alcoholic patients. *Drug and Alcohol Review 21:*73–76, 2002.
126. Sassine, M. P., Mergler, D., Bowler, R., & Hudnell, H. K. Manganese accentuates adverse mental health effects associated with alcohol use disorders. *Biological Psychiatry 51:*909–921, 2002.
127. Lemoine, A., Chanay, H., Cirette, B., & Bouillot, P. Vitamin status and alcohol. *Alcoologie 18:*151–154, 1996.
128. Schwartz, S. M., Doody, D. R., Fitzgibbons, E. D., Ricks, S., Porter, P. L., & Chen, C. Oral squamous cell cancer risk in relation to alcohol consumption and alcohol dehydrogenase-3 genotypes. *Cancer Epidemiology, Biomarkers & Prevention 10:*1137–1144, 2001.
129. Enberg, N., Wolf, J., Ainamo, A., Alho, H., Heinälä, P., & Lenander-Lumikari, M. Dental diseases and loss of teeth in a group of Finnish alcoholics: A radiological study. *Acta Odontologica Scandinavica 59:*341–347, 2001.
130. Hiratsuka, Y., & Li, G. Alcohol and eye diseases: A review of epidemiologic studies. *Journal of Studies on Alcohol 62:*397–402, 2001.
131. Epstein, M. Alcohol's impact on kidney function. *Alcohol Health & Research World 21:*84–91, 1997.
132. Faunce, D. E., Garner, J. L., Llanas, J. N., Patel, P. J., Gregory, M. S., Duffner, L. A., Garnelli, R. L., & Kovacs, E. J. Effect of acute ethanol exposure on the dermal inflammatory response after burn injury. *Alcoholism: Clinical and Experimental Research 27:*1199–1206, 2003.

133. Hoefkens, P., Higgins, E. M., Ward, R. J., & Van Eijk, H. G. Isoforms of transferrin in psoriasis patients abusing alcohol. *Alcohol & Alcoholism 32:*195–199, 1997.
134. Green, J. E., Saveanu, R. V., & Bornstein, R. A. The effect of previous alcohol abuse on cognitive function in HIV infection. *American Journal of Psychiatry 161:*249–254, 2004.
135. Waller, P. F., Hill, E. M., Maio, R. F., & Blow, F. C. Alcohol effects on motor vehicle crash injury. *Alcoholism: Clinical and Experimental Research 27:*695–703, 2003.
136. Zador, P. L., Krawchuk, S. A., & Voas, R. B. Alcohol-related relative risk of driver fatalities and driver involvement in fatal crashes in relation to driver age and gender: An update using 1996 data. *Journal of Studies on Alcohol 61:*387–395, 2000.
137. Yu, J., & Shacket, R. W. Drinking-driving and riding with drunk drivers among young adults: An analysis of reciprocal effects. *Journal of Studies on Alcohol 60:*615–621, 1999.
138. Li, G., Baker, S. P., Sterling, S., Smialek, J. E., Dischinger, P. C., & Soderstrom, C. A. A comparative analysis of alcohol in fatal and nonfatal bicycling injuries. *Alcoholism: Clinical and Experimental Research 20:*1153–1559, 1996.
139. Cook, C. C. H. Alcohol and aviation. *Addiction 92:*539–555, 1997.
140. Soderstrom, C. A., Smith, G. S., Dischinger, P. C., McDuff, D. R., Hebel, J. R., Gorelick, D. A., Kerns, T. J., Ho, S. M., & Read, K. M. Psychoactive substance use disorders among seriously injured trauma center patients. *Journal of the American Medical Association 277:*1769–1774, 1997.
141. Zink, B. J., Maio, R. F., & Chen, B. Alcohol, central nervous system injury, and time to death in fatal motor vehicle crashes. *Alcoholism: Clinical and Experimental Research 20:*1518–1522, 1996.
142. Currie, S. R., Clark, S., Rimac, S., & Malhotra, S. Comprehensive assessment of insomnia in recovering alcoholics using daily sleep diaries and ambulatory monitoring. *Alcoholism: Clinical and Experimental Research 27:*1262–1269, 2003.
143. Irwin, M., Gillin, J. C., Dang, J., Weissman, J., Phillips, E., & Ehlers, C. L. Sleep deprivation as a probe of homeostatic sleep regulation in primary alcoholics. *Biological Psychiatry 51:*632–641, 2002.
144. Kühlwein, E., Hauger, R. L., & Irwin, M. R. Abnormal nocturnal melatonin secretion and disordered sleep in abstinent alcoholics. *Biological Psychiatry 54:*1437–1443, 2003.
145. Crum, R. M., Ford, D. E., Storr, C. L., & Chan, Y.-F. Association of sleep disturbance with chronicity and remission of alcohol dependence: Data from a population-based prospective study. *Alcoholism: Clinical and Experiment Research 28:*1533–1540, 2004.
146. Slutske, W. S., Plasecki, T. M., & Hunt-Carter, E. E. Development and initial validation of the hangover symptoms scale: Prevalence and correlates of hangover symptoms in college students. *Alcoholism: Clinical and Experimental Research 27:*1442–1450, 2003.
147. Verster, J. C., van Duin, D., Volkerts, E. R., Schreuder, A. H. C. M. L., & Verbaten, M. N. Alcohol hangover effects on memory functioning and vigilance performance after an evening of binge drinking. *Neuropsychopharmacology 28:*740–746, 2003.
148. Hartzler, B., & Fromme, K. Fragmentary blackouts: Their etiology and effect on alcohol expectancies. *Alcoholism: Clinical and Experimental Research 27:*628–637, 2003.
149. Nelson, E. C., Heath, A. C., Bucholz, K. K., Madden, P. A. F., Fu, Q., Knopik, V., Lynskey, M. T., Whitfield, J. B., Statham, D. J., & Martin, N. G. Genetic epidemiology of alcohol-induced blackouts. *Archives of General Psychiatry 61:*157–263, 2004.
150. Charney, D. S., Mihic, J., & Harris, R. A. Hypnotics and sedatives. In J. G. Hardman, L. E. Limbird, & A. G. Goodman (Eds.), *The Pharmacological Basis of Therapeutics* (10th ed.). New York: McGraw-Hill, 2001, pp. 399–427.
151. Correa, M., Sanchis-Segura, C., & Aragon, C. M. G. Influence of brain catalase on ethanol-induced loss of righting reflex in mice. *Drug and Alcohol Dependence 65:*9–15, 2001.
152. Quartemont, E., Grant, K. A., Correa, M., Arizzi, M. N., Salamone, J. D., Tambour, S., Aragon, C. M. G., McBride, W. J., Rodd, Z. A., Goldstein, A., Zaffaroni, A., Li, T.-K., Pisano, M., & Diana, M. The role of acetaldehyde in the central effects of ethanol. *Alcoholism: Clinical and Experimental Research 29*:221–234, 2005.

153. Li, T.-K., Beard, J. D., Orr, W. E., Kwo, P. Y., Ramchandani, V. A., & Thomasson, H. R. Variation in ethanol pharmacokinetics and perceived gender and ethnic differences in alcohol elimination. *Alcoholism: Clinical and Experimental Research 24:*415–416, 2000.
154. Baraona, E., Abittan, C. S., Dohmen, K., Moretti, M., Pozzato, G., Chayes, Z. W., Schaefer, C., & Lieber, C. S. Gender differences in pharmacokinetics of alcohol. *Alcoholism: Clinical and Experimental Research 25:*502–507, 2001.
155. Thomasson, H. Alcohol elimination: Faster in women? *Alcoholism: Clinical and Experimental Research 24:*419–420, 2000.
156. Hasin, D., Aharonovich, E., Liu, X., Mamman, Z., Matseoane, K., Carr, L. G., & Li, T.-K. Alcohol dependence symptoms and alcohol dehydrogenase 2 polymorphism: Israeli Ashkenazis, Sephardics, and recent Russian immigrants. *Alcoholism: Clinical and Experimental Research 26:*1315–1321, 2002.
157. Cook, T. A. R., Luczak, S. E., Shea, S. H., Ehlers, C. L., Carr, L. G., & Wall, T. L. Associations of ALDH2 and ADH1B genotypes with response to alcohol in Asian Americans. *Journal of Studies on Alcohol 66*:196–204, 2005.
158. Schuckit, M. A. Alcohol and alcoholism. In D. L. Kasper, E. Braunwald, A. S. Fauci, *et al.* (Eds.), *Harrison's Principles of Internal Medicine* (16th ed.). New York, NY: McGraw-Hill, 2004, pp. 2562–2567.
159. Nestler, E. J. Molecular neurobiology of addiction. *The American Journal on Addictions 10:*201–217, 2001.
160. Anthony, J. C., & Echeagaray-Wagner, F. Epidemiologic analysis of alcohol and tobacco use: Patterns of co-occurring consumption and dependence in the United States. *Alcohol Research & Health 24:*201–208, 2000.
161. Johnston, L. D., O'Malley, P. M., Bachman, J. G., & Schulenberg, J. E. Monitoring the Future National Survey Results on Drug Use, 1973–2003. Vol II: College Students and Adults Ages 19–40 (NIH Publication No. 04-5506), Bethesda, MD: National Institute on Drug Abuse, 2004.
162. Substance Abuse and Mental Health Services Administration. Overview of Findings from the 2002 National Survey on Drug Use and Health (Office of Applied Studies, NHSDA Series H-21, DHHS Publication No. SMA 03-3774). Rockville, MD, 2003.
163. Schuckit, M. A., Smith, T. L., & Kalmijn, J. Findings across subgroups regarding the level of response to alcohol as a risk factor for alcohol use disorders (AUDs): A college population of women and Latinos. *Alcoholism: Clinical and Experimental Research 28:*1499–1508, 2004.
164. Spicer, P., Beals, J., Croy, C. D., Mitchell, C. M., Novins, D. K., Moore, L., Manson, S. M., & the American Indian Service Utilization, Psychiatric Epidemiology, Risk and Protective Factors Project Team. The prevalence of DSM-III-R alcohol dependence in two American Indian populations. *Alcoholism: Clinical and Experimental Research 27:*1785–1797, 2003.
165. Holdcraft, L. C., & Iacono, W. G. Cohort effects on gender differences in alcohol dependence. *Addiction 97:*1025–1036, 2002.
166. Knight, J. R., Wechsler, H., Kuo, M., Seibring, M., Weitzman, E. R., & Schuckit, M. A. Alcohol abuse and dependence among U.S. college students. *Journal of Studies on Alcohol 63:*263–270, 2002.
167. Schuckit, M. A., Kraft, H. S., Hurtado, S. L., Tschinkel, S. A., Minagawa, R., & Shaffer, R. A. A measure of the intensity of response to alcohol in a military population. *American Journal of Drug and Alcohol Abuse 27:*749–757, 2001.
168. Mandell, W., Eaton, W. W., Anthony, J. C., & Garrison, R. Alcoholism and occupations: A review and analysis of 104 occupations. *Alcoholism: Clinical and Experimental Research 16:*734–746, 1992.
169. Cassell, S., Pledger, M., & Hooper, R. Socioeconomic status and drinking patterns in young adults. *Addiction 98:*601–610, 2003.
170. Hesselbrock, M. N., Hesselbrock, V. M., Segal, B., Schuckit, M. A., & Bucholz, K. Ethnicity and psychiatric comorbidity among alcohol-dependent persons who receive inpa-

tient treatment: African Americans, Alaska Natives, Caucasians, and Hispanics. *Alcoholism: Clinical and Experimental Research 27:*1368–1373, 2003.

171. Neumark, Y. D., Friedlander, Y., Durst, R., Leitersdorf, E., Jaffe, D., Ramchandani, V. A., O'Connor, S., Carr, L. G., & Li, T.-K. Alcohol dehydrogenase polymorphisms influence alcohol-elimination rates in a male Jewish population. *Alcoholism: Clinical and Experimental Research 28:*10–14, 2004.
172. McGue, M., Iacono, W. G., Legrand, L. N., & Elkins, I. Origins and consequences of age at first drink. I. Associations with substance-use disorders, disinhibitory behavior and psychopathology and P2 amplitude. *Alcoholism: Clinical and Experimental Research 25:*1156–1165, 2001.
173. deWit, D. J., Adlaf, E. M., Offord, D. R.., & Ogborne, A. C. Age at first alcohol use: A risk factor for the development of alcohol disorders. *American Journal of Psychiatry 157:*745–750, 2000.
174. Hingson, R. W., Heeren, T., Zakocs, R. C., Kopstein, A., & Wechsler, H. Magnitude of alcohol-related mortality and morbidity among U.S. college students ages 18–24. *Journal of Studies on Alcohol 63:*136–144, 2002.
175. Rivara, F. P., Garrison, M. M., Ebel, B., McCarty, C. A., & Christakis, D. A. Mortality attributable to harmful drinking in the United States, 2000. *Journal of Studies on Alcohol 65:*530–536, 2004.
176. Fillmore, K. M., Kerr, W. C., & Bostrom, A. Changes in drinking status, serious illness and mortality. *Journal of Studies on Alcohol 64:*278–285, 2003.
177. Dawson, D. A. Alcohol and mortality from external causes. *Journal of Studies on Alcohol 62:*790–797, 2001.
178. Andreasson, W., & Brandt, L. Mortality and morbidity related to alcohol. *Alcohol & Alcoholism 32:*173–178, 1997.
179. Skog, O. J., & Duckert, F. The development of alcoholics' and heavy drinkers' consumption: A longitudinal study. *Journal of Studies on Alcohol 54:*178–188, 1993.
180. Schuckit, M. A., Tipp, J. E., Smith, T. L., & Bucholz, K. K. Periods of abstinence following the onset of alcohol dependence in 1,853 men and women. *Journal of Studies on Alcohol 58:*581–589, 1997.
181. Wallace, J. M., Jr., Bachman, J. G., O'Malley, P. M., Schulenberg, J. E., Cooper, S. M., & Johnston, L. D. Gender and ethnic differences in smoking, drinking and illicit drug use among American 8th, 10th, and 12th grade students, 1976–2000. *Addiction 98:*225–234, 2003.
182. Lynskey, M. T., Day, C., & Hall, W. Alcohol and other drug use disorders among older-aged people. *Drug and Alcohol Review 22:*125–133, 2003.
183. Satre, D. D., Mertens, J., Arean, P. A., & Weisner, C. Contrasting outcomes of older versus middle-aged and younger adult chemical dependence patients in a managed care program. *Journal of Studies on Alcohol 64:*520–530, 2003.
184. Bischof, G., Rumpf, H.-J., Hapke, U., Meyer, C., & John, U. Remission from alcohol dependence without help: How restrictive should our definition of treatment be? *Journal of Studies on Alcohol 63:*229–236, 2002.
185. Tucker, J. A., Vuchinich, R. E., & Rippens, P. D. Environmental contexts surrounding resolution of drinking problems among problem drinkers with different help-seeking experiences. *Journal of Studies on Alcohol 63:*334–341, 2002.
186. Tarter, R. E. Etiology of adolescent substance abuse: A developmental perspective. *American Journal of Addictions 11:*171–191, 2002.
187. Windle, M., & Windle, R. C. Depressive symptoms and cigarette smoking among middle adolescents: Prospective associations and intrapersonal and interpersonal influences. *Journal of Consulting & Clinical Psychology 60:*215–226, 2001.
188. Goodwin, R. D., Fergusson, D. M., & Horwood, L. J. Association between anxiety disorders and substance use disorders among young persons: Results of a 21-year longitudinal study. *Journal of Psychiatric Research 38:*295–304, 2004.

189. Schuckit, M. A., Smith, T. L., Danko, G. P., Anderson, K. G., Brown, S. A., Kuperman, S., Kramer, J., Hesselbrock, V., & Bucholz K. K. Evaluation of a "level of response to alcohol based" structural equation model in adolescents, *Journal of Studies on Alcohol 44:*174–184, 2005.

190. Schuckit, M. A., Smith, T. L., Anderson, K. G., Brown, S. A. Testing the level of response to alcohol-social information processing model of the alcoholism risk: A 20-year prospective study, *Alcohol: Clinical and Experimental Reserch 28:*1881–1889, 2004.

191. Sutherland, I., & Shepherd, J. P. Social dimensions of adolescent substance use. *Addiction 96:*445–458, 2001.

192. D'Amico, E. J., McCarthy, D. M., Appelbaum, M., Metrik, J., Frissell, K. C., & Brown, S. A. Progression into and out of binge drinking among high school students. *Psychology of Addictive Behaviors 15:*341–349, 2001.

193. Leonard, K. E., Eiden, R. D., Wong, M. M., Zucker, R. A., Puttler, L. I., Fitzgerald, H. E., Hussong, A., Chassin, L., & Mudar, P. Developmental perspectives on risk and vulnerability in alcoholic families. *Alcoholism: Clinical and Experimental Research 24:*238–240, 2000.

194. Patock-Peckham, J. A., Cheong, J.-W., Balhorn, M. E., & Nagoshi, C. T. A social learning perspective: A model of parenting styles, self-regulation, perceived drinking control, and alcohol use and problems. *Alcoholism: Clinical and Experimental Research 25:*1284–1292, 2001.

195. Kuperman, S., Schlosser, S. S., Kramer, J. R., Bucholz, K., Hesselbrock, V., Reich, T., & Reich, W. Developmental sequence from disruptive behavior diagnosis to adolescent alcohol dependence. *American Journal of Psychiatry 158:*2022–2026, 2001.

196. Sayette, M. A., Martin, C. S., Perrott, M. A., Wertz, J. M., & Hufford, M. R. A test of the appraisal-disruption model of alcohol and stress. *Journal of Studies on Alcohol 62:*247–256, 2001.

197. Averna, S., & Hesselbrock, V. The relationship of perceived social support to substance use in offspring of alcoholics. *Addictive Behaviors 26:*363–374, 2001.

198. Longabaugh, R., Wirtz, P. W., & Rice, C. Social functioning, in project match hypotheses: Results and causal chain analyses. In R. Longabaugh, P. W. Wirtz (Eds.), NIAAA Project MATCH Monograph Series (Vol. 8). NIH Publication No. 01-4238, 2001, Bethesda, MC, pp. 285.

199. Shen, S. A., Locke-Wellman, J., & Hill, S. Y. Adolescent alcohol expectancies in offspring from families at high risk for developing alcoholism. *Journal of Studies on Alcohol 62:*763–772, 2001.

200. Noar, S. M., LaForge, R. G., Maddock, J. E., & Wood, M. D. Rethinking positive and negative aspects of alcohol use: Suggestions from a comparison of alcohol expectancies and decisional balance. *Journal of Studies on Alcohol 64:*60–69, 2003.

201. Griffin, K. W., Botvin, G. J., Epstein, J. A., Doyle, M. M., & Diaz, T. Psychosocial and behavioral factors in early adolescence as predictors of heavy drinking among high school seniors. *Journal of Studies on Alcohol 61:*603–606, 2000.

202. Holahan, C. J., Moos, R. H., Holahan, C. K., Cronkite, R. C., & Randall, P. K. Drinking to cope, emotional distress and alcohol use and abuse: A ten-year model. *Journal of Studies on Alcohol 62:*190–198, 2001.

203. Poikolainen, K., Tuulio-Henriksson, A., Aalto-Setala, T., Marttunen, M., & Lonnqvist, J. Predictors of alcohol intake and heavy drinking in early adulthood: A 5-year follow-up of 15–19-year-old Finnish adolescents. *Alcohol & Alcoholism 36:*85–88, 2001.

204. Mason, W. A., & Windle, M. A longitudinal study of the effects of religiosity on adolescent alcohol use and alcohol-related problems. *Journal of Adolescent Psychiatry 17:*346–363, 2002.

205. Casswell, S., Pledger, M., & Hooper, R. Socioeconomic status and drinking patterns in young adults. *Addiction 98:*601–610, 2003.

206. Demers, A., & Kairouz, S. A multilevel analysis of change in alcohol consumption in Quebec, 1993–98. *Addiction 98:*205–213, 2003.

207. Enoch, M.-A., Schuckit, M. A., Johnson, B. A., & Goldman, D. Genetics of alcoholism using intermediate phenotypes. *Alcoholism: Clinical and Experimental Research. 27:*169–176, 2003.

208. Li, T.-K. Pharmacogenetics of responses to alcohol and genes that influence alcohol drinking. *Journal of Studies on Alcohol 61:*5–12, 2000.
209. Crabbe, J. C. Use of genetic analyses to refine phenotypes related to alcohol tolerance and dependence. *Alcoholism: Clinical and Experimental Research 25:*288–292, 2001.
210. Osier, M. V., Pakstis, A. J., Soodyall, H., Comas, D., Goldman, D., Odunsi, A., Okonofua, F., Parnas, J., Schulz, L. O., Bertranpetit, J., Bonne-Tamir, B., Lu, R.-B., Kidd, J. R., & Kidd, K. K. A global perspective on genetic variation at the *ADH* genes reveals unusual patterns of linkage disequilibrium and diversity. *American Journal of Human Genetics 71:*84–99, 2002.
211. Dick, D. M., Edenberg, H. J., Xuei, X., Goate, A., Kuperman, S., Schuckit, M., Crowe, R., Smith, T. L., Porjesz, B., Begleiter, H., & Foroud, T. Association of *GABRG3* with alcohol dependence. *Alcoholism: Clinical and Experimental Research 28:*4–9, 2004.

CHAPTER 4

Alcoholism: Acute Treatment

4.1. INTRODUCTION

Alcohol is one of the most commonly misused substances; with abuse and dependence creating serious medical and psychological difficulties.[1,2] This chapter presents an overview of *emergency problems* associated with alcohol, while rehabilitation is extensively discussed in Chapter 14. Substantial background material on alcohol has already been given in Chapter 3.

4.1.1. Identifying the Alcoholic

4.1.1.1. The Clinician's Preconceptions

The usual alcohol-dependent person is vastly different from the public stereotype. He or she is a middle-class individual who often presents to the clinician with rather nonspecific complaints, including insomnia, sadness, nervousness, or interpersonal problems. Because 10–20% of adult men develop dependence on alcohol, an additional 5–10% have alcohol abuse at some time in their lives (the rate for women being approximately half of these figures), and the rate of such serious alcohol problems in medical and surgical inpatients may be over 25%, it is important to consider alcoholism as a part of the differential diagnosis for every individual.

4.1.1.2. Physical Findings and Laboratory Tests

Several medical conditions should heighten the suspicion that alcohol problems are present. These include moderate high blood pressure, gastric or peptic ulcer disease, or cancers of the head and neck, gastrointestinal, or respiratory systems.[3–5] It may be worthwhile to reread Chapter 3 in order to review the many medical problems that are associated with repeated intake of high levels of alcohol.

Another indication of alcohol problems comes from temporary alterations in several blood tests in persons with a regular intake of six to eight or more drinks per day.[6] These "state markers of heavy drinking" reverse toward normal within several weeks of abstinence, and thus, can also be useful in monitoring abstention on an ongoing basis.[7,8] The most commonly used and widely available of these state markers is gamma glutamyltransferase (GGT), an enzyme important in amino acid transport, which is found in many body tissues, and is produced at higher levels in the liver in several conditions, including heavy drinking.[6,9] The usual GGT levels in the blood are <35 units, and while values of 50 or higher are indicative of a variety of conditions including liver disease, GGTs over 35 can indicate heavy drinking, even in the absence of damage to liver cells. The sensitivity and specificity of GGT as a screening tool for heavy drinking (and thus, for a high risk for an alcohol-use disorder) are estimated to be between 70 and 80%.

A second useful state marker is a blood protein responsible for the transport of iron. In the cases of heavy drinking, an abnormal form of a protein, called "carbohydrate deficient transferrin" (CDT), is produced.[6,10–12] Values higher than 20 g/l also have sensitivities and specificities in the range of 70–80%, and can be used both to identify heavier drinkers and to monitor abstinence. The combination of CDT and GGT appears to be better than either of them being alone, and has applicability to a broader range of patients.

There are a number of other tests that can be clinically useful as state markers of heavy drinking.[10,13–15] These include a modest increase in the size of red blood cells, with subsequent mean corpuscular volumes (MCV) higher than 90 cubic microns, as well as high normal values of uric acid (e.g., 6.4 mg/dl or higher). The usual liver function tests such as alanine aminotransferase (ALT-formerly known as SGPT) and aspartate aminotransferase (AST—formerly SGOT) are indicative of a slightly advanced liver impairment, hepatocellular damage, regardless of the source, and therefore, are neither very sensitive nor very specific for alcohol-related problems.

4.1.1.3. Potentially Useful Questionnaires

A diagnosis of alcohol dependence can only be reliably established through an interview with the patient establishing that clinically relevant levels of problems associated with at least three of the seven DSM-IV dependence criteria regarding alcohol are clustered together.[16] On the other hand, several relatively brief questionnaires can be helpful as preliminary screening tools in busy clinical settings.[17,18] Perhaps the most appropriate of these are the two ten-item instruments, that take only a minute or two for the average patient to fill up. The Alcohol Use Disorders Identification Test (AUDIT) is a highly reliable questionnaire with a sensitivity of 70% and a specificity of 80% in identifying individuals with more severe alcohol-related problems.[19,20]

Here, individuals use a four-point scale (from never, to increasing frequencies), to answer questions regarding the usual number of drinks consumed, the frequency of heavy intake, and a variety of problems as demonstrated in Table 4.1. A second useful measure is the ten-item version of the Michigan Alcohol Screening Test (MAST), which covers similar questions. At the same time, shorter measures are, not surprisingly, not likely to perform as well as the ten-item questionnaires.[21–24] The CAGE, for example, asks individuals to rate whether they have ever "cut-down" on their drinking, felt that they have "annoyed" others with their drinking behavior, felt "guilty" about drinking, or taken an "eye-opener" first thing in the morning. An additional and similarly brief questionnaire is the Tweak.[23]

Despite the assets of some of these tools, it is the history from the patient that is most important. Therefore, I take 2 or 3 min necessary to query *every* patient about alcohol-related life problems. I begin by asking about *general* areas of difficulty, including such questions as "How are things going with your spouse?" "Have you had any accidents since I last saw you?" "How are things going on the job?" or "Have you had any arrests or traffic

Table 4.1
The Alcohol Use Disorders Identification Test

Item	5-point scale (least to most)
1. How often do you have a drink containing alcohol?	Never (0) to 4+ per week (4)
2. How many drinks containing alcohol do you have on a typical day?	1 or 2 (0) to 10+ (4)
3. How often do you have six or more drinks on one occasion?	Never (0) to daily or almost daily (4)
4. How often during the last year have you found that you were not able to stop drinking once you had started?	Never (0) to daily or almost daily (4)
5. How often during the last year have you failed to do what was normally expected from you because of drinking?	Never (0) to daily or almost daily (4)
6. How often during the last year have you needed a first drink in the morning to get yourself going after a heavy drinking session?	Never (0) to daily or almost daily (4)
7. How often during the last year have you had a feeling of guilt or remorse after drinking?	Never (0) to daily or almost daily (4)
8. How often during the last year have you been unable to remember what happened the night before because you had been drinking?	Never (0) to daily or almost daily (4)
9. Have you or someone else been injured as a result of your drinking?	No (0) to yes, during the last year (4)
10. Has a relative, friend, doctor, or other health worker been concerned about your drinking or suggested that you should cut down?	No (0) to yes, during the last year (4)

The AUDIT is scored by simply summing the values associated with the endorsed response. (Adapted from Reinert, D.F., & Allen, G.P. The alcohol use disorders identification test (AUDIT): A review of recent research, *Alcoholism: Clinical and Experimental Research 26*:272–279, 2002.)

tickets?"[25] If there is a general life problem, I try to determine what role, if any, alcohol may have played in that difficulty and then go on to questions about the quantity and frequency of drinking. If the patient appears evasive, or if I have any further doubts, I separately interview an additional informant such as the spouse.

4.1.2. Obtaining a History

The essential element in establishing a diagnosis is to gather a good clinical history that demonstrates repetitive problems with alcohol in multiple areas of life.[16,26] Because the diagnosis rests with repetitive problems and not the specific pattern of quantity and frequency, I begin by asking a patient about a series of life problems, looking for the age at which three or more of these problems appeared to have clustered together. To help with this chronology-based history, I establish ages of major life events, including the time of graduation from high school, ages of entering and leaving the military, college years, marriage, birth of children, and so on. This not only builds rapport and gives useful information about an individual's background, but also focuses as a series of markers of major life events that can be used to identify the ages of onset of a series of alcohol-related problems. Next, I briefly review the seven DSM-IV dependence criteria, defining each as I go along, and asking for the age at which the criterion item represented a repetitive problem. This might begin with a question about a time in life when the individual noted that more alcohol was needed to achieve the effects they used to experience from fewer drinks—an indication of tolerance; I then might ask about periods of anxiety, insomnia, and tremor lasting for 24 h or more after cutting down on alcohol—establishing the age of first occurrence of withdrawal; additional questions can relate to times in life when the person gave up important events such as family gatherings or other important social experiences in order to drink; continued to use alcohol despite the recognition that problems were occurring, and so on, using the time line to establish the approximate age of repetitive occurrence of problems. From this history, I am able to establish the approximate age of the onset of alcohol dependence (or alcohol abuse) as the time by which, for dependence, the third of the potential seven items had developed.

The next step in establishing a diagnosis is to determine whether the person is currently experiencing symptoms of a major psychiatric disorder, severe and persistent enough for the clinician to consider an additional diagnosis. For example, I might focus on whether the individual has been depressed almost all day every day for two or more weeks at a time, with depressive symptoms interfering with functioning or, I might evaluate a history of possible panic disorder by focusing on classical panic attacks unrelated to stress occurring multiple times a month with a frequency high enough to interfere with life functioning. If the patient presents with alcohol dependence, on one hand, and appears to meet the criteria for another major psychiatric disorder, on the other, I next take steps to determine whether it appears as if the psychiatric condition (e.g., a major depressive episode) had ever occurred at a time unrelated to substances such as alcohol, that might mimic the major psychiatric syndrome. Details about this approach are presented in greater depth in Section 3.1.2.3. Briefly, having established the approximate age of onset of alcohol dependence, I next turn to reviewing whether the major psychiatric disorder (for example, major depressive episodes) ever occurred prior to the onset of alcohol dependence, or were clearly established during a period of abstinence of at least a month or more. If no history of major depressions (or other psychiatric syndromes) is apparent either before the onset of alcohol dependence or during a period of abstinence, the working diagnosis is a substance-induced mood, anxiety, psychotic, etc. disorder.

The last step in the diagnostic workup for individuals, who meet criteria for both alcohol dependence and a current psychiatric syndrome potentially mimicked by heavy doses of alcohol, is to observe the patient's psychiatric symptoms over a period of abstinence of a month or more. This can be done either as an inpatient or outpatient, where I am trying to determine whether the syndrome (e.g., major depression) is improving over the month, and that the severity and persistence of the disorder has dropped below the diagnostic threshold. In two out of three instances of major depression and alcohol dependence, the depressive disorders appear to be substance induced, with the full psychiatric syndrome likely to disappear with abstinence more rapidly than one might expect with the prescription of antidepressant medications.

These steps are well worth the 5–10 min required, as complex and perplexing medical and psychological problems associated with alcoholism can be confusing and can lead to serious complications through improper diagnosis and treatment.

4.2. EMERGENCY PROBLEMS

The most frequent emergency problems for alcoholics involve toxic overdose reactions and accidents. Almost 10% of all emergency room patients have alcohol problems as part of their mode of presentation, rates that increase upto 33–50% for accident victims.[27] Recognition of the presence of high blood-alcohol levels is important, as this drug alters the patient's reactions to emergency procedures.

4.2.1. Toxic Reactions or Overdose

See Sections 1.7.1, 2.2.1, 6.2.1, and 13.2.1

Toxic reactions to alcohol can be life-threatening because of the narrow range between the intoxicating, anesthetic, and lethal doses of this drug. These conditions can be especially dangerous when alcohol and other drugs are combined (see Section 12.2.1).[28–30]

4.2.1.1. Clinical Picture

The overdose of alcohol, which can be lethal at blood-alcohol concentrations of 350–400 mg% (0.4 g/l), results into CNS depression to the point of respiratory and circulatory failure.[28,31] The danger is heightened when alcohol is taken in combination with other depressing drugs, such as any of the hypnotics or antianxiety drugs, but serious problems can also occur with drugs of other classes, such as the opioids. The clinical picture of an ethanol overdose is similar to that described for the depressants in Section 2.2.1.

4.2.1.1.1. History

The patient usually smells of alcohol with a history of recent ingestion of high doses of it. It can be lethal with alcohol alone, and even more dangerous if accompanied by other depressants, such as sleeping pills [e.g., the barbiturates such as secobarbital (Seconal)] or the antianxiety drugs [e.g., chlordiazepoxide (Librium) or diazepam (Valium)]. If no history can be obtained directly from the patient, a friend or relative might supply the relevant information, or there may be obvious evidence of drug ingestion (e.g., empty bottles).

4.2.1.1.2. Physical Signs and Symptoms

These are similar to the physical manifestations reported for other depressants in Section 2.2.1. Basically, the patient presents with depressed vital signs, including a lowered respiratory rate, reduced body temperature, and a low blood pressure.[32]

4.2.1.1.3. Psychological State

This also resembles the description for other depressants given in Section 2.2.3, including signs of severe intoxication such as nystagmus along with confusion, irritability, and coma.

4.2.1.1.4. Relevant Laboratory Data

The diagnosis, resting with the history and the physical examination, is aided by a toxicological screen (10 cc blood or 50 ml urine) for both alcohol and other depressants. The remaining laboratory tests are those necessary to properly exclude other causes of stupor (e.g., low glucose or electrolyte abnormalities) and to monitor the physical status (e.g., blood counts, BUN, createnine), as well as a chest film and EKG, and, if the patient is stuporous, blood gases, as shown in Table 1.6.[32,33]

4.2.1.2. Treatment

A fatal toxic reaction has been reported with blood-alcohol levels as low as 350 mg% in non-tolerant individuals. The treatments generally follow those outlined for depressants in Section 2.2.1.2. Once again, it is important to emphasize the lack of detail offered here, and the need to carefully review a text of emergency medicine.[34]

1. As always, it is imperative to follow the ABCs of emergency care to guarantee adequate airway, breathing, and circulation. Additional basic steps include control of shock and careful evaluation to rule out ancillary medical problems such as electrolyte disturbances, cardiac disorders, associated infections, and subdural hematomas. Then, general supportive measures should be established while the body metabolizes the alcohol.
2. Take special care to rule out hypoglycemia.
3. Consider establishing an IV line in case shock develops.
4. If you suspect that opioids were also ingested, naloxone (Narcan, beginning at 0.4 mg, IM or IV) should be given. If, as outlined in Section 6.2.1.2, the patient does not respond to two doses given in 30 min, opioids were probably not part of the respiratory and cardiac depression. There is some anecdotal evidence that symptoms of shock accompanying alcohol overdoses, uncomplicated by opioid misuse, may themselves improve with 0.4 mg of naloxone IV, which can be repeated twice in 10 min. However, laboratory experiments have failed to confirm these findings in animals.
5. It is also appropriate to consider the possibility that a Bz might have been involved in the overdose and to prescribe flumazenil (Romazicon) at 0.2 mg IV every minute up to 3 min. However, special care must be taken regarding precipitating seizures or increasing intracranial pressure (see Section 2.2.1.2).[32,35]
6. Activated charcoal is not likely to be of use for alcohol overdoses.

4.2.2. Alcoholic Withdrawal (291.8 and 291.0 in DSM-IV)

See Sections 2.2.2, and 6.2.2.

4.2.2.1. Clinical Picture

This is an example of a *depressant withdrawal syndrome*, as discussed in Section 2.2.2. Although the direct effects of alcohol over an extended period of time are responsible for the vulnerability toward an abstinence syndrome, the severity of the symptoms also reflects the presence of additional drug withdrawals, medical problems, the level of acidosis and to disturbances in electrolytes.[31,36–38] Figure 4.1 gives a simplified outline of the symptoms expected during withdrawal.

4.2.2.1.1. History

A history of withdrawal symptoms, usually mild in nature, are reported in the histories of 50% or more of men and women who are alcohol dependent.[31,38,39] This rebound phenomenon, or withdrawal syndrome, reflects the body's adaptation to alcohol over periods of time, leaving a

Symptoms	*Treatment*
Begin in hours, peak day 2 or day 3, Subside day 4 or 5	Thiamine
Anxiety Malaise ANS dysfunction Insomnia	Physical exam Multiple vitamins Food and rest
Convulsions State of confusion Hallucination (visual or tactile)	Depressant drugs

Figure 4-1. Alcohol detoxification. Abbreviation: ANS, autonomic nerve system

vulnerability toward symptoms that are the opposite of the original acute effects of the drug when blood-alcohol levels decrease. It is hypothesized that some of this rebound hyperactivity might relate to augmentation of brain excitation from overactivity of the NMDA receptor system, as well as decreases in activity in the GABA system.[38–41]

It is wise to consider possible alcoholic withdrawal in all patients with autonomic hyperactivity, tremor, and anxiety, especially for those who present with any of the more obvious signs of alcoholism, ranging from a high GGT, CDT, CTD, or MCV (see Table 1.6), liver enlargement, to cancer of the esophagus or head and neck.[31,38,42,43]

4.2.2.1.2. Physical Signs and Symptoms

For 95% of people with alcoholism, the withdrawal is of mild to moderate severity and is limited to elevated pulse and blood pressure, tremors, insomnia, and anxiety, as described in Section 2.2.2. Additional symptoms include increased deep tendon reflexes, anorexia or nausea and vomiting, and emotional complaints, including sadness.

Fewer than 5% of alcohol-dependent men and women ever experience more severe withdrawal with delirium or grand-mal convulsions.[38] The convulsions are likely to develop within the first 24–48 h of abstinence, although they can be delayed in the context of inadequate treatment with benzodiazepenes.[36,44] An enhanced risk for withdrawal seizures might relate to preexisting brain damage, an independent seizure disorder, or associated severe medical problems. The risk appears to increase with repeated episodes of alcohol withdrawal, where the seizure threshold might decrease through a mechanism known as kindling.

Alcohol withdrawal delirium, also known as delirium tremens or DTs,[38,45,46] is characterized by severe overactivity of the ANS (i.e., pulse rates of 120 or more, marked elevation in blood pressure, marked increase in respiratory rate, an oral temperature of 101°F, etc.), an intense hand tremor, and severe agitated confusion. In the context of any state of severe confusion, especially with associated agitation, temporary hallucinations (usually visual) can develop. Fortunately, DTs are observed in less than 1% of alcohol withdrawals, and the rate might actually be one in 1,000 patients. The risk for DTs increases in the context of severe medical problems or of other intense physiological stresses such as recent surgery. Although death can occur in the context of severe DTs, especially with associated seizures, the mortality rate during such alcohol withdrawal is exceedingly low (e.g., 1 in 500 or less), especially when the concomitant medical abnormality is treated. Once DTs begin, they are likely to continue for 5 days or so, and the treatments discussed in Section 4.2.2.2 are aimed primarily at improving the general condition during the withdrawal, minimizing the probability of seizures, and controlling behaviors until the severe agitated, confused state passes.

Reflecting the relatively short half-life of alcohol, the acute withdrawal syndrome begins within 12 h or less of the decrease in blood-alcohol level, symptoms are then likely to peak in intensity by 48–72 h, and are usually greatly reduced by 4–5 days. As is true of withdrawal conditions from other depressants, opioids, and stimulants, following acute withdrawal, a condition that might be described as protracted abstinence is observed.[47] Here the blood pressure is likely to be mildly elevated for weeks to months, a mild tremor might be observed, there may be moodiness, and sleep patterns remain abnormal with frequent awakenings. The discomfort might contribute to the propensity to return to the use of alcohol or other drugs. Thus, education about these lingering symptoms as well as the high probability that these problems will disappear over the subsequent months can be an important aspect of the treatment of men and women who are alcohol dependent.

4.2.2.1.3. Psychological State

This aspect of withdrawal is as dramatic as the physical problems and consists of nervousness, a feeling of decreased self-worth, and a high drive to continue drinking. For less than 1%, it can include an obvious state of confusion, sometimes accompanied by hallucinations.

4.2.2.1.4. Relevant Laboratory Tests

There are no laboratory tests that are uniquely diagnostic for alcoholic withdrawal. However, research has demonstrated evidence of dysregulation of several hormones, including abnormally high values for antidiuretic hormone and high cortisol values.[48,49] For an individual entering an abstinence syndrome, it is necessary to rule out serious physical problems. Thus, it is important to perform an adequate neurological examination, to determine the cardiac status through an EKG, and carry out some of the relevant laboratory procedures outlined in Table 1.6. Abnormalities in liver and kidney function as well as in glucose levels should be monitored throughout withdrawal.

4.2.2.2. Treatment

The array of variations in therapeutic approaches proposed for withdrawal, reflects the relatively mild nature of most withdrawal syndromes as well as the need to balance cost and efficacy. Although the comments that follow are based on clinical trials whenever possible, the relatively large number of therapeutic evaluations for alcoholic withdrawal include only about one third that incorporate random controls.

4.2.2.2.1. Physical Examination

In recognition of the increased risk for medical problems among people with alcoholism, EKG, and a thorough physical examination is an essential first step. Special emphasis must be placed on searching for evidence of cardiac arrhythmias or of heart failure; the possibility of upper or lower GI bleeding; infections, including pneumonias; problems with liver failure or associated ascites; or neurological impairment, including peripheral neuropathies.

In people with alcoholism who otherwise appear relatively healthy, dehydration is relatively uncommon, and there is evidence that overhydration may exist.[50] Therefore, in the absence of severe or prolonged vomiting, bleeding, or significant failure of other systems, oral fluids, not IV infusions, should be used.

4.2.2.2.2. Vitamins and Minerals

Alcohol is absorbed primarily from the proximal small intestine, the same site as many vitamins.[51] Because of direct interference with absorption as well as increased excretion of these nutrients in the course of heavy drinking, in the past even well-nourished alcoholics were assumed to be deficient in folic acid, thiamine, and perhaps niacin.[52] In the absence of stigmata of severe vitamin deficiencies, however, these problems are usually easily corrected with oral multiple vitamins for several weeks, making sure that folic acid and thiamine are included. It has also been reported that some people with alcoholism might develop deficiencies in magnesium, and others might present with decreased body stores of Vitamin D. However, it is not clear that there is a need for more supplementation than can be offered with multiple vitamins.

4.2.2.2.3. Non-pharmacological Approaches to Treating Withdrawal

All detoxification programs offer general supports including a physical evaluation, reassurance, and reality-orientation techniques (e.g., reminders of day, date, and time) for patients showing mild levels of confusion, as well as the opportunity for sleep and adequate nutrition. Taking advantage of the usual mild nature of the withdrawal syndrome and the probable rapid recovery, 75% of detoxification patients improve markedly with these steps alone as part of a "social-model" treatment regimen.[37,38] To be optimally effective, these programs need close medical backup, so that the patients who demonstrate medical problems, severe confusion, or convulsions can be properly evaluated and treated.

4.2.2.2.4. Medications for the General Treatment of Withdrawal

Medications are used to decrease overall symptoms (especially ANS dysfunction), increase comfort, and decrease the risk for convulsions and DTs. In light of the fact that depressant withdrawal syndromes occur because physical dependence has developed and the alcohol was decreased too quickly, re-institution of the specific drug of abuse or of any drug with cross-tolerance (e.g., another depressant) should help ameliorate symptoms. Any brain depressant, including barbiturates, chloral hydrate, paraldehyde, and the benzodiazepines, can help people with alcoholism during withdrawal. If they all work, the choice rests mostly with considerations of safety and cost.

Almost all reviews of alcoholic withdrawal agree that the optimal medicinal treatment utilizes the Bzs.[36–38] The Bzs are less likely than other depressant drugs, such as paraldehyde, to cause neurotoxicity when injected IM, are less likely than barbiturates to decrease respiratory rates or produce hypotention, and carry less dangers of adverse drug reactions than anticonvulsants. As a result, when the clinician decides that pharmacological therapies should be added to general supportive care, the treatment of choice is a Bz.

Within this class of medications, one can select either a longer acting drug, such as diazepam (Valium) or chlordiazepoxide (Librium), or a shorter acting Bz such as oxazepam (Serax) or lorazepam (Ativan). An asset of the longer acting drugs is their relatively smooth withdrawal, because, reflecting the long half-life, drug blood levels decrease slowly over time. Therefore, it is not necessary to be certain that medications are administered every 4 h. The dangers of the longer acting drugs, however, include the problem of drug accumulation in individuals with clinically significant liver impairment (e.g., cirrhosis), and with subsequent severe lethargy, drowsiness, and ataxia. On the other hand, the shorter acting drugs, although safer in severe liver disease and less likely to accumulate, have their own problems in that doses must be given every 4 h for the fear that falling Bz blood levels might add to the preexisting alcoholic withdrawal syndrome and might even precipitate seizures.

The recommended approach takes advantage of the assets and liabilities of both long-acting and short-acting drugs. Short-acting Bzs should be reserved for patients with evidence of liver failure or for those in whom cognition is severely impaired at the time therapy is begun. For the average alcohol-dependent person going through withdrawal, longer acting drugs should be used. The appropriate dose is determined on day 1 as the level needed to diminish symptoms, decreased by 20% of the day 1 dose with each subsequent 24 h, i.e., stopping the drug by day 4 or 5. In addition to the rapid tapering of drugs, an important safeguard against toxicity is to skip a dose when the patient is lethargic or asleep. For example, chlordiazepoxide can be begun as 25 mg by mouth [PO (Latin *per os*)] (this drug is not well absorbed IM) given QID, with an additional 25 mg dose on day 1 if needed because of increased tremor or other signs of ANS dysfunction. This establishes the dose on day 1, which is then subsequently cut to zero over the next 4–5 days.

Although fewer data are available, other authors have suggested alternative possible medicinal approaches to treat alcoholic withdrawal, but most data do not support their superiority to Bzs.[37,38,53] These include the alpha-adrenergic agonists such as clonidine (Catapres), or beta-blockers such as propranolol (Inderal) and atenolol (Tenormin). The beta-blockers and alpha-agonists decrease symptoms of tremor, fast heart rate, and hypertension, but do little to address the anxiety and drug craving or the propensity to seizures, and can mask impending seizures or DTs. Nor do data support the use of antipsychotic drugs for alcoholic withdrawal.

Finally, the 1% or so prevalence of seizures during withdrawal raises the question whether anticonvulsant medications should be added to the Bzs. The data to date do not indicate that anticonvulsants are needed for the treatment of the average person with alcoholism going through withdrawal, except for patients with evidence of an independent seizure disorder.

4.2.2.2.5. Optimal Setting for the Treatment of Mild to Moderate Withdrawal

Common sense dictates that the most thorough physical examination, the best opportunity for close observation, and the largest number of treatment options are provided by supervision of withdrawal in an inpatient treatment setting. On the other hand, the high cost of inpatient care would result in a rapid consumption of the limited monies available for treatment, if all people with alcoholism were detoxified in a hospital. Reflecting the usual mild nature of the withdrawal syndrome, many public administrators have opted to establish a series of levels of care, ranging from outpatient to "social-model" detoxification facilities to inpatient care, when needed.[54]

The plan calls for a careful physical examination and gathering of the past history to identify patients best detoxed as inpatients. These include individuals with signs of impending severe withdrawal, histories of withdrawal seizures, or those with medical or psychiatric symptoms that might impair their ability to function outside the hospital.[54,55] The latter include severe and suicidal depression, confusion, and evidence of psychotic symptoms without insight. In our own outpatient setting, the remaining individuals—or preferably their "significant others"—are given a 1- or 2-day supply of a Bz for the person with alcoholism (e.g., four to six 25 mg tablets of chlordiazepoxide), the patient is offered the opportunity of spending part of the day at the rehabilitation center as an outpatient (perhaps participating in lectures or groups), and is asked to return daily over the next 3–5 days, for a readjustment of medications and brief physical evaluation centered on ANS functioning. He is warned to visit the emergency room if symptoms of withdrawal rapidly escalate, and a drug dose is to be omitted if the patient is sleepy or lethargic. The approach appears to be well accepted by most patients. Social-model detoxification programs incorporate much of the same philosophy, but offer greater day and night supervision.

4.2.2.2.6. Treatment of Delirium Tremens

The optimal treatment for full-blown DTs has not been clearly established. Fortunately, this intense medical syndrome, characterized by severe confusion and agitation (i.e., delirium) along with hallucinations and delusions and ANS dysfunction, is relatively rare. The first and potentially most important step in treatment is to carry out a thorough physical examination, because the stress of DTs added to a preexisting medical problem can have lethal consequences. The second step involves the usual general supportive measures (using IV fluids carefully and only if there is objective evidence of dehydration) as well as the prescription of multiple vitamins including thiamine and folic acid.

Finally, while medications may not shorten the usual 3–5-day course of DTs, they can help control symptoms. Some clinicians recommend using Bzs, sometimes in high doses (e.g., 200 mg or more of chlordiazepoxide per day), to control behavior while decreasing the number of individuals who will develop seizures and sedating patients so they are less dangerous to themselves and to those around them.[45] Other clinicians, fearing the possible excessive sedation and hypotension that could be expected with the high levels of Bzs that can be required for DTs, recommend antipsychotic drugs such as haloperidol (Haldol) or risperidone (Risperdal). This group of medications might actually lower the seizure threshold and, at least theoretically, would have no major direct effect on depressant withdrawal syndromes, but can be used in doses titrated to decrease agitation, wandering about the ward, and threats to other patients.

4.2.3. Delirium, Dementia, and Other Cognitive Disorders

See Sections 1.7.3 and 2.2.3.

4.2.3.1. Clinical Picture

Alcohol intoxication can include mental confusion and clouding of consciousness, and similar symptoms can result from vitamin deficiencies, and indirect consequences of alcohol intake, such as trauma and metabolic disturbances. Therefore, temporary but serious states of confusion can be seen during both alcohol intoxication and during withdrawal from alcohol.[56] Longer lasting syndromes can develop as a complication of vitamin deficiency (e.g., thiamine), as the result of trauma (e.g., a subdural hematoma), and probably as a consequence of many years of heavy drinking.

4.2.3.1.1. Direct Effects of Alcohol (291.2 in DSM-IV)

1. *Acute and subacute intoxication.* At relatively low doses (i.e., one or two drinks), judgment and performance can be mildly impaired.[28,57] At blood-alcohol levels in excess of 150 mg% (roughly seven to eight drinks), more intense confusion and disorientation can occur in most non-tolerant people. This condition can be seen at even lower doses for older people and for individuals with preexisting brain disorders, such as those with prior serious head trauma. The course is *usually* relatively benign, with a clearing of confusion over a matter of hours as blood-alcohol levels decrease. However, in older people and in those with prior brain damage, the confusion may last for days or even longer, and alcohol intoxication may thus, be an important part of the differential diagnosis of acute-onset deleria and dementias in the elderly.
2. *Chronic heavy drinking.* As noted previously, 15–30% of nursing home patients with chronic dementias have histories of alcoholism. This may result in part from the deleterious effects of alcohol on nerve cells, but it is also probably the combined result of alcohol, hormonal imbalances, vitamin deficiencies, trauma, and symptoms of additional dementias such as Alzheimer's disease.[58–60] Perhaps one third to as many as 50% of individuals with long-term alcohol dependence also demonstrate changes on brain-imaging tests including an increased size of the brain ventricles along with evidence of changes in the corpus callosum and possible shrinkage of brain material in the cortex.[61] Fortunately, many of these physiological changes, as well as the alterations in cognitive functioning, are likely to partially or fully reverse with prolonged abstinence.[62] The clinical picture and treatment for these cognitive deficits are similar to those for the rare vitamin-related deliria in alcoholics discussed in the next section.

4.2.3.1.2. Vitamin Deficiencies (291.1 in DSM-IV)

In the context of alcohol, thiamine is not absorbed adequately and is used up faster. This is of special importance in individuals with inefficient thiamine-dependent enzymes such as transketolase deficiencies.[63] The result is a syndrome consisting of a mixture of neurological problems, such as ataxia, nystagmus, and the paralysis of certain ocular muscles, which characterize *Wernicke's syndrome* (labeled an alcohol amnestic disorder in DSM-IV).[64,65] As briefly discussed in Chapter 3, the pathology involves shrinkage and microhemorrhages in the mammillary bodies, in the dorsomedial nucleus of the thalamus, and in the periventricular grey matter. The syndrome runs an unpredictable course, with a tendency toward rapid and complete improvement of most neurological signs with the administration of adequate thiamine, but with a slower resolution of the mental clouding and some level of a permanent cognitive deficit in almost two thirds of such patients.[66]

4.2.3.1.3. Other Causes of Dementia in People with Alcoholism

Any alcohol-dependent individual presenting with confusion, disorientation, and decreased intellectual functioning should receive a thorough evaluation for trauma (and resultant subdural hematomas), infections, and for metabolic abnormalities (especially glucose, and electrolyte-related problems). Regarding glucose, alcohol interferes with gluconeogenesis (sugar production) as well as with the action of insulin, and may cause pancreatic damage. Thus, people with alcoholism may show hyper- or, more frequently, hypoglycemia when they enter treatment. These problems tend to revert toward normal after several weeks of abstinence.

4.2.3.2. Treatment

1. The cornerstone of treatment for cognitive disorders is finding and treating the physical causes (e.g., infection, electrolyte abnormalities, and consequences of trauma).
2. All such patients should receive oral thiamine and if Wernicke-Korsakoff's is suspected, IM thiamine in doses of 100 mg IM daily for several months, followed by oral multiple-vitamin preparations.
3. Patients should be given good general nutrition and ample opportunity to rest.
4. Although improvement in the level of cognitive impairment is to be expected, the mental confusion may clear slowly, and it may not be possible to establish the exact degree of permanent intellectual deterioration for several months.

4.2.4. Psychosis (291.5 and 291.3 in DSM-IV) and Violence

See Sections 1.7.4, 2.2.4, and 5.2.4.

4.2.4.1. Clinical Picture

The chronic ingestion of high doses of alcohol can cause suspiciousness without insight that can progress to the point of frank paranoid delusions.[67] This was referred to as *alcoholic paranoia* in some manuals, and is labeled *alcohol-induced psychotic disorder* in DSM-IV. Similarly, alcohol can cause persistent hallucinations, usually voices accusing the patient of being a bad person, although the hallucinations can also be visual or tactile. This is an example of *alcoholic hallucinosis*, which is a second variant of an alcohol-induced psychotic disorder in DSM-IV.[68] Both of these can develop in the midst of a drinking bout, occur in an otherwise clear sensorium (i.e., there is no delirium or dementia), and might not be noticed until the cessation of drinking. Both are very likely to run a course of complete recovery within several days to perhaps a month if no further drinking occurs. Clinically, the syndrome resembles the stimulant-induced psychosis (see Section 5.2.4) and psychoses associated with other depressant drugs (see Section 2.2.4). This is not a form of schizophrenia, as there is no increased family history of that disorder in these individuals, and there is no evidence that alcoholic paranoia or hallucinosis progresses to schizophrenia.

4.2.4.2. Treatment

1. If the patient has delusions or hallucinations without insight (i.e., believes that they are real), the clinician should consider hospitalization to protect him or her from acting out delusions.
2. Treatment should be aimed at giving the patient insight and at evaluating and treating any medical problems associated with his heavy intake of alcohol.
3. Although any psychotic picture is likely to clear spontaneously within a few days to a month, an antipsychotic agent such as haloperidol (Haldol) at 1–5 mg/day (but up to 20 mg each day, if needed) by mouth, may help keep the patient comfortable until the psychosis clears. There is no indication for continued use of these drugs, and they should be stopped within 2–4 weeks. If the patient has demonstrated delusions and/or hallucinations before the onset of heavy drinking or has a history of persistence of the psychosis despite abstinence, the diagnosis of schizophrenia with secondary alcohol problems should be entertained and antipsychotic medications should be continued.[69]

4.2.5. Flashbacks

Flashbacks are not noted with alcohol.

4.2.6. Anxiety and Depression (291.8 and 291.3 in DSM-IV)

See Section 1.7.6.

4.2.6.1. Clinical Picture

Regarding anxiety, as discussed in Section 4.2.2, the signs and symptoms of alcoholic withdrawal do not end on day 4 or 5, and some symptoms, including anxiety, are likely to be observed at decreasing levels for several months.[25,47,70] In this condition of protracted abstinence, the patient can demonstrate irritability, restlessness, hyperventilation, insomnia, and distractibility, problems that will diminish as the period of abstinence lengthens. Thus, low levels of almost any form of increased anxiety, ranging from panic to general nervousness, can be seen for 3 or more months after cessation of heavy drinking. This may not be a true independent major anxiety syndrome such as social phobia, panic disorder, or generalized anxiety disorder because the anxiety is not likely to have been observed before the alcohol-related life problems and is likely to disappear or at least improve greatly with time alone.

A similar case can be made regarding symptoms of depression.[70–74] In the context of heavy drinking, the majority of men and women develop mood swings.[75] If the period of heavy drinking continues, the depressions can (and in perhaps one third of the cases do) resemble major depressive episodes.[70] These individuals can demonstrate the full range of severe depressive symptoms including feelings of hopelessness and serious suicidal ideas and plans. However, unless the patient has demonstrated periods of severe depressive episodes independent of his heavy drinking in the past, it is highly likely that this depression will markedly improve over the first several days to weeks of abstinence, reaching relatively mild levels of depressive symptoms by 4 weeks of sobriety.[70,76,77] Although some level of mood swings is likely to continue for several months as part of a protracted withdrawal syndrome, this condition is unlikely to fulfill criteria for major depressive episodes beyond the first several weeks to 1 month of abstinence. Thus, similar to what is described in Chapter 3 and in the immediately preceding brief discussion regarding anxiety disorders, depressive episodes are likely to be observed during severe intoxication, and can be identified as an alcohol-induced mood disorder by the absence of a history of major depression episodes when sober and observation of the patient over time. Alcohol-induced mood (or anxiety) disorders are not likely to run a course of independent major depressions requiring antidepressant medications. In fact, the depressive symptoms are likely to improve markedly before antidepressants would start working.[70,75]

The first and the most important step in treatment is to evaluate the patient carefully for any history of independent anxiety or depressive disorders.[70,75] If it appears that severe major depressions and lifelong major anxiety disorders are present, it is important to plan for the possible need for longer term treatments for these conditions.

The second important step is to take care to offer the patient appropriate emergency treatments, especially if the individual is suffering from a depression. The lifetime risk for suicide among people with alcoholism is perhaps as high as 10%[78], and suicide precautions, which can include hospitalization in a locked ward, may be important for the first several days to several weeks of abstinence, after which the depression is likely to disappear on its own. Of course, people with severe anxiety conditions must be carefully evaluated for the possibility of physiological causes such as thyroid disease.

If the workup indicates an alcohol-induced mood or anxiety disorder, the cornerstone of treatment is reassurance and education for both the patient and significant people in their lives. Cognitive-behavioral treatments can be very effective in decreasing symptoms.[79,80] The individuals must understand that these symptoms, although severe, are likely to be complications of the alcohol-use disorder. They must also realize that the problems are likely to improve fairly rapidly over the first month, and then continue to disappear more slowly over the subsequent months. If independent psychiatric conditions are present, they must be aggressively treated as described in Chapters 1, 3, and 14. The co-occurrence of alcoholism with manic depressive disease, schizophrenia, or any other independent psychiatric condition makes treatment of both disorders challenging.[69,81] The optimal therapeutic approach involves common-sense combinations of the therapeutic regimens appropriate for each of the independent disorders.[82,83]

4.2.7. Medical Problems

4.2.7.1. General Comments

The deleterious physical effects of alcohol on people with alcoholism are so ubiquitous that it is impossible to adequately discuss all the resulting medical conditions in this short handbook.[5,84–87] The clinician must be able to recognize the complications described in Section 3.2.

It is also important to consider alcohol-induced complications in *nonalcoholics* with chronic disorders. Examples include the increased chance of bleeding in individuals with ulcer disease, respiratory depression in people with emphysema, the adverse effects of alcohol on the livers of people with infectious hepatitis, the interference with normal pancreatic functioning in those who already have pancreatitis, the deterioration in sugar metabolism that might adversely affect people with diabetes, and the impairment of cardiac functioning in individuals with heart disease. The impairment in immune functioning with heavy drinking also can exacerbate the clinical course and treatment of immune deficiencies states, including AIDs.[88,89]

Alcohol also adversely affects the metabolism and the efficacy of a wide variety of medications, including potentiation of the adverse effects of analgesics, adverse interactions with antidepressants, and interference with the proper actions of all psychotropic medications. The problems extend to antihypertensive drugs, as alcohol can potentiate orthostatic drops in blood pressure, and to hypoglycemic agents and anticoagulants because of the induction of liver metabolic enzymes.

4.2.7.2. Fetal Alcohol Syndrome

4.2.7.2.1. Clinical Picture

Heavy drinking during pregnancy can cause a number of problems, including multiple spontaneous abortions. Alcohol intake can also produce fetal alcohol effects such as a baby with a low birth weight for gestational stage (a smaller size that is never "caught up"); malformations in facial structure, including shortened palpebral fissures, a flattened bridge of the nose, and an absent philtrum; ventricular septal defects of the heart; malformations of the hands and feet (especially syndactyly); and levels of mental retardation that may be mild or moderately severe.[90] Problems in behavior and in learning are also likely to persist into at least later childhood, and the interpersonal difficulties can exceed those predicted from the level of intelligence. The amount of ethanol consumed, the timing of the drinking, the possible role of associated nutritional deficiencies, and other aspects of the clinical situation required to produce the fetal alcohol syndrome (FAS) are not fully understood. However, some level of general cognitive deficit, much milder than the true FAS, has been reported after an average of as low as three drinks per day during pregnancy.[91–93]

There are other manifestations of the fetal alcohol effect (FAE) or the full-blown FAS. These include reports of clinically significant levels of hearing loss in FAS children, which might reflect a vulnerability toward otitis media, a central hearing loss, or a developmental delay in auditory maturation.[94] Cognitive difficulties are prominent, and in school these children are likely to have problems in reading, spelling, and arithmetic, deficiencies that are likely to persist in upper grades.[93] In light of the history of alcohol problems in their mothers, it is not surprising that as they grow older these children have an enhanced risk for developing alcohol abuse and dependence.[95] They are also at elevated risk for a wide range of externalizing symptoms and other psychiatric conditions.[96,97]

The exact mechanism through which alcohol produces specific impairment in the developing fetus has not been conclusively proved, nor is it certain whether alcohol's effect on sperm from fathers with alcoholism contributes to these phenomena.[91,98] However, the information available to date favors both a direct and an indirect role of alcohol in problems in fetal development, and some effects on the egg even before fertilization. There is ample evidence, described in Section 3.2.3, that alcohol is capable of causing bodily damage in almost all systems, including the heart, the muscles, and the nervous system. Ethanol and acetaldehyde [the first breakdown product of ethanol (see Section 3.2.4)] readily cross to the fetus. The developing baby does not have efficient alcohol- or acetaldehyde-metabolizing systems, and the result is that these substances are likely to stay with the baby over an extended period of time. Most prudent parents recognize that it is unwise for pregnant women to drink and the possible harm that could occur to the newborn baby from the transfer of alcohol in breast milk. Some authors[99] also argue against the use of alcohol while breast-feeding.

4.2.7.2.2. Treatment

The only treatment for FAS is prevention. Women should be advised not to drink at any time during pregnancy or, if they must drink, to keep their alcohol intake as low as possible. The cost of caring for children with the syndrome in the United States is estimated to be at least $75 million per year, making almost any preventive effort cost-effective.

REFERENCES

1. Johnston, L. D., O'Malley, P. M., Bachman, J. G., & Schulenberg, J. E. *Monitoring the Future National Survey Results on Drug Use, 1975–2003. Vol. II: College Students and Adults Ages 19–40* (NIH Publication No. 04-5506). Bethesda, MD: National Institute on Drug Abuse, 2004.
2. Substance Abuse and Mental Health Services Administration. Results from the 2002 National Survey on Drug use and Health: National Findings (Office of Applied Studies, NHSDA Series H-22, DHHS Publication No. SMA 03-3836). Rockville, MD, 2003.
3. Bardou, M., Montembault, S., Giraud, V., Balian, A., Borotto, E., Houdayer, C., Capron, F., Chaput, J. C., & Naveau, S. Excessive alcohol consumption favors high risk polyp or colorectal cancer occurrence among patients with adenomas: A case control study. *Gut 50:*38–42, 2002.
4. Minami, J., Yoshii, M., Todoroki, M., Nichikimi, T., Ishimitsu, T., Fukunaga, T., & Matsuoka, H. Effects of alcohol restriction on ambulatory blood pressure, heart rate, and heart rate variability in Japanese men. *American Journal of Hypertension 15:*125–129, 2002.
5. Theobald, H., Johansson, S.-E., Bygren, L.-O., & Engfeldt, P. The effects of alcohol consumption on mortality and morbidity: A 26-year follow-up study. *Journal of Studies on Alcohol 62:*783–789, 2001.
6. Anton, R. F., Lieber, C., & Tabakoff, B. Carbohydrate-deficient transferring and γ-glutamyltransferase for the detection and monitoring of alcohol use: Results from a multisite study. *Alcoholism: Clinical and Experimental Research 26:*1215–1222, 2002.
7. Anttila, P., Järvi, K., Latvala, J., & Niemelä, O. Method-dependent characteristics of carbohydrate-deficient transferrin measurements in the follow-up of alcoholics. *Alcohol & Alcoholism 39:*59–63, 2004.
8. Pfefferbaum, A., Rosenbloom, M. J., Serventi, K. L., & Sullivan, E. V. Brain volumes, RBC status, and hepatic function in alcoholics after 1 and 4 weeks of sobriety: Predictors of outcome. *American Journal of Psychiatry 161:*1190–1196, 2004.
9. Martinez, L. D., Barón, A. E., Helander, A., Conigrave, K. M., & Tabakoff, B. The effect of total body water on the relationship between alcohol consumption and carbohydrate-deficient transferrin. *Alcoholism: Clinical and Experimental Research 26:*1097–1104, 2002.
10. Javors, M. A., & Johnson, B. A. Current status of carbohydrate deficient transferring, total serum sialic acid, sialic acid index of apolipoprotein J and serum β-hexosaminidase as markers for alcohol consumption. *Addiction 98:*45–50, 2003.
11. Sillanaukee, P., van der Gaag, M. S., Sierksma, A., Hendriks, H. F. J., Strid, N., Pönniö, M., & Nikkari, S. T. Effect of type of alcoholic beverages on carbohydrate-deficient transferrin, sialic acid, and liver enzymes. *Alcoholism: Clinical and Experimental Research 27:*57–60, 2003.
12. Chen, J., Conigrave, K. M., Macaskill, P., Whitfield, J. B., & Irwin, L. on behalf of the World Health Organization and the International Society for Biomedical Research on Alcoholism Collaborative Group. Combining carbohydrate-deficient transferrin and gamma-glutamyltransferase to increase diagnostic accuracy for problem drinking. *Alcohol & Alcoholism 38:*574–582, 2003.
13. Whitfield, J. B., Zhu, G., Heath, A. C., Powell, L. W., & Martin, N. G. Effects of alcohol consumption on indices of iron stores and of iron stores on alcohol intake markers. *Alcoholism: Clinical and Experimental Research 25:*1037–1045, 2001.
14. Alte, D., Lüdemann, J., Piek, M., Adam, C., Rose, H.-J., & John, U. Distribution and dose response of laboratory markers to alcohol consumption in a general population: Results of the Study of Health in Pomerania (SHIP). *Journal of Studies on Alcohol 64:*75–82, 2003.
15. Conigrave, K. M., Degenhardt, L. J., Whitfield, J. B., Saunders, J. B., Helander, A., & Tabakoff, B. on behalf of the WHO/ISBRA Study Group. CDT, GGT, and AST as markers of alcohol use: The WHO/ISBRA Collaborative Project. *Alcoholism: Clinical and Experimental Research 26:*332–339, 2002.
16. American Psychiatric Association. *Diagnostic and Statistical Manual of Mental Disorders* (DSM-IV-TR) (4th ed., Text Revision). Washington, DC: American Psychiatric Association, 2000.

17. Aertgeerts, B., Buntinx, F., Baude-Knops, J., Vandermeulen, C., Roelants, M., Ansoms, S., & Fevery, J. The value of CAGE, CUGE, and AUDIT in screening for alcohol abuse and dependence among college freshmen. *Alcoholism: Clinical and Experimental Research 24:*53–57, 2000.
18. Maisto, S. A., & Saitz, R. Alcohol use disorders: Screening and diagnosis. *The American Journal on Addictions 12:*S12–S25, 2003.
19. Chen, C.-H., Chen, W. J., & Cheng, A. T. A. New approach to the validity of the Alcohol Use Disorders Identification Test: Striatum-specific likelihood ratios analysis. *Alcoholism: Clinical and Experimental Research 29:*602-608, 2005.
20. Hermansson, U., Helander, A., Brandt, L., Huss, A., & Rönnberg, S. The alcohol use disorders identification test and carbohydrate-deficient transferrin in alcohol-related sickness absence. *Alcoholism: Clinical and Experimental Research 26:*328–335, 2002.
21. Saremi, A., Hanson, R. L., Williams, D. E., Roumain, J., Robin, R. W., Long, J. C., Goldman, D., & Knowler, W. C. Validity of the CAGE questionnaire in an American Indian population. *Journal of Studies on Alcohol 62:*294–300, 2001.
22. Bradley, K. A., Kivlahan, D. R., Bush, K. R., McDonell, M. B., & Fihn, S. D. Variations on the CAGE alcohol screening questionnaire: Strengths and limitations in VA general medical patients. *Alcoholism: Clinical and Experimental Research 25:*11472–11478, 2001.
23. Bush, K. R., Kivlahan, D. R., Davis, T. M., Dobie, D. J., Sporleder, J. L., Epler, A. J., & Bradley, K. A. The TWEAK is weak for alcohol screening among female veterans affairs outpatients. *Alcoholism: Clinical and Experimental Research 27:*1971–1978, 2003.
24. Friedmann, P. D., Saitz, R., Gogineni, A., Zhand, J. X., & Stein, M. D. Validation of the screening strategy in the NIAAA "Physicians' Guide to Helping Patients with Alcohol Problems". *Journal of Studies on Alcohol 62:*234–238, 2001.
25. Schuckit, M. A. *Educating Yourself About Alcohol and Drugs.* New York: Plenum Publishing Co., 1998.
26. Campbell, T. C., Hoffmann, N. G., Madson, M. B., & Melchert, T. P. Performance of a brief assessment tool for identifying substance use disorders. *Addiction Disorder and Their Treatment 2:*113–117, 2003.
27. Waller, P. F., Hill, E. M., Maio, R. F., & Blow, F. C. Alcohol effects on motor vehicle crash injury. *Alcoholism: Clinical and Experimental Research 27:*695–703, 2003.
28. Charney, D. S., Mihic, S. J., & Harris, R. H. Hypnotics and sedatives. In J. G. Hardman, L. E. Limbird, & A. G. Goodman (Eds.), *The Pharmacological Basis of Therapeutics* (10th ed.). New York: McGraw-Hill, 2001, pp. 399–427.
29. Gossop, M., Stewart, D., Treacy, S., & Marsden, J. A prospective study of mortality among drug misusers during a 4-year period after seeking treatment. *Addiction 97:*39–47, 2002.
30. Poikolainen, K., Leppänen, K., & Vuori, E. Alcohol sales and fatal alcohol poisonings: A time-series analysis. *Addiction 97:*1037–1040, 2002.
31. Schuckit, M. A. Alcohol and alcoholism. In D. G. Kramer, E. Braunwald, A. S. Fauci, *et al.* (Eds.), *Harrison's Principles of Internal Medicine* (16th ed.). New York: McGraw-Hill, 2004, pp. 2562–2566.
32. Mausner, K. L., Analgesics. In O. J. Ma & D. M. Cline (Eds.), *Emergency Medicine Manual* (6th ed.). New York: McGraw-Hill Medical Publishing Div., 2004, pp. 505–511.
33. Kefer, M. P. Alcohols. In O. J. Ma & D. M. Cline (Eds.), *Emergency Medicine Manual* (6th ed.). New York: McGraw-Hill Medical Publishing Div., 2004, pp. 494–498.
34. Ma, O. J., & Cline, D. M. (Eds.). *Emergency Medicine Manual* (6th ed.). New York: McGraw-Hill Medical Publishing Div., 2004.
35. Maxa, J. L., Ogu, C. C., Adeeko, M. A., & Swaner, T. G. Continuous-infusion flumazenil in the management of chlordioazepoxide toxicity. *Pharmacotherapy 23:*1513–1516, 2003.
36. Becker, H. C., & Veatch, L. M. Effects of lorazepam treatment for multiple ethanol withdrawals in mice. *Alcoholism: Clinical and Experimental Research 26:*371–380, 2002.
37. Krystal, J. H., & Tabakoff, B. Ethanol abuse, dependence, and withdrawal: Neurobiology and clinical implications. In K. L. Davis, D. Charney, J. T. Coyle, & C. Nemeroff (Eds.), *Neuropsychopharmacology: The Fifth Generation of Progress*, Williams & Wilkins, 2002.

38. Schuckit, M. A., Tipp, J. E., Reich, T., Hesselbrock, V. M. & Bucholz, K. K. The histories of withdrawal convulsions and delirium tremens in 1648 alcohol dependent subjects. *Addiction 90:*1335–1347, 1995.
39. Johnson, B. A., & Ait-Daoud, N. Alcohol: Clinical aspects. In J. H. Lowinson, P. Ruiz, R. B. Millman, & J. G. Langrod (Eds.), *Substance Abuse: A Comprehensive Textbook* (4th ed.). Baltimore, MD: Williams & Wilkins, 2004, pp. 151–163.
40. Haugbol, S. R., Ebert, B., & Ulrichsen, J. Upregulation of glutamate receptor subtypes during alcohol withdrawal in rats. *Alcohol & Alcoholism 40:*89-95, 2005.
41. Krystal, J. H., Petrakis, I. L., Limoncelli, D., Webb, E., Gueorgueva, R., D'Souza, D. C., Boutros, N. N., Trevisan, L., & Charney, D. S.: Altered NMDA glutamate receptor antagonist response in recovering ethanol-dependent patients. *Neuropsychopharmacology 28:*2020–21028, 2003.
42. Schuckit, M. A., Smith, T. L., Danko, G. P., Reich, T., Bucholz, K. K., & Bierut, L. J. Similarities in the clinical characteristics related to alcohol dependence in two populations. *The American Journal on Addictions 11:*1–9, 2002.
43. Martin, M. J., Heymann, C., Neumann, T., Schmidt, L., Soost, F., Mazurek, B., Bohm, B., Marks, C., Heilig, K., Lenzenhuber, E., Muller, C., Kox, W. J., & Spies, C. D. Preoperative evaluation of chronic alcoholics assessed for surgery of the upper digestive tract. *Alcoholism: Clinical and Experimental Research 26:*836–840, 2002.
44. Reoux, J. P., Saxon, A. J., Malte, C. A., Baer, J. S., & Sloan, K. L. Divalproex sodium in alcohol withdrawal: A randomized double-blind placebo-controlled clinical trial. *Alcoholism: Clinical and Experimental Research 25:*1324–1329, 2001.
45. Wasilewski, D., Matsumoto, H., Kur, E., Dziklinska, A., Wozny, E., Stencka, K., Skalski, M., Chaba, P., & Szelenberger, W. Assessment of diazepam loading dose therapy of delirium tremens. *Alcohol & Alcoholism 31:*273–278, 1996.
46. Wojnar, M., Bizoń, Z., & Wasilewski, D. The role of somatic disorders and physical injury in the development and course of alcohol withdrawal delirium. *Alcoholism: Clinical and Experimental Research 23:*209–213, 1999.
47. Rasmussen, D. D., Mitton, D. R., Green, J., & Puchalski, S. Chronic daily ethanol and withdrawal: 2. Behavioral changes during prolonged abstinence. *Alcoholism: Clinical and Experimental Research 25:*999–1005, 2001.
48. Trabert, W., Caspari, D., Bernhard, P., & Biro, G. Inappropriate ADH secretion in severe alcohol withdrawal. *Acta Psychiatrica Scandinavica 85:*376–379, 1992.
49. Adinoff, B., Risher-Flowers, D., De Jong, J., Ravitz, B., Bone, G. H., Nutt, D. J., Roehrich, L., Martin, P. R., & Linnoila, M. Disturbances of hypothalamic–pituitary–adrenal axis functioning during ethanol withdrawal in six men. *American Journal of Psychiatry 148:*1023–1025, 1991.
50. Knott, D. H., & Beard, J. D. A diuretic approach to acute withdrawal from alcohol. *Southern Medical Journal 62:*485–488, 1969.
51. Forsander, O. A. Dietary influences on alcohol intake: A review. *Journal of Studies on Alcohol 59:*26–31, 1998.
52. Ambrose, M. L., Bowden, S. C., & Whelan, G. Thiamin treatment and working memory function of alcohol-dependent people: Preliminary findings. *Alcoholism: Clinical and Experimental Research 25:*112–116, 2001.
53. Alho, H., Methuen, T., Paloheimo, M., Strid, N., Seppä, K., Tiainen, J., Salaspuro, M., & Roine, R. Long-term effects of and physiological responses to nitrous oxide gas treatment during alcohol withdrawal: A double-blind, placebo-controlled trial. *Alcoholism: Clinical and Experimental Research 26:*1816–1822, 2002.
54. Fleeman, N. D. Alcohol home detoxification: A literature review. *Alcohol & Alcoholism 32:*649–656, 1997.
55. Bennie, C. A comparison of home detoxification and minimal intervention strategies for problem drinkers. *Alcohol & Alcoholism 33:*157–163, 1998.
56. Duka, T., Townshend, J. M., Collier, K., & Stephens, D. N. Impairment in cognitive functions after multiple detoxifications in alcoholic inpatients. *Alcoholism: Clinical and Experimental Research 27:*1563–1572, 2002.

57. Pihl, R. O., Paylan, S. S., Gentes-Hawn, A., & Hoaken, P. N. S. Alcohol affects executive cognitive functioning differentially on the ascending versus descending limb of the blood alcohol concentration curve. *Alcoholism: Clinical and Experimental Research 27:*773–779, 2003.
58. Schulte, T., Meuller-Oehring, E. M., Rosenbloom, M. J., Pfefferbaum, A., & Sullivan, E. V. Differential effect of HIV infection and alcoholism on conflict processing, attentional allocation, and perceptual load: Evidence from a Stroop Match-to-Sample Task. *Biological Psychiatry 57:*67-75, 2005.
59. Errico, A. L., King, A. C., Lovallo, W. R., & Parsons, O. A. Cortisol dysregulation and cognitive impairment in abstinent male alcoholics. *Alcoholism: Clinical and Experimental Research 26:*1198–1204, 2002.
60. Harris, C. R., Albaugh, B., Goldman, D., & Enoch, M. A. Neurocognitive impairment due to chronic alcohol consumption in an American Indian community. *Journal of Studies on Alcohol 64:*458–466, 2003.
61. Bjork, J. M., Grant, S. J., & Hommer, D. W. Cross-sectional volumetric analysis of brain atrophy in alcohol dependence: Effects of drinking history and comorbid substance use disorder. *American Journal of Psychiatry 160:*2038–2045, 2003.
62. O'Neill, J. J., Cardenas, V. A., & Meyerhoff, D. J. Effects of abstinence on the brain: Quantitative magnetic resonance imaging and magnetic resonance spectroscopic imaging in chronic alcohol abuse. *Alcoholism: Clinical and Experimental Research 26:*1673–1682, 2001.
63. Wang, J. J.-L., Martin, P. R., & Singleton, C. K. A transketolase assembly defect in a Wernicke-Korsakoff syndrome patient. *Alcoholism: Clinical and Experimental Research 21:*576–580, 1997.
64. Reuster, T., Buechler, J., Winiecki, P., & Oehler, J. Influence of reboxetine on salivary MHPG concentration and cognitive symptoms among patients with alcohol-related Korsakoff's syndrome. *Neuropsychopharmacology 28:*974–978, 2003.
65. Oscar-Berman, M., Kirkley, S. M., Gansler, D. A., & Couture, A. Comparisons of Korsakoff and non-Korsakoff alcoholics on neuropsychological tests of prefrontal brain functioning. *Alcoholism: Clinical and Experimental Research 28:*667–675, 2004.
66. Thomson, A. D., & Cook, C. C. H. Parenteral thiamine and Wernicke's encephalopathy: The balance of risks and perception of concern. *Alcohol & Alcoholism 32:*207–209, 1997.
67. Soyka, M. Pathophysiological mechanisms possibly involved in the development of alcohol hallucinosis. *Addiction 90:*289–294, 1995.
68. Tsuang, J. W., Irwin, M. R., Smith, T. L., & Schuckit, M. A. Characteristics of men with alcoholic hallucinosis. *Addiction 89:*73–78, 1994.
69. Soyka, M. Alcoholism and schizophrenia. *Addiction 95:*1613–1618, 2000.
70. Schuckit, M. A., Tipp, J. E., Bergman, M., Reich, W., Hesselbrock, V. M., & Smith, T. L. Comparison of induced and independent major depressive disorders in 2,945 alcoholics. *American Journal of Psychiatry 154:*948–957, 1997.
71. Brook, D. W., Brook, J. S., Zhang, C., Cohen, P., & Whiteman, M. Drug use and the risk of major depressive disorder, alcohol dependence, and substance use disorders. *Archives of General Psychiatry 59:*1039–1044, 2002.
72. Caldwell, T. M., Rodgers, B., Jorm, A. F., Christensen, H., Jacomb, P. A., Korten, A. E., & Lynskey, M. T. Patterns of association between alcohol consumption and symptoms of depression and anxiety in young adults. *Addiction 97:*583–594, 2002.
73. de Graaf, R., Bijl, R. V., Smith, F., *et al.* Risk factors for 12-month comorbidity of mood, anxiety, and substance use disorders: Findings from the Netherlands mental health survey and incidence study. *American Journal of Psychiatry 159:*620–629, 2002.
74. Hasin, D. S., & Grant, B. F. Major depression in 6050 former drinkers. *Archives of General Psychiatry 59:*794–800, 2002.
75. Raimo, E. B., & Schuckit, M. A. Alcohol dependence and mood disorders. *Addictive Behaviors 23:*933–946, 1998.
76. Biederman, J., Faraone, S. V., Wozniak, J., & Monuteaux, M. C. Parsing the association between bipolar, conduct, and substance use disorders: A familial risk analysis. *Biological Psychiatry 48:*1037–1044, 2000.

77. Kahler, C. W., Ramsey, S. E., Read, J. P., & Brown, R. A. Substance-induced and independent major depressive disorder in treatment-seeking alcoholics: Associations with dysfunctional attitudes and coping. *Journal of Studies on Alcohol 63:*363–371, 2002.
78. Preuss, U. W., Schuckit, M. A., Smith, T. L., Danko, G. P., Dasher, A. C., Hesselbrock, M. N., Hesselbrock, V. M., & Nurnberger, J. I., Jr. A comparison of alcohol-induced and independent depression in alcoholics with histories of suicide attempts. *Journal of Studies on Alcohol 63:*498–502, 2002.
79. Morgenstern, J., Blanchard, K. A., Morgan, T. J., Labouvie, E., & Hayaki, J. Testing the effectiveness of cognitive-behavioral treatment for substance abuse in a community setting: Within treatment and post-treatment findings. *Journal of Consulting Clinical Psychology 69:*1007–1017, 2001.
80. Zarkin, G. A., Bray, J. W., Davis, K. L., Babor, T. F., & Higgins-Biddle, J. C. The costs of screening and brief intervention for risky alcohol use. *Journal of Studies on Alcohol 64:*849–857, 2003.
81. Frye, M. A., Altshuler, L. L., McElroy, S. L., Suppes, T., Keck, P. E., Denicoff, K., Nolen, W. A., Kupka, R., Leverich, G. S., Pollio, C., Grunze, H., Walden, J., & Post, R. M. Gender differences in prevalence, risk, and clinical correlates of alcoholism comorbidity in bipolar disorder. *American Journal of Psychiatry 160:*883–889, 2003.
82. Barrowclough, C., Haddock, G., Tarrier, N., Lewis, S. W., Moring, J., O'Brien, R., Schofield, N., & McGovern, J. Randomized controlled trial of motivational interviewing, cognitive behavior therapy, and family intervention for patients with comorbid schizophrenia and substance use disorders. *American Journal of Psychiatry 158:*1706–1713, 2001.
83. Ritsher, J. B., McKellar, J. D., Finney, J. W., Otilingam, P. G., & Moos, R. H. Psychiatric comorbidity, continuing care and mutual help as predictors of five-year remission from substance use disorders. *Journal of Studies on Alcohol 63:*709–715, 2002.
84. Fatjo, F., Fernandez-Sola, J., Lluis, M., Elena, M., Badia, E., Sacanella, E., Estruch, R., & Nicolas, J.-M. Myocardial antioxidant status in chronic alcoholism. *Alcoholism: Clinical and Experimental Research 29:*864-870, 2005.
85. Albertsen, K., & Gronbaek, M. Does amount or type of alcohol influence the risk of prostate cancer? *Prostate 52:*297–304, 2002.
86. Mukamal, K. J., Conigrave, K. M., Mittleman, M. A., Camargo, C. A., Jr., Stampfer, M. J., Willett, W. C., & Rimm, E. B. Roles of drinking pattern and type of alcohol consumed in coronary heart disease in men. *New England Journal of Medicine 348:*109–118, 2003.
87. Perreira, K. M., & Sloan, F. A. Excess alcohol consumption and health outcomes: A 6-year follow-up of men over age 50 from the health and retirement study. *Addiction 97:*301–310, 2002.
88. Green, J. E., Saveanu, R. V., & Bornstein, R. A. The effect of previous alcohol abuse on cognitive function in HIV infection. *American Journal of Psychiatry 161:*249–254, 2004.
89. Samet, J. H., Horton, N. J., Traphagen, E. T., Lyon, S. M., & Freedberg, K. A. Alcohol consumption and HIV disease progression: Are they related? *Alcoholism: Clinical and Experimental Research 27:*862–867, 2003.
90. Schonfeld, A. M., Mattson, S. N., Lang, A. R., Delis, D. C., & Riley, E. P. Verbal and nonverbal fluency in children with heavy prenatal alcohol exposure. *Journal of Studies on Alcohol 62:*239–246, 2001.
91. Schneider, M. L., Moore, C. F., & Kraemer, G. W. Moderate alcohol during pregnancy: Learning and behavior in adolescent rhesus monkeys. *Alcoholism: Clinical and Experimental Research 25:*1383–1392, 2001.
92. Larroque, B., & Kaminski, M. Prenatal alcohol exposure and development at preschool age: Main results of a French study. *Alcoholism: Clinical and Experimental Research 22:*295–303, 1998.
93. Day, N. L., Leech, S. L., Richardson, G. A., Cornelius, M. D., Robles, N., & Larkby, C. Prenatal alcohol exposure predicts continued deficits in offspring size at 14 years of age. *Alcoholism: Clinical and Experimental Research 26:*1584–1591, 2002.

94. Church, M. W., & Kaltenbach, J. A. Hearing, speech, language, and vestibular disorders in the fetal alcohol syndrome: A literature review. *Alcoholism: Clinical and Experimental Research 21:*495–512, 1997.
95. Baer, J. S., Sampson, P. D., Barr, H. M., Connor, P. D., & Streissguth, A. P. A 21-year longitudinal analysis of the effects of prenatal alcohol exposure on young adult drinking. *Archives of General Psychiatry 60:*377–385, 2003.
96. Lynch, M. E., Coles, C. D., Corley, T., & Falek, A. Examining delinquency in adolescents differentially prenatally exposed to alcohol: The role of proximal and distal risk factors. *Journal of Studies on Alcohol 64:*678–686, 2003.
97. O'Connor, M. J., Shah, B., Whaley, S., Cronin, P., Gunderson, B., & Graham, J. Psychiatric illness in a clinical sample of children with prenatal alcohol exposure. *The American Journal of Drug and Alcohol Abuse 28:*743–754, 2002.
98. Bielawski, D. M., Zaher, F. M., Svinarich, D. M., & Abel, E. L. Paternal alcohol exposure affects sperm cytosine methyltransferase messenger RNA levels. *Alcoholism: Clinical and Experimental Research 26:*347–351, 2002.
99. Mennella, J. A. Regulation of milk intake after exposure to alcohol in mothers' milk. *Alcoholism: Clinical and Experimental Research 25:*590–593, 2001.

CHAPTER 5

Stimulants: Amphetamines and Cocaine

5.1. INTRODUCTION

Stimulants, including all forms of amphetamines and cocaine, are widely prescribed and greatly misused medications that have only a few bona fide medical uses. It is important that the clinician knows these drugs well, as their misuse can mimic a variety of medical and psychiatric syndromes.

Nonmedicinal use of stimulants, such as ephedrine in Ma-Huang (see Chapter 10), has occurred for many centuries, increasing with the discovery of coca leaves by natives of the Andes in their effort to decrease hunger and fatigue.[1–4] Cocaine itself was first isolated in Germany in 1857, and its local anesthetic properties were applied in ophthalmology in the 1880s. Amphetamine was first synthesized in 1887, its clinical assets were recognized in about 1930, and until the mid-1950s or early 1960s, many people considered stimulants to be generally safe. Such claims were made despite evidence of their widespread misuse in Germany after World War I and epidemics of misuse in Japan after World War II, perhaps reflecting the ready availability of amphetamines as "wake-up" pills for US Army troops.

In more recent times, a series of steps have been taken by governments to attempt to control the use of these drugs. In 1914, President Taft named cocaine "Public Enemy Number One," a concern that contributed to the passage of the Harrison Act, which attempted to control the distribution and sale of these drugs. Yet, 100 mg of cocaine cost only 25 cents in the 1920s, and amphetamines were still available in over-the-counter benzedrine inhalers until 1971. In the mid-1960s, the Food and Drug Administration placed amphetamines under more strict regulation, and over the years the United States has taken escalating steps to control diversion of pharmaceutical products into illegal markets.

Stimulants are highly lucrative on the black market. It has been estimated that a $700 investment in phenylacetic acid can produce amphetamines with a street value of almost $250,000. These numbers have contributed to the widespread development of kitchen laboratories to produce these drugs. As a result, stimulants remain a major health hazard in many parts of the world.

5.1.1. Pharmacology

See Section 11.2.2 and Chapter 11.

5.1.1.1. The Relevant Drugs

The stimulants encompass a variety of drugs, including all forms of cocaine and amphetamines (some of which are listed in Table 5.1), which share the ability to stimulate the CNS at many levels. These include some interesting substances engineered, or designed, to circumvent legal sanctions, such as 4-methylaminorex or 4 MAM and methcathinone.[5] This discussion is limited to those substances that are the most relevant to misuse, avoiding other stimulants (such as strychnine). Two other important stimulants, nicotine and caffeine, are consumed in large amounts, but because of their relatively low potency and different mechanisms of action, they are presented in Chapter 11. Other more "exotic" drugs with stimulant properties are used in specific areas of the world and can produce the patterns of problems typical of stimulants in general. Two examples are khat, a stimulant from the Catha edulis plant, used in leaf form in North Africa and

Table 5.1
Some Commonly Abused Stimulants

Generic name	Trade name
Amphetamine	Adderall
Atomoxetine	Strattera[a]
Caffeine	(see Chapter 11)
Cocaine	—
Dexmethylphenidate	Focalin[a]
Dextroamphetamine	Dexedrine
Diethylpropion	Tenuate
Fenfluramine	Pondimin[a]
Methamphetamine	Desoxyn
Methylphenidate	Ritalin
Phenmetrazine	Preludin
Phentermine	Adipex-P
Pemoline	Cylert[a]
Sibutramine	Meridia[a]

[a]These drugs may be less reinforcing, and there are few data on misuse in humans.

in the Middle East, and ayahuasca, which is used in South America. Both are reported to be capable of inducing intense overactivity and even psychoses.[6,7] Also, methylenedioxy methamphetamine (MDMA), or ecstasy, is used mostly as a stimulating hallucinogen, as described in Chapter 8, while ephedrine, a stimulating drug which is sold over the counter, is presented in Chapter 10.

The clinical effects of stimulants are similar across various forms of amphetamine (including the crystalline amphetamines sold as ice) and forms of cocaine.[8–10] Several other amphetamine-like drugs are capable of causing similar types of intoxication, including the prescription stimulants and weight-reducing pills (Preludin), diethylpropion (Tenuate), and phentermine (Adipex-P).[11,12]

Finally, in this brief review of additional stimulant-like drugs, it is important to mention methylphenidate (Ritalin) and related drugs. These agents are capable of causing intoxication similar to amphetamine and cocaine but are less often misused. Perhaps this reflects the fact that, although methylphenidate is distributed in the brain in a manner similar to cocaine, a lower level of subjective feelings of reinforcement might be related to a slower clearance from brain areas rich in dopamine.

5.1.1.2. Mechanisms of Action

As a group, the stimulants, including all forms of amphetamine and all varieties of cocaine, work at least in part by causing the release or blocking the reuptake of neurotransmitters (chemicals that stimulate neighboring neurons), such as dopamine (DA) and norepinephrine (NE), from nerve cells.[13–16] Cocaine is thought to have more prominent actions on DA and to cause release of stored, rather than newly synthesized, catecholamines when compared to amphetamines. Some stimulants also mimic the actions of transmitters like NE through a direct effect on the nerve cells themselves. In general, stimulants also have effects on other neurotransmitter systems, including serotonin (especially at higher doses), NMDA, acetylcholine, substance P, endogenous opioids, and GABA.[17–23] The combination of these changes results in alterations in brain metabolism and in blood flow (especially in the prefrontal, frontal, temporal, and subcortical grey areas), causes a shift to higher frequency waves on the EEG, and is associated with feelings of stimulation and euphoria.

The recent data regarding the prominent actions on DA are of particular interest.[24–27] Using clinically relevant doses of cocaine, several studies have confirmed an increase of 20% or more in DA activity in the mesolimbic and mesocortical brain areas in both humans and animals, with similar results regarding amphetamines. There is also evidence that the level of euphoria experienced with cocaine (and presumably with amphetamines) correlates with the degree of DA change in the corpus striatum. The effects on DA appear to differ in different areas of the brain, and variations occur between acute and chronic drug administration.

The clinical effects of the stimulants and impact on DA and on other neurochemicals are also influenced by an organism's genetic makeup. Animals engineered to lack the DA transporter, which therefore lack a mechanism of action for the stimulants, demonstrate little or no effect of either amphetamines or cocaine.[28] There are also data demonstrating that some specific types of DA receptors are particularly sensitive to the effects of cocaine.

5.1.1.3. Drug Combinations

Cocaine is often taken in conjunction with heroin, where it is used IV as a "speed-ball."[29–31] Clinicians have hypothesized that this combination might be popular because the stimulant effects of the cocaine offset some of the more sedating actions of the opioid, and vice versa. It is also possible that the effects of the cocaine–heroin combination might reflect stimulant-related changes in mu opioid receptors, a speculation that might apply to mixtures of amphetamines and alcohol as well.

It is estimated that 60–80% of cocaine users, and many people with amphetamine abuse or dependence, simultaneously drink alcohol.[32,33] When taken in the usual street doses, these stimulants have been reported to attenuate some of the cognitive performance impairments observed with low to moderate doses of alcohol. However, with repeated administration of cocaine and alcohol, alcohol appears to have the effect of increasing the body's sensitivity to subsequent doses of cocaine, and cocaine might attenuate the rate of development of tolerance to alcohol, thus contributing to a more intense alcohol response. At least some of these effects occur because the combination of alcohol and cocaine produces a third active substance, cocaethylene.[34] This compound has a longer half-life than cocaine (2 h as opposed to less than 1 h for cocaine), and also appears to function by increasing DA release and blocking its reuptake from presynaptic cells.[4] This longer lasting and more intense intoxication has been theorized to contribute to as much as a 20-fold increased risk for sudden cardiac deaths with individuals with preexisting coronary artery disease.[4,35]

5.1.1.4. Cocaine and Amphetamines

Cocaine, derived from a plant that contains about 0.5% active drug, is sold "on the street" in a variety of forms, including an impure hydrochloride powder, most frequently "cut" or expanded with glucose, lactose, and mannitol. Resulting purity levels of this form of cocaine are between 0 and 17% in the average street sample, though much higher purity is seen for crack.[4] Cocaine is well absorbed through all modes of administration, but the powder is most often injected IV or "snorted" [intranasally (IN)]. For snorting, powder is usually arranged on a glass plate in thin lines, 3–5 cm long, each with approximately 25 mg of the active substance, which are then inhaled into the nostrils through a straw or rolled paper.[2] The "average" dose used by the usual non-tolerant person is between 20 and 100 mg.

The drug can also be smoked in tobacco, although such use is inefficient, as cocaine sulfate has a melting point of almost 200°C. As a result, cocaine "freebase" was developed to lower the melting point to 98'C for use sprinkled over tobacco or smoked in special pipes. The freebase is produced by adding a strong base (e.g., buffered ammonia) to an aqueous solution of cocaine and then extracting the alkaline freebase precipitate.

Similar changes in the salt structure have also resulted in a crystallized form of cocaine known on the streets as "crack" (reflecting the crackling sound when it is burned)[11] or "rock." The relatively low melting point and the ready solubility of this form in water have contributed to the widespread use of this form of cocaine.[1,2,36] Whether freebase or crack, the smoked product is usually 40% or more pure.

The predominant actions of cocaine are similar, no matter what the salt-form. Thus, the same pattern of problems is likely to appear with crack as is seen with freebase or with other forms of cocaine, although because of the rapid onset and intense effects with smoking, crack may be particularly likely to precipitate a psychosis.

The pattern of blood levels of this stimulant differ a bit depending on whether it is taken IV or IN, smoked, or taken orally. The peak levels develop rapidly (within 5–30 min), after which most of the cocaine disappears over 2 h: cocaine has a half-life of approximately 1.5–1 h. The longest lasting effects are probably seen after IN ingestion (though the onset is slower), as the active drug remains in the nasal mucosa for 3 h or longer, probably reflecting local constriction of the blood vessels.[4]

Most of the active drug is metabolized in the liver, but some is acted on by plasma esterases, and a small amount is excreted unchanged in the urine.[1,4] Cocaine does not completely disappear from the body rapidly, and traces are likely to be found in urine samples for 3 days or longer, and up to 14 days if high doses were taken.[37]

Oral administration of *amphetamines* produces a much slower onset of intoxication than smoking, snorting, or IV use. For any of these methods of taking the drug into the body, it is likely that half or more of the active substance is destroyed by the liver soon after intake, with a half-life of amphetamines of 7 h or more, but the intoxication usually lasts 30–45 min.[2,11] Especially at high doses, much of the amphetamine is also excreted directly through the urine, with a possibility that acidifying the urine (by giving vitamin C, for example) might speed up the rate of disappearance of this drug from the bloodstream.[2]

A number of cocaine "substitutes" (not truly related to cocaine itself) have been developed. Some (e.g., "iceberg" and "snort") contain benzocaine and/or procaine, whereas others contain about 75 mg of caffeine (e.g., "cocaine snuff," "coca snow," and "incense"), ephedrine, or other stimulants (e.g., "zoom"). The effects of these drugs would be expected to resemble those of caffeine. (Refer Chapter 11 for further information.)

5.1.1.5. Predominant Effects of Intoxication (303.00 and 292.89 in DSM-IV)

The most obvious actions of stimulants are on the CNS, the peripheral nervous system (outside the CNS), and the cardiovascular system.[2,10,38] Clinically, the drugs cause euphoria, decrease fatigue and the need for sleep, may increase feelings of sexuality, prolong orgasm, interfere with normal sleep patterns, decrease appetite, increase energy, and tend to decrease the level of distractibility.[2,11,22] The heightened energy can combine with increased levels of anxiety to precipitate violence. The impairment of judgment and the psychological changes seen with stimulants might also pose problems in the operation of motor vehicles, although these have been difficult to document.

Physically, the drugs produce adrenaline-like actions that yield a tremor of the hands, restlessness, a rapid heart rate, increased muscle tension, and increased blood pressure and body temperature.[1] Most of the substances have actions similar to those of amphetamine, although methamphetamine (Desoxyn) has fewer cardiac effects (especially at low doses), and methylphenidate and phenmetrazine are less potent.[1,2]

Using cocaine as an example, it is possible to look more closely at the predominant effects of intoxication. The CNS actions show a biphasic response, lower doses tending to improve motor performance but higher doses causing deterioration, with subsequent severe tremors and possible convulsions.[1,2] Additional CNS effects can include nausea and vomiting, dilated pupils, and an increased body temperature that probably reflects both direct actions on the brain and indirect effects through muscle contractions. While cocaine might not increase muscle strength, there is a decrease in fatigue, probably mediated through CNS effects. The cardiovascular changes are also biphasic, with lower doses tending to produce a decrease in heart rate via actions on the vagus nerve, but higher doses causing both an increased heart rate and vasoconstriction, with a resulting elevation in blood pressure. The actions on the heart may produce arrhythmias both directly through the effects of the drug and indirectly through catecholamine release.

The time course of effects also differs with the route of administration.[1] Oral drugs (e.g., amphetamine) can take 45 min for peak effects, which are subsequently less intense with other modes. IN use of amphetamines or cocaine has an onset of about 3–5 min, with peak effects at 10–20 min, and a fading high by 45 min or less. IV use gives almost an instant high that lasts 10–20 min or less.

5.1.2. Tolerance, Sensitization, Abuse, and Dependence (Abuse and Dependence on Amphetamines and Cocaine are 305.70, 304.40, 305.60, and 304.20 in DSM-IV)

5.1.2.1. Tolerance and Sensitization

Tolerance to some of the actions of stimulant drugs develops within hours to days.[39] It is the result of *metabolic* tolerance [an alteration in drug distribution and metabolism perhaps related to increased acidity of the body (acidosis) or an increased rate of metabolism], *pharmacodynamic* tolerance (as exemplified by toleration of injections of 1 g and more of methamphetamine or cocaine IV every 2 h), and *behavioral* tolerance.[1,2] An additional example of pharmacodynamic tolerance is the demonstration that even when constant cocaine-blood levels are maintained through an IV infusion, the euphoric effects tend to disappear rapidly, while the feelings of anxiety and heightened energy remain.

Acute tolerance is likely to develop quite rapidly, and the euphoric and the cardiovascular manifestations of the substance diminish more rapidly than the plasma levels.[1,2] This phenomenon can be pronounced with tolerant humans capable of taking up to 3–10 g of cocaine every day, and monkeys will repeatedly self-administer doses that produce convulsions and cardiorespiratory complications in naive animals.

An important additional phenomenon for depressants is *sensitization*.[40–43] Here, users demonstrate some increasing effects with repeated doses, perhaps related to a CNS process similar to enhanced cellular sensitivity, or kindling. This phenomenon has been observed for both cocaine and amphetamine regarding a broad array of actions including behavioral changes and alterations in moods.

5.1.2.2. Abuse and Dependence

For decades, diagnostic manuals have recognized the likelihood that people will continue to take stimulants despite legal, interpersonal, occupational, and social problems. Therefore, there is little argument about the clinical relevance of cocaine or amphetamine misuse.

However, in the past, some clinicians and researchers did not understand the psychological and physiological problems that can be associated with dependence. It was not until the late 1980s that a substantial body of evidence developed to demonstrate that heavy use of stimulants often produces dependence.[44] Now there are plentiful data demonstrating that high levels of tolerance can develop. Almost 90% of people who are cocaine and amphetamine dependent describe a prominent and disturbing physiological withdrawal syndrome involving depression, somnolence, and intense hunger, which is experienced for several days following abstinence, as is described further in Section 5.2.2.[45] Withdrawal symptoms are most intense for 3–5 days, but remain at decreasing intensity for many weeks, and perhaps months after cessation of stimulant use, following a time course consistent with protracted withdrawal. Other dependence criteria that often occur with stimulant use include using despite consequences, spending much time using, giving up important events, and so on.

The withdrawal phase is also characterized by EEG changes, usually involving an excess of alpha power along with a decrease in the faster delta and theta frequency bands,[46] with at least one report of a continuation of these findings in some individuals for 6 months.[47] Animal models also support the existence of a stimulant withdrawal syndrome with changes in dopamine activity in several brain areas, including the amygdala.[48] Additional changes observed in humans and animals during withdrawal included alterations in cerebral glucose utilization and changes in the normal hormonal alterations, including prolactin.[11]

5.1.3. Purported Medical Uses

This section and Table 5.2 reinforce the fact that, despite the claim that stimulants are effective for many medical disorders, in most instances the potential benefit might not outweigh the potential harm. This is true, at least in part, because of a rapid development of tolerance to stimulants that seriously limits their ability to maintain a level of clinical usefulness.

Problems for which stimulants have been prescribed include those described in the following sections.

5.1.3.1. Narcolepsy

This disorder—characterized by falling asleep without warning through the development of rapid-eye-movement (REM) or "dream-type" sleep at

Table 5.2
Purported Medical Uses of Stimulants

Use	Comment
Narcolepsy	A rare disorder that responds to other REM-suppressing drugs as well. The preferred treatment is modafinil (Provigil).
Attention deficit disorder with hyperactivity	Responds to stimulants or antidepressants.
Obesity	Stimulants result in *temporary* relief. Dangers far outweigh assets.
Fatigue	Rule out medical diseases or depression. Stimulants do not work.
Depression	Stimulants sometimes can make the picture worse, and the preferred treatment is antidepressants.
Dysmenorrhea	No proven usefulness.

any time of the day or night—can also be associated with falling attacks (catalepsy). Stimulants can both modify and prevent attacks, in part by decreasing REM sleep.[2,49] However, narcolepsy may be a rare disorder and should be diagnosed only with confirmatory EEG studies. Also, other less dangerous REM-decreasing drugs are available, including modafinil and most of the antidepressants. Classical stimulants such as amphetamines should be used carefully, if at all, for this disorder.

5.1.3.2. Attention Deficit/Hyperactivity Disorder (ADHD)

This syndrome of children, which can persist into adulthood, is characterized by a short attention span, a problem focusing attention, and an inability to sit quietly, with resultant difficulty in learning, and it may be associated with signs of minimal brain damage.[44,50] However, hyperactivity and problems with attention in children can be a temporary reaction to stress, and the diagnosis of ADHD should not rest solely with the symptom of overactivity, especially when it occurs in relation to a life problem. True ADHD, which usually develops before age 6, becomes more incapacitating once school begins. For a person with a bona fide ADHD, stimulants decrease symptoms and enhance learning. When used carefully, moderate potency drugs like methylphenidate (Ritalin) and pemoline (Cylert) can be very effective, and do not predispose the child to go on to drug dependence. This is one of the few disorders for which stimulants are the drug treatment of choice, but alternate modes of pharmacotherapy, including antidepressants, are available.[51]

5.1.3.3. Obesity

Stimulants do decrease the appetite, but only temporarily, with activity lasting *at most* for 3 or 4 weeks. In most controlled investigations, weight lost while on stimulants reappears within a relatively short time after the drugs are stopped. Some newer antiappetite drugs with fewer stimulant side effects (e.g., subutramine (Meridia) and phentermine (Adipex P) appear to produce fewer heart and possible CNS dangers. However, considering these dangers and the potential for dependence on these drugs, the long-term use of stimulants for weight reduction may not be justified.

5.1.3.4. Other Problems

The stimulants have also been used for fatigue, depression, menstrual pain or dysmenorrhea, and some neurological disorders. Controlled studies have not demonstrated that the drugs are effective for most of these problems, and their potential dangers outweigh their usefulness.

5.1.4. Epidemiology and Patterns of Use

It is difficult to establish the accurate prevalence of the nonmedical use of stimulants in the United States. This reflects the wide range of stimulant drugs produced each year, such as methylphenidate and the weight-reducing pills, as well as the drugs available in the illegal market.

Among the illegal stimulants, both cocaine and amphetamines have been popular in the United States. According to the 2002 National Survey on Drug Use and Health (formerly the National Household Survey), 15% of people aged 12 or older admitted to ever having used cocaine.[52] These data reflected about 1% of the population who reported using cocaine in the previous month and perhaps a higher rate in college students.[53]

The 1997 National Household Survey indicated slightly lower levels for other "stimulants," a category of drugs assumed to be predominantly amphetamines. Here, about 5% of the general population had taken such stimulant drugs (about 6% of men and 3% of women), including 1% who used them in the prior year (0.5% and 1% across the genders), and 0.3% (0.4% for men and 0.2% for women) who took these drugs over the prior month. Similar to cocaine, the age of highest lifetime prevalence was 26–34 years (5%), and the group most likely to have taken the prior year was 18–25 years old (2%), with that same age group indicating that 1% had taken them in the prior month. Useful information regarding the pattern of use of stimulants among young adults can also be found in the Monitoring the Future study.[36] Regarding cocaine, in 2003 about 8% of high school seniors and almost 14% of young adults have ever used cocaine in any form, including about 4% of each group who took crack cocaine. Basically 5% of both age groups had used any form of cocaine in the prior year, including about 2% in the prior 30 days. The lifetime prevalence of having used amphetamines in any form was about 14% in high school seniors, and almost 15% in young adults, figures that included approximately 10% of each group in the prior year, and almost 5% who had used amphetamines in the prior month.

Although the prevalence of stimulant use appears to be lower in other countries, the rates are still appreciable. In 1997, approximately 3% of adults in Spain and 2–3% of teenagers in Chile reported that they had ever used a stimulant. Among high school students in Northern Mexico, 1% reported that they had ever used cocaine, and 2% reported ever using amphetamines.[54]

Recognizing that any use of these substances for intoxication is likely to be dangerous, these high levels of prevalence are cause for concern. However, few surveys give adequate information to determine the actual rate of abuse or dependence. The National Comorbidity Survey estimated a lifetime prevalence of abuse or dependence on these substances of approximately 2%.[11]

Focusing on cocaine, several reports reveal that repeated use is likely to cost the user between $500 and $2000+ per month. Subsequently, half or more of users report problems with their families related to stimulants, trouble at work, neglect of usual activities, and feelings of being unable to stop use when desired.[55–57] About half of the users are likely to report periods of at least some level of paranoia or hallucinations associated with stimulants, and 80–90% indicate that they have tried to develop strategies to control use, although only 15–30% of those actually sought help.[1,58] The average individual with cocaine problems admits to experience with between three and four additional drugs, and a quarter or more fulfill criteria for antisocial personality disorder.[29] It is not surprising that the death rate in people who are stimulant dependent is higher than the general population.

5.1.5. Establishing the Diagnosis

Substances that so easily mimic other medical and psychiatric emergencies and that are readily available both on prescription and "on the street" must be considered part of the differential diagnosis in most psychiatric symptoms. As with the other drugs of abuse, one must keep stimulant-related diagnoses in mind or they will be missed.[59] It is important to gather a careful history from both the patient and any available resource person about the use of stimulant drugs, ask each person about patterns of life problems, and then go on to the patterns of use of prescription and illegal drugs. The clinician should be especially suspicious of stimulants when an individual presents with any of the following problems.

1. A restless, hyperalert state
2. An anxiety attack, i.e., a 15 min or so episode of intense nervousness and a rapid pulse
3. Intense emotional lability or irritability
4. Aggressive or violent outbursts
5. Paranoia or increased suspiciousness
6. Hallucinations, especially auditory
7. Depression
8. Fatigue
9. Evidence of IV drug use, such as needle marks or skin abscesses
10. Abnormalities in the nasal lining (mucosa) as might be expected after inhaling stimulants
11. Worn-down teeth (from tooth grinding while intoxicated)

Also, in an emergency room, anyone presenting with *dilated pupils*, *an increased heart rate*, *dry mouth*, *increased reflexes*, *elevated temperature*, *sweating*, or *hyperactive behavioral abnormalities* should be considered a possible stimulant-drug misuser. If there is a hint of stimulant use, it may be worthwhile to take blood or urine sample for a toxicological screen.

5.2. EMERGENCY PROBLEMS

Drug-induced psychiatric disturbances are probably more prevalent among people dependent on stimulants than among the users of any other type of drug.[1,2] The difficulties can include manic-like states, psychoses resembling schizophrenia, depressions almost identical to major mood disorders (especially during withdrawal), and anxiety conditions including panic states (most prevalent during intoxication). These all tend to be transitory and disappear over a period of days or weeks (perhaps up to a month) after the drug is stopped. The most frequently seen clinical problems associated with stimulant abuse and dependence are anxiety conditions, a temporary psychosis, and medical problems. Although DSM-IV lists cocaine and amphetamine problems separately, the clinical patterns are so similar that the two drugs are discussed together here.

5.2.1. Toxic Reactions

See Sections 2.2.1, 4.2.1, 6.2.1, and 13.2.

5.2.1.1. Clinical Picture

5.2.1.1.1. History

Cocaine-related overdoses accounted for almost 75% of the overdose deaths in New York City in the early 1990s, either alone or in conjunction with heroin.[60] The clinical picture of stimulant overdose may develop within minutes (e.g., with IV use or with snorting) or more slowly over hours, as with oral use of amphetamines.

5.2.1.1.2. Physical Signs and Symptoms

Evidence of sympathetic nervous system overactivity dominates the clinical picture for toxic reactions of all stimulants, including cocaine.[2,61,62] The patient presents with a rapid pulse, an increased respiratory rate, and an elevated body temperature. At high drug doses, the picture progresses to grand mal convulsions, markedly elevated blood pressure, chest pain sometimes related to myocardial ischemia, and a body temperature as high as 41'C rectally—all of which can lead to cardiovascular shock. Cardiac effects can include a fatal arrhythmia or a myocardial infarction secondary to arterial spasm or direct damage to heart muscle from continued stimulant use. It has been estimated that between 100 and 200 mg of dextroamphetamine (Dexedrine) and similar doses of cocaine can be lethal in a non-tolerant individual, but chronic users may tolerate 1 g or more, and the use of up to 10 g of cocaine per day has been reported.[2]

Death is often related to a stroke-like vascular picture, cardiac arrhythmias, or to high body temperature, and is likely to be associated with muscle rigidity, delirium, and agitation. The biological mechanisms are complex and probably involve acute changes in catecholamine levels and perhaps alterations in opioid receptors.[63]

5.2.1.1.3. Psychological State

High doses of stimulants produce restlessness, dizziness, irritability, and insomnia. These may be associated with headache, palpitations, and the physical signs and symptoms listed in Section 5.2.1.1.2. As the dose increases, toxic behavioral signs develop, including suspiciousness, repetitive stereotyped behaviors, bruxism (grinding of the teeth), and stereotypy (repetitive touching and picking at various objects and parts of the body).

5.2.1.1.4. Relevant Laboratory Tests

With the exception of a toxicological screen and the usual vital-sign changes expected with stimulants, there are no specific laboratory test results. However, the usual blood tests include a panel of electrolytes along with liver, cardiac and muscle enzymes (a chem. panel), BUN, creatinine, and creatinine kinase (CK), along with an EKG and chest film.[62]

5.2.1.2. Treatment

Treatment depends on the clinical condition.

1. Emergency care to ensure a clear *airway*, *circulatory* stability, and treatment of *shock* should be carried out as described in Sections 2.2.1.2, 6.2.1.2, and 13.2.1.2.
2. For an *oral overdose*, gastric lavage should be considered via either a nasogastric tube (for a conscious patient) or after intubation (for a comatose patient).
3. Elevated *body temperature* must be controlled, with levels above 102°F orally treated with cold water, ice packs, or, at higher temperatures, a hypothermic blanket (see also item 7). Some authors suggest using dantroline (Dantrium) in doses that can be built up to 4–8 mg/kg/day in 4 divided doses similar to the regimen given for the neuroleptic malignant syndrome.
4. Repeated *seizures* should be treated with doses of IV diazepam (Valium) of 5–20 mg injected *very slowly* over a minute and repeated in 15–20 min as needed. In this instance, intubation should be strongly considered, as IV diazepam could result in laryngospasm or apnea.
5. A major elevation in *blood pressure* (e.g., a diastolic pressure of over 120 mm) lasting for over 15 min requires the usual medical regimen

for malignant hypertension, which may include a phentolamine (Regitine) IV drip of 2–5 mg given over 5–10 min.

6. Evidence of cardiac ischemia should be treated with aspirin, nitrates, morphine, or benzodiazepines, *not* beta blockers.[62]
7. *Hyperthermia* and marked *agitation* can also be treated with a dopamine-blocking agent such as haloperidol (Haldol), beginning with doses of 5 mg orally per day, but the dose might have to be a good deal higher for some individuals. Other authors recommend treating agitation and elevated pulse with lorazepam (Ativan) 2 mg IV.
8. Recent research is evaluating the potential benefits of enhancing drug metabolizing enzymes (e.g., butyrylcholinesterase for cocaine) or dopamine agonists (e.g., for D_3 and D_2 receptors) to diminish some overdose symptoms, but the routine clinical use of these approaches has not been established.[61,64]
9. Blood and urine should be drawn for baseline studies and for toxicological tests, which will help to rule out the concomitant use of other medications.

5.2.2. Withdrawal (292.0 and 292.89 in DSM-IV)

5.2.2.1. Clinical Picture

5.2.2.1.1. History

Depending on the pattern of stimulant use, withdrawal symptoms may be acute and more dramatic or intense or begin more insidiously, with the patient having no idea why he is depressed, lethargic, or irritable.

5.2.2.1.2. Physical Signs and Symptoms

For cocaine, amphetamines, and other stimulants, there are usually few obvious physical signs. The withdrawal syndrome can begin while the individual continues to take stimulants as tolerance develops, or start following abstinence.

The absence of obvious physiological changes does not mean that the body is normal during amphetamine and cocaine withdrawal.[65] The prominent dopamine boosting effects of the stimulants result in a decrease in the hormone prolactin during acute administration. Thus, it is not surprising that during the first several weeks following withdrawal, persisting dopamine abnormalities and possible elevations in prolactin have been documented. Similarly, dopamine is an important neurochemical in the perception of pleasure and reward, and during withdrawal patients often complain of moodiness, irritability, and lack of motivation.[24,66–68] Similar symptoms are likely to be seen during amphetamine withdrawal. Changes in EEG activity patterns can also be seen for a month or more following abstinence.[47]

5.2.2.1.3. Psychological State

The clinical syndrome for withdrawal might be divided into several phases, although not all studies agree.[11] In this scheme, during the first 9 h to several days, the "crash" is characterized by intense craving and cocaine-seeking behavior. In this early phase, the person experiences intense agitation, depression, and a decreased appetite which give way to fatigue with associated insomnia and continued depression. All of these result in a final experience of exhaustion, a rebound in appetite, and a need to sleep. Early in the next phase, sleep patterns begin to normalize, feelings of cocaine craving remain but at lower levels, and the mood is still impaired but more normal. This is followed by a period of months during which there is improvement in mood and in the ability to enjoy life experiences, but feeling of craving and problems concentrating improve slowly.

5.2.2.1.4. Relevant Laboratory Tests

There are no specific laboratory tests for stimulant withdrawal. IV drug users should be screened for possible hepatitis (e.g., the liver function tests listed in Table 1.6), signs of occult infection (a WBC as listed in Table 1.6), and possible AIDS. They should also be given a thorough neurological examination.

5.2.2.2. Treatment

Treatment of withdrawal involves addressing the *symptoms*, as the most intense syndrome improves with 2–5 days on its own (although moodiness, problems concentrating, and lethargy may remain for several months). It is often possible to treat the syndrome in an outpatient setting, offering general supports as follows.

1. The patient must be given a careful neurological and physical examination.
2. The possibility of the concomitant dependence on other drugs, especially opioids or depressants, must be considered. Blood or urine samples should be sent for toxicological screening, and the patient should be carefully queried about additional drug use.
3. For the first day or so, the patient should be advised to sleep as much as possible.
4. If he or she is markedly despondent, temporary suicide precautions should be considered.
5. Once again, I prefer to avoid medications, as there are no convincing data that they are better than the passage of time. Education and reassurance, along with cognitive therapy, are the mainstay of treatment.[69] Evaluations have been carried out with dopamine-boosting drugs and with antidepressants, but the results are not impressive.[70]

5.2.3. Delirium, Dementia, and Other Cognitive Disorders (292.81 in DSM-IV)

Confusion and disorientation can develop when an individual takes so much of the drug that his normal mental processes are disturbed (i.e., as part of a toxic reaction). The symptoms can also represent CNS ischemia which, while usually reversible as the drug levels drop, can cause permanent sequelae of strokes.[71-75]

5.2.3.1. Clinical Picture

See Section 1.7.1.

Clinically relevant doses of stimulants can cause constriction of blood vessels in the brain, thus raising the possibility of subsequent brain damage. Also, several brain-wave and imaging changes observed during withdrawal do not disappear quickly, and perhaps 80% of people who are cocaine dependent demonstrate at least a temporary, diffuse, global hyperfusion on dynamic brain imaging techniques, especially in brain areas rich in dopamine.[4,11,73,76,77] Although obvious long-term neuronal damage has not been proven, there are data indicating the persistence of a hand tremor and what appears to be mild impairments in memory and attention for at least several months after abstinence, findings that might be correlated with the severity of dependence,but which might continue to clear with longer abstinence.[73,78,79]

5.2.3.2. Treatment

1. Because the acute confusion tends to be transient, the general approach is to give supportive care following the guidelines offered in Section 5.2.4.2.
2. However, one must be certain to carry out an adequate neurological examination to rule out possible causes of a delirium or dementia, including a focal CNS lesion or intracranial bleeding.

5.2.4. Psychosis or Delusional Disorder (292.81, 292.11, and 292.12 in DSM-IV)

See Sections 1.7.4, 2.2.4, and 4.2.4.

Intoxication with stimulants is associated with a problem filtering out irrelevant stimuli, and with evidence of hypervigilance and suspiciousness.[80–82] As the dose escalates, these symptoms can progress to a full-blown (but temporary) stimulant-induced psychosis, probably related to changes in the dopamine activity in mesolimbic and in negro-striatal areas. The clinical state can be seen with *any* of the major stimulants, including methylphenidate, pemoline, the amphetamines, prescription (and some nonprescription) weight-reducing products, and cocaine. Many of the psychological changes seen in stimulant psychoses resemble those in schizophrenia.

5.2.4.1. Clinical Picture

Intense suspiciousness and paranoid delusions in a *clear sensorium* (the patient is alert and oriented) developing after an individual takes stimulants is called an amphetamine or cocaine induced psychosis.[1,11] This picture develops fairly rapidly, over a few hours or days, and can even occur following a single very large dose. The paranoia is usually associated with hallucinations, either auditory or tactile (e.g., the individual feels things crawling on him), but it can also include visual hallucinations or illusions, and is usually accompanied by a very labile mood.[11]

The paranoid delusions can be very frightening to the patients and to those around them. There is usually little or no insight, and the suspiciousness has been known to result in unprovoked violence. In fact, it has been reported that in the midst of the epidemic of amphetamine abuse in Japan, half of the convicted murder cases were related to the misuse of amphetamines.

With cessation of stimulants, the psychosis usually clears within a few days to a week (sometimes remaining for as long as a month), the hallucinations tending to disappear first and the delusions later. This is followed by increased need for sleep (often accompanied by disturbing dreams) and a temporary depression. It has been reported that some patients originally presenting with amphetamine or stimulant psychosis might have some residual symptoms for up to 1 year or more. However, this persistence of symptoms may represent a triggering or uncovering of a preexisting psychotic state or a marked vulnerability to psychotic disorders such as schizophrenia.

The stimulant induced psychosis must be differentiated from other diagnoses. Schizophrenia usually has a relatively slow onset and tends to be associated with a stable, somewhat bland mood. Also, while a person with schizophrenia rarely shows such abnormal physical findings, the person with a stimulant psychosis can reveal evidence of weight loss, excoriations from scratching at nonexistent bugs (a condition known as *formication* which is a term derived from the Latin word for "ant"), needle marks, nasal irritation or sores from snorting, and elevated blood pressure, heart rate, and temperature. However, these physical findings are variable, and their absence does not rule out stimulant-induced psychosis.

5.2.4.2. Treatment

Treatment of the stimulant psychoses is relatively straightforward. The prognosis is good, as even without active therapy the pathological picture tends to disappear within a few days to a month of abstinence.

1. Hospitalization should be considered for patients out of contact with reality.
2. They must be carefully screened for physical pathology, as psychotic symptoms can be temporary during an overdose. See Section 5.2.1.2.

3. Vital signs must be carefully recorded, and elevated blood pressure, especially if over 120 diastolic, should be treated with drugs such as phentolamine (Regitine) in doses of 2–5 mg given over 5–10 min. Special care must be given to avoid precipitating hypotension.
4. In evaluating the clinical picture, consider the possibility that the individual may have also been dependent on a depressant, and check for signs of depressant withdrawal.
5. When possible, the patient should be placed in a quiet, nonthreatening atmosphere and treated with the general precautions one would extend to any paranoid patient (e.g., do not perform any procedures without thorough explanation, do not touch the patient without permission, and avoid any rapid movements in the patient's presence).[11]
6. The possibility of assaultive behavior based on paranoid delusions should be noted.
7. A careful history of preexisting psychoses, especially schizophrenia, should be taken from the patient and from available resource persons. Such conditions indicate the need for long-term (potentially even lifelong) medication.
8. a. Some authors recommend an antipsychotic drug such as chlorpromazine (Thorazine) in doses of 50–150 mg by mouth or 25–50 mg IM, to be repeated up to four times a day, if needed, with special care to avoid anticholinergic problems or hypotension.[2,3,11] I avoid this drug and other classical antipsychotics, as they have been reported to increase the half-life of amphetamine, and might produce enhanced craving or drug use.[83]
   b. The newer generation of antipsychotics may avoid these problems while offering beneficial effects for stimulant psychoses.[83,84] One study suggested the use of quetiapine (Seroquel) up to 50–250 mg PO three times a day.[83]
   c. An alternative approach is to use another newer generation antipsychotic drug such as risperidone (Risperdal) in doses of 2–3 mg by mouth daily, increasing by 1 mg/day if needed up to 16 mg/day.
   d. Some authors recommend the use of diazepam (Valium) in doses of 10–30 mg orally or 10–20 mg IM to control anxiety or overactivity. However, I feel that there is little role for depressant drugs in treating the stimulant psychoses, and the Bzs may increase the risk of violence by contributing to disinhibition.
9. As is true for most drug related problems described in this text, patients should be referred after discharge to a drug treatment center to help them deal with their drug problems and to rule out the existence of other psychiatric disorders.

5.2.5. Flashbacks

The relatively short length of action and the rapid metabolism of stimulants do not make them conducive to the development of flashbacks.

5.2.6. Anxiety and Depression (292.84 and 292.89 in DSM-IV)

5.2.6.1. Clinical Picture

See Sections 1.2.6, 7.2.6, 8.2.6, and 13.7.

Perhaps two out of three men and women who are stimulant dependent give histories of depression and/or anxiety symptoms[8,85–90] during the course of their disorder. Regarding anxiety, intoxication can cause a rapid heart rate, palpitations, nervousness, and hyperventilation. High doses of stimulants can be associated with obsessive–compulsive-like pictures with a compulsive desire to take mechanical objects apart and reassemble them.

Intense depressive symptoms are often temporarily related to the stimulant withdrawal syndrome. Initial symptoms in heavy users of stimulants (especially amphetamine and cocaine, but also with weight-reducing products and other less potent stimulants) can resemble the "atypical depressions" involving impaired mood accompanied by sleepiness and an excessive appetite. Even when this more dramatic clinical picture is absent, many (perhaps most) men and women who use stimulants demonstrate mood swings for weeks to months following cessation of stimulant use, perhaps as part of a protracted withdrawal syndrome.

Thus, it has been said that the stimulants are the group of drugs most likely to mimic major psychiatric syndromes. These include panic attacks and states that resemble generalized anxiety disorder during intoxication, obsessive–compulsive symptoms during periods of high levels of drug use, and withdrawal states that resemble atypical depressions, cyclothymia, and dysthymia as defined in DSM-IV.[89] When these clinical conditions are observed, counseling, behavioral, and cognitive approaches should be used. However, there are few, if any, data to indicate that substance-induced depressions run a long-term course indicative of an independent psychiatric disorder, and medications are not usually required.[82,89]

5.2.6.2. Treatment

Treatment involves careful evaluation to rule out medical or psychiatric disorders, while offering reassurance, and allowing for the passage of time.

1. For panic conditions, the patient should be evaluated for any medical illness that can cause panic symptoms (e.g., a heart attack or hyperthyroidism).
2. A careful history should be taken to rule out preexisting psychiatric disorders, especially panic or major depressive disorders.

3. Blood (10 cc) should be drawn or a urine sample should be taken (50 ml) for toxicological tests.
4. If the points in the first two items are negative, the patient should be told that his reaction is likely to be a result of the drug, and that the symptoms should improve quickly.
5. Of course, if stimulant misuse is a regular occurrence, he should be referred for evaluation and counseling for his substance-use disorder.
6. Medications should be used sparingly, if at all. If needed, antianxiety drugs [e.g., chlordiazepoxide (Librium), 10–25 mg by mouth, repeated several times in 30–60 min, if necessary] may be helpful.[91]

5.2.7. Medical Problems

The medical problems associated with overdose were described in Section 5.2.1. Additional problems that must be considered are as follows:

1. Complications from the use of contaminated needles include endocarditis, tetanus, hepatitis, emboli, abscesses, AIDS, and so on (see Section 6.2.7).
2. Apparent signs of a stroke can accompany the strong contraction of blood vessels caused by stimulants. These can progress to an ischemic stroke, with some data indicating that aspirin can be helpful for residual ischemic effects.[92–94]
3. A related phenomenon occurs in those individuals who snort cocaine. The constriction of blood vessels in the nasal mucosa can be so severe that the nasal septum is destroyed.
4. Another problem after snorting or smoking is possible aspiration subsequent to laryngeal or pharyngeal anesthesia.
5. Pulmonary problems can also develop after smoking stimulants, including cocaine. These range from localized irritation, such as bronchitis, through possible decreases in pulmonary diffusion abilities. Data also demonstrate a potentially lethal pulmonary hypertension and heart valve abnormalities as a consequence of some diet pills similar to fenfluramine.[95]
6. The elevated blood pressure that can accompany the use of stimulant drugs can cause an intracranial hemorrhage.
7. As briefly noted in Section 5.2.1, the rapid intake of any of these drugs, especially cocaine or methamphetamine, results in an increased heart rate and can progress to cardiac fibrillation, respiratory arrest, and death.[1,11] An associated phenomenon that occurs as a consequence of the stimulation of the heart as well as the spasms in cardiac blood vessels is the possibility of a myocardial infarction or heart attack, with numerous cases documented in otherwise healthy young adults.[96] These potentially lethal cardiac complications are likely to occur in both naive and in regular stimulant abusers.

8. Cocaine and other brain stimulants are also likely to cross the placenta to the fetus.[97] This can contribute to a decrease in the delivery of oxygen to the baby, and the direct effects of the stimulant might produce small-vessel and cardiac changes in the baby similar to those reported previously. Cocaine use during pregnancy contributes to an increase in spontaneous abortions, premature labor, and abruptio placentae, as well as in infants born with a low weight and an apparent (temporary) diminished response to the environment.[1,11,98] It should be noted that stimulants can be passed to a baby through breast milk.[99]
9. Some authors have discussed a possible "neonatal cocaine exposure syndrome" with poor feeding, tremor, irritation, and abnormal sleep patterns that can appear on day 2 and last 7–14 days. This might be followed by subtle behavioral changes of aggressiveness, impulsivity, and attention deficits lasting into the school years.[100]
10. The stereotyped behavior during intoxication can include bruxism (grinding of the teeth), which can wear down the teeth and cause dental difficulties.
11. A variety of skin problems, including scratches (secondary to delusions about bugs on the skin) and skin ulcers, can be noted.
12. Stimulant use is associated with an increased risk for violent death. These can occur through accidents, suicide, and homicide.
13. Other medical problems associated with cocaine or amphetamine include the possibility of liver damage, alterations in brain areas that control hormonal responses, impaired immune functioning, and enhanced replication of the HIV virus.[101]

REFERENCES

1. King, G. R., & Ellinwood, E. H. Amphetamines and other stimulants. In J. H. Lowinson, P. Ruiz, R. B. Millman, & J. G. Langrod (Eds.), *Substance Abuse: A Comprehensive Textbook* (4th ed.). Baltimore, MD: Lippincott, Williams & Wilkins, 2004, pp. 277–301.
2. O'Brien, C. P. Drug addiction and drug abuse. In J. G. Hardman, L. E. Limbird, A. G. Gilman (Eds.), *The Pharmacological Basis of Therapeutics* (10th ed.). New York: McGraw-Hill, 2001, pp. 621–642.
3. Gold, M. S., & Jacobs, W. S. Cocaine and crack: Clinical aspects. In J. H. Lowinson, P. Ruiz, R. B. Millman, & J. G. Langrod (Eds.), *Substance Abuse: A Comprehensive Textbook* (4th ed.). Baltimore, MD: Lippincott, Williams & Wilkins, 2004, pp. 218–251.
4. Repetto, M., & Gold, M. S. Cocaine and crack: Neurobiology. In J. H. Lowinson, P. Ruiz, R. B. Millman, & J. G. Langrod (Eds.), *Substance Abuse: A Comprehensive Textbook* (4th ed.). Baltimore, MD: Lippincott, Williams & Wilkins, 2004, pp. 195–217.
5. Morgan, J. P. Designer drugs. In J. H. Lowinson, P. Ruiz, R. B. Millman, & J. G. Langrod (Eds.), *Substance Abuse: A Comprehensive Textbook* (4th ed.). Baltimore, MD: Lippincott, Williams & Wilkins, 2004, pp. 367–373.
6. Numan, N. Exploration of adverse psychological symptoms in Yemeni khat users by the Symptoms Checklist-90 (SCL-90). *Addiction 99:*61–65, 2004.

7. Freedland, C. S., & Mansbach, R. S. Behavioral profile of constituents in ayahuasca, an Amazonian psychoactive plant mixture. *Drug and Alcohol Dependence 54:*183–194, 1999.
8. Toomey, R., Lyons, M. J., Eisen, S. A., Xian, H., Chantarujikapong, S., Seidman, L. J., Faraone, S. V., & Tsuang, M. T. A twin study of the neuropsychological consequences of stimulant abuse. *Archives of General Psychiatry 60:*303–310, 2003.
9. Strakowski, S. M., Sax, K. W., Rosenberg, H. L., DelBello, M. P., & Adler, C. M. Human response to repeated low-dose *d*-amphetamine: Evidence for behavioral enhancement and tolerance. *Neuropsychopharmacology 25:*548–554, 2001.
10. Taylor, J. R., & Jentsch, J. D. Repeated intermittent administration of psychomotor stimulant drugs alters the acquisition of Pavlovian approach behavior in rats: Differential effects of cocaine, *d*-amphetamine and 3,4-methylenedioxymethamphetamine ("Ecstasy"). *Biological Psychiatry 50:*137–143, 2001.
11. Jaffe, J. H. Amphetamine (or amphetaminelike)-related disorders. In B. J. Sadock & V. A. Sadock (Eds.), *Kaplan and Sadock's Comprehensive Textbook of Psychiatry* (7th ed.). Baltimore, MD: Williams & Wilkins, 2000, pp. 971–981.
12. Mendelson, J. H., & Mello, N. K. Cocaine and other commonly abused drugs. In D. L. Kasper, E. Braunwald, A. S. Fauci, *et al.* (Eds.), *Harrison's Principles of Internal Medicine* (16th ed.). New York: McGraw-Hill, 2004, pp. 2570–2572.
13. Harris, G. C., & Aston-Jones, G. Critical role for ventral tegmental glutamate in preference for a cocaine-conditioned environment. *Neuropsychopharmacology 28:*73–76, 2003.
14. Duarte, C., Lefebvre, C., Chaperon, F., Hamon, M., & Thiébot, M.-H. Effects of a dopamine D_3 receptor ligand, BP 897, on acquisition and expression of food-, morphine-, and cocaine-induced conditioned place preference, and food-seeking behavior in rats. *Neuropsychopharmacology 28:*1903–1915, 2003.
15. Lott, D. C., Kim, S.-J., Cook, E. H. Jr., & de Wit, H. Dopamine transporter gene associated with diminished subjective response to amphetamine. *Neuropsychopharmacology 30:*602-609, 2005.
16. DiCiano, P., Underwood, R. J., Hagan, J. J. & Everitt, B. J. Attenuation of cue-controlled cocaine-seeking by a selective D_3 dopamine receptor antagonist SB-277011-A. *Neuropsychopharmacology 28:*329–338, 2003.
17. DiCiano, P., & Everitt, B. J. Dissociable effects of antagonism of NMDA and AMPA/KA receptors in the nucleus accumbens core and shell on cocaine-seeking behavior. *Neuropsychopharmacology 25:*341–360, 2001.
18. Porras, G., DiMatteo, V., Fracasso, C., Lucas, G., DeDeurwaerdere, P., Caccia, S., Esposito, E., & Spampinato, U. 5-HT_{2A} and 5-$_{HtsC/2B}$ receptor subtypes modulate dopamine release induced in vivo by amphetamine and morphine in both the rat nucleus accumbens and striatum. *Neuropsychopharmacology 26:*311–324, 2002.
19. Centonze, D., Picconi, B., Baunez, C., Borrelli, E., Pisani, A., Bernardi, G., & Calabresi, P. Cocaine and amphetamine depress striatal GABAergic synaptic transmission through D2 dopamine receptors. *Neuropsychopharmacology 26:*164–175, 2002.
20. Hall, F. S., Drgonova, J., Goeb, M., & Uhl, G. R. Reduced behavioral effects of cocaine in heterozygous brain-derived neurotrophic factor (BDNF) knockout mice. *Neuropsychopharmacology 28:*1485–1490, 2003.
21. Fletcher, P. J., Chintoh, A. F., Sinyard, J., & Higgins, G. A. Injection of the 5-HT_{2C} receptor agonist Ro60-0175 into the ventral tegmental area reduced cocaine-induced locomotor activity and cocaine self-administration. *Neuropsychopharmacology 29:*308–318, 2004.
22. Volkow, N. D., Wang, G.-J., Fowler, J. S., Telang, F., Maynard, L., Logan, J., Gatley, S. J., Pappas, N., Wong, C., Vaska, P., Zhu, W., Swanson, J. M. Evidence that methylphenidate enhances the saliency of a mathematical task by increasing dopamine in the human brain. *American Journal of Psychiatry 161:*1173–1180, 2004.
23. Sekine, Y., Minabe, Y., Ouchi, Y., Takei, N., Iyo, M., Nakamura, K., Suzuki, K., Tsukada, H., Okada, H., Yoshikawa, E., Futatsubashi, M., & Mori, N. Association of dopamine transporter loss in the orbitofrontal and dorsolateral prefrontal cortices with

methamphetamine-related psychiatric symptoms. *American Journal of Psychiatry 160:*1699–1701, 2003.

24. Sora, I., Hall, F. S., Andrews, A. M., Itokawa, M., Li, X.-F., Wei, H.-B., Wichems, C., Lesch, K.-P., Murphy, D. L., & Uhl, G. R. Molecular mechanisms of cocaine reward: Combined dopamine and serotonin transporter knockouts eliminate cocaine place preference. *PNAS 98:*5300–5305, 2001.
25. Weiss, R. D., Griffin, M. L., Mazurick, C., *et al.* The relationship between cocaine craving, psychosocial treament, and subsequent cocaine use. *American Journal of Psychiatry 160:*1320–1325, 2003.
26. Martinez, D., Broft, A., Foltin, R. W., Slifstein, M., Hwang, D.-R., Huang, Y., Perez, A., Frankel, W. G., Cooper, T., Kleber, H. D., Fischman, M. W., Laruelle, M. Cocaine dependence and D_2 receptor availability in the functional subdivisions of the striatum: Relationship with cocaine-seeking behavior. *Neuropsychopharmacology 29:*1190–1202, 2004.
27. Neisewander, J. L., Fuchs, R. A., Tran-Nguyen, L. T. L., Weber, S. M., Coffey, G. P., Joyce, J. N. Increases in dopamine D_3 receptor binding in rats receiving a cocaine challenge at various time points after cocaine self-administration: Implications for cocaine-seeking behavior. *Neuropsychopharmacology 29:*1479–1487, 2004.
28. Giros, B., Jaber, M., Jones, S. R., *et al.* Hyperlocomotion and indifference to cocaine and amphetamine in mice lacking the dopamine transporter. *Nature 379:*606–612, 1996.
29. Coffin, P. O., Galea, S., Ahern, J., Leon, A. C., Vlahov, D., & Tardiff, K. Opiates, cocaine and alcohol combinations in accidental drug overdose deaths in New York City, 1990–98. *Addiction 98:*739–747, 2003.
30. Sizemore, G. M., Davies, H. M. L., Martin, T. J., & Smith, J. E. Effects of 2-propanoyl-3-(4-tolyl)-tropane (PTT) on the self-administration of cocaine, heroin, and cocaine/heroin combinations in rats. *Drug and Alcohol Dependence 73:*259–265, 2004.
31. DeVries, T. J., Schoffelmeer, A. N. M., Binnekade, R., Raaso, H., & Vanderschuren, L. J. M. J. Relapse to cocaine- and heroin-seeking behavior mediated by dopamine D2 receptors is time-dependent and associated with behavioral sensitization. *Neuropsychopharmacology 26:*18–26, 2002.
32. Pennings, E. J. M., Leccese, A. P., & de Wolff, F. A. Effects of concurrent use of alcohol and cocaine. *Addiction 97:*773–783, 2002.
33. Heil, S. H., Badger, G. J., & Higgins, S. T. Alcohol dependence among cocaine-dependent outpatients: Demographics, drug use, treatment outcome and other characteristics. *Journal of Studies on Alcohol 62:*14–22, 2001.
34. Harris, D. S., Everhart, E. T., Mendelson, J., & Jones, R. T. The pharmacology of cocaethylene in humans following cocaine and ethanol administration. *Drug and Alcohol Dependence 72:*169–182, 2003.
35. McCance-Katz, E. F., Kosten, T. R., & Jatlow, P. Concurrent use of cocaine and alcohol is more potent and potentially more toxic than use of either alone—a multiple-dose study. *Biological Psychiatry 44:*250–259, 1998.
36. Johnston, L. D., O'Malley, P. M., Bachman, J. G., & Schulenberg, J. E. *Monitoring the Future National Survey Results on Drug Use, 1975–2003, Vol. II: College Students and Adults Ages 19–40* (NIH Publication No. 04-5506). Bethesda, MD: National Institute on Drug Abuse, 2004.
37. Dolan, K., Rouen, D., & Kimber, J. An overview of the use of urine, hair, sweat, and saliva to detect drug use. *Drug and Alcohol Review 23:*213–217, 2004.
38. Oswald, L. M., Wong, D. F., McCaul, M., Zhou, Y., Kuwabara, H., Choi, L., Brasic, J., & Wand, G. S. Relationships among ventral striatal dopamine release, cortisol secretion, and subjective responses to amphetamine. *Neuropsychopharmacology 30:*821-832, 2005.
39. Mendelson, J. H., Sholar, M., Mello, N. K., *et al.* Cocaine tolerance: Behavioral, cardiovascular, and neuroendochrine function in men. *Neuropsychopharmacology 18:*263–271, 1998.

40. Barr, A. M., Hofmann, C. E., Weinberg, J., & Phillips, A. G. Exposure to repeated, intermittent *d*-amphetamine induces sensitization of HPA Axis to a subsequent stressor. *Neuropsychopharmacology 26:*286–294, 2002.
41. Segal, D. S., Kuczenski, R., O'Neil, M. L., Melega, W. P., & Cho, A. K. Escalating dose methamphetamine pretreatment alters the behavioral and neurochemical profiles associated with exposure to a high-dose methamphetamine binge. *Neuropsychopharmacology 28:*1730–1740, 2003.
42. Magendzo, K., & Bustos, G. Expression of amphetamine-induced behavioral sensitization after short- and long-term withdrawal periods: Participation of μ- and δ-opioid receptors. *Neuropsychopharmacology 28:*468–477, 2003.
43. Abarca, C., Albrecht, U., & Spanagel, R. Cocaine sensitization and reward are under the influence of circadian genes and rhythm. *PNAS 99:*9026–9030, 2002.
44. O'Brien, M. S. & Anthony, J. C. Risk of becoming cocaine dependent: Epidemiological estimates for the United States, 2000-2001. *Neuropsychopharmacology 30:*1006-1018, 2005.
45. Orsini, C., Koob, G. F., & Pulvirenti, L. Dopamine partial agonist reverses amphetamine withdrawal in rats. *Neuropsychopharmacology 25:*789–792, 2001.
46. Herning, R. I., Guo X., Better, W. E., *et al.* Neurophysiological signs of cocaine dependence: Increased electroencephalogram beta during withdrawal. *Biological Psychiatry 41*:1087–1094, 1997.
47. Alper, K. R., Prichep, L. S., Kowalik, S., *et al.* Persistent EEG abnormalities in crack cocaine users at 6 months of drug abstinence. *Neuropsychopharmacology 19*:1–9, 1998.
48. Tran-Nguyen, T. L., Fuchs, R. A., Coffey, G. P., *et al.* Time-dependent changes in cocaine-seeking behavior and extracellular dopamine levels in the amygdala during cocaine withdrawal. *Neuropsychopharmacology 19*:48–59, 1998.
49. Mitler, M. M., Guilleminault, E., Harsh, C., & Hirshkowitz, M. Randomized trial of moodafinil for the treatment of narcolepsy. *Annals of Neurology 43*:88–97, 1998.
50. Faraone, S. V., Biederman, J., Spencer, T., Wilens, T., Seidman, L. J., Mick, E., & Doyle, A. E. Attention-deficit/hyperactivity disorder in adults: An overview. *Biological Psychiatry 48:*9–20, 2000.
51. Wilens, T. E., Spencer, T. J., Biederman, J., Girard, K., *et al.* A controlled clinical trial of bupropion for attention deficit hyperactivity disorder in adults. *American Journal of Psychiatry 158:*282–288, 2001.
52. Substance Abuse and Mental Health Services Administration. *Overview of Findings from the 2002 National Survey on Drug Use and Health* (Office of Applied Studies, NHSDA Series H-21, DHHS Publication No. SMA 03-3774). Rockville, MD, 2003.
53. McCabe, S. E., Knight, J. R., Teter, C. J., & Wechsler, H. Non-medical use of prescription stimulants among US college students: Prevalence and correlates from a national survey. *Addiction 99:*96-106, 2005.
54. Mora, M. E., Villatoro, J., & Rojas, E. Drug use among students in Mexico's northern border states. In Department of Health and Human Services (Ed.), *Epidemiologic Trends in Drug Abuse.* Washington, DC: U.S. Government Printing Office, 1996, pp. 367–375.
55. Shaffer, H. J., & Eber, G. B. Temporal progression of cocaine dependence symptoms in the US National Comorbidity Survey. *Addiction 97:*543–554, 2002.
56. Baker, A., Boggs, T. G., & Lewin, T. J. Characteristics of regular amphetamine users and implications for treatment. *Drug and Alcohol Review 20:*49–56, 2001.
57. Brandon, C. L., Marinelli, M., Baker, L. K., & White, F. J. Enhanced reactivity and vulnerability to cocaine following methylphenidate treatment in adolescent rats. *Neuropsychopharmacology 25:*651–661, 2001.
58. Castner, S. A., & Goldman-Rakie, P. S. Amphetamine sensitization of hallucinatory-like behaviors is dependent on prefrontal cortex in nonhuman primates. *Biological Psychiatry 54:*105–110, 2003.
59. Schuckit, M. A. *Educating Yourself About Alcohol and Drugs.* New York: Plenum Publishing Co., 1998.

60. Tardiff, K., Marzuk, P. M., Leon, A. C., *et al.* Accidental fatal drug overdoses in New York City: 1990–1992. *American Journal of Drug and Alcohol Abuse 22*:135–146, 1996.
61. Witkin, J. M., Dijkstra, D., Levant, B., Akunne, H. C., Zapata, A., Peters, S., Shannon, H. E., & Gasior, M. Protection against cocaine toxicity in mice by the dopamine D_3/D_2 agonist *R*-(+)-*trans*-3,4*a*,10*b*-tetrahydro-4-propyl-2*H*,5*H*-[1]benzopryrano[4,3-*b*]-1,4-oxazin-9-ol [(+)-PD 128,907]. *The Journal of Pharmacology and Experimental Therapeutics 308:* 957–964, 2004.
62. Najarian, S. L. General management of the poisoned patient. *Emergency Medicine Manual* (6th ed.). New York: McGraw Hill Medical Publishing Division, 2004, pp. 467–475.
63. Witkin, J. M., Johnson, R. E., Jaffe, J. H., *et al.* The partial opioid agonist, buprenorphine, protects against lethal effects of cocaine. *Drug and Alcohol Dependence 27*:177–184, 1991.
64. Gao, Y., & Brimijoin, S. An engineered cocaine hydrolase blunts and reverses cardiovascular responses to cocaine in rats. *JPET* Fast Forward, Published on April 20, 2004.
65. Mello, N. K., & Mendelson, J. H. *Cocaine, Hormones, and Behavior: Clinical and Preclinical Studies, in Hormones, Brain and Behavior* (Vol. 5). Elsevier Science, 2002, pp. 665–745.
66. Drevets, W. C., Gautier, C., Price, J. C., Kupfer, D. J., Kinahan, P. E., *et al.* Amphetamine-induced dopamine release in human ventral striatum correlates with euphoria. *Biological Psychiatry 49:*81–96, 2001.
67. Suto, N., Tanabe, L. M., Austin, J. D., *et al.* Previous exposure to VTA amphetamine enhances cocaine self-administration under a progressive ratio schedule in an NMDA, AMPA/Kainate, and metabotropic glutamate receptor-dependent manner. *Neuropsychopharmacology 28:*629–639, 2003.
68. Tong, J., Ross, B. M., Schmunk, G. A., Peretti, F. J., Kalasinsky, K. S., Furukawa, Y., Ang, L. C., Aiken, S. S., Wickham, D. J., & Kish, S. J. Decreased striatal dopamine D_1 receptor-stimulated adenylyl cyclase activity in human methamphetamine users. *American Journal of Psychiatry 160:*896–903, 2003.
69. Carroll, K. M., Fenton, L. R., Ball, S. A., Nich, C., Frankforter, T. L., Shi, J., & Rounsaville, B. J. Efficacy of disulfiram and cognitive behavior therapy in cocaine-dependent outpatients: A randomized placebo-controlled trial. *Archives of General Psychiatry 61:*264–272, 2004.
70. Kampman, K. M., Volpicelli, J. R., Alterman, A. I., Cornish, J., *et al.* Amantadine in the treatment of cocaine-dependent patients with severe withdrawal symptoms. *American Journal of Psychiatry 157:*2052–2054, 2000.
71. Kaufman, M. J., Levin, J. M., Maas, L. C., Kukes, T. J., Villafuerte, R. A., Dostal, K., Lukas, S. E., Mendelson, J. H., Cohen, B. M., & Renshaw, P. F. Cocaine-induced cerebral vasoconstriction differs as a function of sex and menstrual cycle phase. *Biological Psychiatry 49:*774–781, 2001.
72. Lawton-Craddock, A., Nixon, S. J., & Tivis, R. Cognitive efficiency in stimulant abusers with and without alcohol dependence. *Alcoholism: Clinical and Experimental Research 27:*457–464, 2003.
73. Dalley, J. W., Theobald, D. E. H., Berry, D., Milstein, J. A., Laane, K., Everitt, B. J., & Robbins, T. W. Cognitive sequelae of intravenous amphetamine self-administration in rats: Evidence for selective effects on attentional performance. Neuropsychopharmacology 30:525-537, 2005.
74. Matsuzaki, H., Namikawa, K., Kiyama, H., Mori, N., & Sato, K. Brain-derived neurotrophic factor rescues neuronal death induced by methamphetamine. *Biological Psychiatry 55:*52–60, 2004.
75. Simon, S. L., Domier, C., Carnell, J., Brethen, P., Rawson, R., & Ling, W. Cognitive impairment in individuals currently using methamphetamine. *American Journal on Addictions 9:*222–231, 2000.
76. Christensen, J. D., Kaufman, M. J., Frederick, B., Rose, S. L., Moore, C. M., *et al.* Proton magnetic resonance spectroscopy of human basal ganglia: Response to cocaine administration. *Biological Psychiatry 48:*685–692, 2000.
77. Franklin, T. R., Acton, P. D., Maldjian, J. A., Gray, J. D., Croft, J. R., Dackis, C. A., O'Brien, C. P., & Childress, A. R. Decreased gray matter concentration in the insular,

orbitofrontal, cingulate, and temporal cortices of cocaine patients. *Biological Psychiatry 51:*134–142, 2002.

78. van Gorp, W. G., Wilkins, J. N., Hinkin, C. H., *et al.* Declarative and procedural memory functioning in abstinent cocaine abusers. *Archives of General Psychiatry 56*:85–89, 1999.
79. Nordahl, T. E., Salo, R., Natsuaki, Y., Galloway, G. P., Waters, C., Moore, C. D., Kile, S., & Buonocore, M. H. Methamphetamine users in sustained abstinence: A proton magnetic resonance spectroscopy study. *Archives of General Psychiatry 62:*444-452, 2005.
80. Chen, C.-K., Lin, S.-K., Sham, P. C., Ball, D., Loh, E.-W., Hsiao, C.-C., Chiang, Y.-L., Ree, S.-C., Lee, C.-H., Murray, R. M. Pre-morbid characteristics and co-morbidity of methamphetamine users with and without psychosis. *Psychological Medicine 33:*1407–1414, 2003.
81. Srisurapanont, M., Ali, R., Marsden, J., Sunga, A., Wada, K., & Monteiro, M. Psychotic symptoms in methamphetamine psychotic in-patients. *International Journal of Neuropsychopharmacology 6:*347–352, 2003.
82. Caton, C. L. M., Drake, R. E., Hasin, D. S., Dominguez, B., Shrout, P. E., Samet, S., & Schanzer, B. Differences between early-phase primary psychotic disorders with concurrent substance use and substance-induced psychoses. *Archives of General Psychiatry 62:*137-145, 2005.
83. Brown, E. S., Nejtek, V. A., Perantie, D. C., Thomas, N. R., & Rush, A. J. Cocaine and amphetamine use in patients with psychiatric illness: a randomized trial of typical antipsychotic continuation of discontinuation. *Journal of Clinical Psychopharmacology 23:*384–388, 2003.
84. Tsuang, J. W., Eckman, T. E., Shaner, A., *et al.* Clozapine for substance-abusing schizophrenic patients, letter. *American Journal of Psychiatry 156:*1119–1120, 1999.
85. Lambkin, F., Constable, P., Jenner, L., & Carr, V. J. Drug use patterns and mental health of regular amphetamine users during a reported 'heroin draught'. *Addiction 99:*875–884, 2004.
86. O'Leary, T. A., Rohsenow, D. J., Martin, R., Colby, S. M., Eaton, C. A., & Monti, P. M. The relationship between anxiety levels and outcome of cocaine abuse treatment. *American Journal of Drug and Alcohol Abuse 26:*179–194, 2000.
87. London, E. D., Simon, S. L., Berman, S. M., Mandelkern, M. A., Lichtman, A. M., Bramen, J., Shinn, A. K., Miotto, K., Learn, J., Dong, Y., Matochik, M. A., Kurian, V., Newton, T., Woods, R., Rawson, R., & Ling, W. Mood disturbances and regional cerebral metabolic abnormalities in recently abstinent methamphetamine abusers. *Archives of General Psychiatry 61:*73–84, 2004.
88. Garlow, S. J. Age, gender, and ethnicity differences in patterns of cocaine and ethanol use preceding suicide. *American Journal of Psychiatry 159:*615–619, 2002.
89. American Psychiatric Association. *The Diagnostic and Statistical Manual of Mental Disorders* (revised text). Washington, DC: American Psychiatric Press, 2000.
90. George, S. & Moselhy, H. Cocaine-induced trichotillomania. *Addiction 100:*255–256, 2005.
91. Hart, C. L., Ward, A. S., Collins, E. D., Haney, M., & Foltin, R. W. Gabapentin maintenance decreases smoked cocaine-related subjective effects, but not self-administration by humans. *Drug and Alcohol Dependence 73:*279–287, 2004.
92. Johnson, B. A., Devous, M. D., Sr., Ruiz, P., & Ait-Daoud, N. Treatment advances for cocaine-induced ischemic stroke: Focus on dihydropyridine-class calcium channel antagonists. *American Journal of Psychiatry 158:*1191–1198, 2001.
93. Kosten, T. R., Gottschalk, P. C., Tucker, K., Rinder, C. S., Dey, H. M., & Rinder, H. J. Aspirin or amiloride for cerebral perfusion defects in cocaine dependence. *Drug and Alcohol Dependence 71:*187–194, 2003.
94. Kosten, T. R., Tucker, K., Gottschalk, P. C., Rinder, C. S., & Rinder, H. M. Platelet abnormalities associated with cerebral perfusion defects in cocaine dependence. *Biological Psychiatry 55:*91–97, 2004.
95. Aurigemma, G. P., & Gaasch, W. H. Valve disease and diet pills—where do we stand? *American Family Physician 57*:659–660, 1998.
96. Lange, R. A., & Hillis, L. D. Cardiovascular complications of cocaine use. *New England Journal of Medicine 345:*351–358, 2001.

97. Smith, L. M., Chang, L., Yonekura, M. L., Gilbride, K., Kuo, J., Poland, R. E., Walot, I., & Ernst, T. Brain proton magnetic resonance spectroscopy and imaging in children exposed to cocaine in utero. *Pediatrics 107:*227–231, 2001.
98. Hulse, G. K., English, D. R, Milne, E., *et al.* Maternal cocaine use and low birth weight newborns: A meta-analysis. *Addiction 92*:1561–1570, 1997.
99. Vogel, G. Cocaine wreaks subtle damage on developing brains. *Science 278*:38–39, 1997.
100. Ito, S. Drug therapy for breast-feeding women. *The New England Journal of Medicine 343:*118–126, 2000.
101. Roth, M. D., Tashkin, D. P., Choi, R., Jamieson, B. D., Zack, J. A., & Baldwin, G. C. Cocaine enhances human immunodeficiency virus replication in a model of severe combined immunodeficient mice implanted with human peripheral blood leukocytes. *The Journal of Infectious Diseases 185:*701–705, 2002.

CHAPTER 6

Opioids and Other Analgesics

6.1. INTRODUCTION

This chapter is focused on painkilling drugs (analgesics). These range from propoxyphene (Darvon) to the synthetic, opiate-like drugs such as fentamyl (Sublimaze) and tramodol (Ultram), on to the more classical opiates such as codeine, morphine, and heroin. The generalizations made here apply to almost all prescription painkillers, with the exception of a few newer prescription anti-inflammatory medications, and are relevant to mixed agonist—antagonists such as butorphanol (Stadol), buprenorphene (Buprenex), and nalbuphene (Nubain).

It is worthwhile to take a moment and briefly review some terminology. The term *opiate* will be used to relate to the several drugs that are derived directly from opium, such as morphine and codeine. An *opioid*, however, is a broader term for all substances that are used as opiate-like analgesics or pain pills, or medications used to antagonize their effects. Therefore, there are at least 20 different prescription medications that fall into the opioid category, most of which are listed in Schedule I or II by the Federal Drug Administration, although several are in Schedule IV.

Opioids are useful and medically important drugs. Even heroin, which is rapidly converted to morphine in the body, has potent painkilling properties. As a group, however, these drugs are liable to be misused.

The use of opiates can be traced back to at least 4000 BC where the products of the opium poppy, *Papaver somniferum*, were taken by Sumerians, and to 2000 BC, when these drugs were used by the Egyptians.[1] The word opium comes from the Greek name for juice, reflecting the extraction of the active ingredients from the opium poppy itself. In 1806, opium was isolated from the juice, and subsequently, morphine (named after the Greek god of dreams) was identified, with codeine extracted in 1832.[2,3] In 1898, the Bayer Pharmaceutical Company synthesized diacetylmorphine (heroin), which was developed as a potentially less dependence-producing substitute for morphine.[4] Naturally occurring opiates were used widely in over-the-counter medicines in the latter part of the nineteenth century.

Problems associated with opiates have been noted since at least 1700, but it was not until around 1890 that physical dependence among opium smokers became an issue of broad concern. These problems were magnified by the more widespread availability of needles and syringes. As a result, the Hague Opium Conference of 1912 urged countries to control availability of these substances, and the Harrison Act of 1914 in the United States attempted to implement controls on availability. Although these steps had some effect, especially on the middle classes, problems continued, and in the early 1930s two federally funded treatment programs, to deal with prisoners with opioid dependence, were established in Ft. Worth, Texas, and in Lexington, Kentucky.

The search for safer and less dependence-producing synthetic opioids resulted in the development of meperidine (Demerol) at the end of World War II, and the recognition of the importance of antagonists and mixed agonist–antagonist drugs, such as nalorphine (Nalline) in the 1950s.

6.1.1. Pharmacology

See Section 10.4 for over-the-counter analgesics.

6.1.1.1. General Characteristics

The opiates include natural substances, such as opium, morphine, and codeine. The broader group of opioids include semisynthetic drugs produced by minor chemical alterations in the basic poppy products [e.g., heroin, hydromorphone (Dilaudid), and oxycodone (Percodan)]; and synthetic analgesics, such as propoxyphene (Darvon) and meperidine (Demerol; Table 6.1). Even some of the over-the-counter drugs such as cough suppressants with dextromethorphan and the antidiarrhea drug loperamide (Imodium), are opioid-like, and the former has been reported to be misused for opiate-like highs.[5,6] The relative potency of some of these drugs has been described in other texts and can be gauged by the usual doses, with a standard of 10 mg of morphine producing analgesia for the average individual.[2] Rough estimates of the relative dose potencies and the half-lives of these drugs are presented in Table 6.1.[1–3,7,8] In addition, there are a number of drugs where structures have been created to avoid legal restraint ("designer drugs"), many of which are variants of meperidine or fentanyl (Sublimaze).

As a group, the opioids undergo similar metabolism in the body but differ in their degree of oral absorption (ranging from low for heroin to high for propoxyphene). They also vary in their lipid solubility (high for heroin), and thus, the rate of transport into the CNS.[2,7] Detoxification occurs primarily in the liver, and the resulting metabolites are excreted through the urine and the

Table 6.1
Rough Analgesic Equivalent Doses and Half-Lives of Opioids

Drug type	Generic name	Trade name	Dose (mg)	Half-life (hours)
Analgesics	Codeine	–	65	3
	Fentanyl	Duragesic	0.1	3–4
	Heroin	–	20	0.05
	Hydromorphone	Dilaudid	2.5	2–3
	Meperidine	Demerol	100	3–4
	Methadone	Dolophine	5–10	15–30
	Morphine	–	20	2–3.5
	Opium	–	–	–
	Oxycodone	Percodan/Oxycontin	10	–
	Propoxyphene	Darvon	–	–
Mixed agonists–antagonists	Buprenorphene	Buprenex	0.4–0.8 Sublingual	3+
	Nalbuphene	Nubain	3–4 IM	5
	Pentazocine	Talwin	60	2–3
Antagonists	Cyclazocine	–	0.2–0.8	1.5–2
	Levallorphan	Lorfan	2–5	–
	Nalmefene	Revex	–	–
	Nalorphine	Nalline	3–5 IV	–
	Naloxone	Narcan	0.2–2 IV	1
	Naltrexone	Trexan/Revia	50–150	3

bile. Over 90% of the excretion of these drugs (with the exception of a very long-acting substance such as methadone) occurs within the first 24 h, although metabolites can be seen for 48 h or more.

6.1.1.2. Brain Mechanisms

There are three major families of endogenous opioid peptides (the endorphins, enkephalins, and dynorphans), and three major receptors (mu, kappa, and delta). Regarding the first type of receptors, all prescription opioids have a major impact on the *mu* receptor systems (named after morphius or morphine).[2,7,9,10] Activation of *mu* 1 or *mu* 2 receptors results in analgesia, euphoria, and a feeling of reinforcement, along with decreases in breathing rate, muscle tone, movement in the digestive tract (and resulting decreased appetite), and changes in hormones.

Kappa receptors, of which there are at least two varieties ($kappa_1$ and $kappa_3$), are named after their response to the substance ketocyclazine, and $kappa_1$ receptors are also responsive to butorphanol (Stadol).[2,7,8,11,12] Both $kappa_1$ and $kappa_3$ are affected by nalbuphene (Nubain) and pentazocine (Talwin), and also by morphine.[2] The activation of these receptors results in changes in analgesia (especially in the spinal cord), sedation, sleep, urine production, and the size of the pupil in the eye (miosis).[13] *Kappa* receptors are also understood to have an impact on the mood states (dysphoria) and appetite, but they do not play a major role in the reinforcement of drug actions in animals.[2,7]

The third major class of these proteins, *delta* receptors, consists of at least the two subgroups of *delta*$_1$ and *delta*$_2$. Their activation appears to have an impact on appetite, hormones, and might also contribute to analgesia.[2]

Research has also pointed toward the possible importance of another family of receptors, designated as *sigma*. Activation of these proteins can produce dysphoria and might contribute to the development of hallucinations. However, reflecting their lack of responsiveness to opioid antagonists such as naloxone, these are not usually considered true opioid receptors.[2]

Pure opioid antagonists can displace opioids from receptors and thus, antagonize, or block, their actions, but have no painkilling, reinforcing, or other properties of their own. Partial antagonists stimulate *mu* receptors, but only incompletely, with less than optimal subsequent receptor activity. Because they occupy the receptor but result in less than maximal actions, at higher doses the partial agonist–antagonists can precipitate withdrawal symptoms in individuals who are already physically dependent on agonists (such as heroin or methadone). As a consequence of their partial agonistic effects, these drugs do not produce as intense sedation or respiratory depression as is produced by the full agonists.

The stimulation of opioid receptors, especially those of the *mu* variety, has an important impact on the neurotransmitter dopamine.[14] This occurs throughout the brain, with a major effect on the "reward" system in the ventral tegmental area or VTA.[15–17] Dopamine pathways from the VTA to the nucleus accumbens and onto the cortex are key to the recognition of pleasure and perception of reward.[17,18] Important additional opioid actions are also observed in the NMDA, cholinergic, GABA, cannabinoid, and serotonin systems.[19–23] These various effects result in significant changes in regional blood flow, especially in the limbic system, when measured on functional brain imaging.

The generalities offered in this section apply fairly well across opioid drugs, even though there are differences in the usual doses, half-lives, and the most appropriate routes of administration as demonstrated in Table 6.1. Clinicians may occasionally need to review the specific pharmacology regarding the receptor subtypes most likely to be affected and the pharmacokinetic properties of the specific drug, to understand the actions that these agents have on specific patients.

6.1.1.3. Predominant Effects [Intoxication (292.89 in DSM-IV)]

All the substances listed in the two top categories of Table 6.1, result in analgesia, drowsiness, changes in mood (usually positive), and at high doses, a clouding of mental functioning through the depression of CNS activity.[2,7,8,24,25] Although there are some major differences in the way these drugs affect specific brain systems, the actions are homogeneous enough to allow for generalizations.

The acute intake of an opioid, especially intravenously (IV), is highly reinforcing.[2,7] The first minute or two after an injection of heroin is characterized as a "kick" or "rush" of feelings in the lower abdomen (resembling an orgasm), accompanied by a warm flushing of the skin. The latter, along with possible itching of the skin and the nose, is at least partially explained by a release of histamines that follows the administration of some *mu* agonists. Opioids also slow down contractions in the digestive tract, making them useful for the treatment of diarrhea [e.g., loperamide (Imodium) and one of the components of the medication Lomotil, diphenoxylate].[2] These drugs also decrease pupillary size (miosis), with the exception of meperidine for which atropine-like effects result in dilated pupils, and can produce twitching muscles and a tremor. The effects of the endorphins on hormones is likely to contribute to some other prominent effects of the opioids, including inhibition of gonadotropin-releasing hormone and of testosterone, as well as changes in menstrual functioning. The opioids also inhibit corticotropin (CRF) release, with resulting decreases in ACTH and cortisol.

6.1.1.4. Tolerance and Dependence (Abuse and Dependence are 305.50 and 304.00 in DSM-IV)

6.1.1.4.1. Tolerance

Tolerance develops rapidly to most opioids, particularly the more potent analgesics, and can increase the dose needs for some effects by as much as 100-fold.[1–3,7] However, the changes in organ sensitivity develop unevenly.[3,7,8] For example, high levels of tolerance can be expected for the opioid effects on respiratory depression, analgesia, sedation, and vomiting, as well as for the euphoric properties, while the same pattern of chronic use is likely to yield little tolerance for pupillary constriction (miosis) or for constipation.[3,7] As is true of most drugs within a class, cross-tolerance is common among the opioids, with a predictable variability depending on the opioid receptor type most prominently affected.

6.1.1.4.2. Dependence

These substances can cause both physical and psychological dependence.[7,8] The degree of dependence varies directly with the potency of the drug, the doses taken, and the length of exposure. Evidence of a rebound (or a withdrawal-like phenomenon) can be seen after a single 15 mg ingestion of morphine followed by an antagonist such as naloxone.[7] Therapeutic doses of morphine given twice a day [BID (Latin *bis in die*)] for 2 weeks or QID for 3 days can result in a mild withdrawal syndrome, especially if precipitated by a narcotic antagonist.[7] Thus, the use of opioids can produce any of the criteria for abuse or dependence listed in the DSM-IV.[26]

6.1.2. Epidemiology, Patterns, and Use

The sale of illicit opioids is a highly profitable business. Most of these drugs enter the United States illegally as part of an intricate economic-manufacturing-marketing complex that begins in Asia, the Middle East, Mexico, or South and Central America, with an estimated profit of sale price over costs of 1600-fold. The resulting drugs are administered through all routes, including oral (primarily the synthetic and semisynthetic opioids), IN (snorting), smoking (usually heating opium or heroin on tin foil and inhaling it through a straw, a process called "chasing the dragon"), and IV (especially heroin).[4,27,28]

After many years of low-level endemic use of opioids in the United States, the proportion of the population that used began to grow after World War II[2,7] and again in the 1960s. The prevalence of opioid misuse stabilized in middle-class population in the 1970s.[29]

Surveys over the past several decades support the importance of use, abuse, and dependence on opioid drugs, although the prevalence of these disorders is a good deal lower than alcohol, and not as high as figures relating to other illicit drugs. The 2002 National Survey on Drug Use and Health indicated that almost 170,000 (about 0.1% of Americans age 12 and older) had used heroin in the prior year, and almost 2 million (0.8%) had used a prescription opioid such as an extended-release form of oxycodone (Oxycontin) for intoxication at some time in their lives. In this survey, in 2002 about 350,000 men and women (0.15% of the population) had received treatment for misuse of an opioid analgesic, and 235,000 (0.12%) entered care for heroin. It was estimated that among those who used heroin, almost 55% developed abuse or dependence, while the same thing was true for an estimated 15% of those who self-administered prescription analgesics for a high.

Additional data come from the yearly, Monitoring the Future Study.[29] In 2003, 17% of young adults admitted to ever having used an analgesic for a high, with almost 2% reported ever having used heroin. These figures included about 8 and 0.4%, respectively who had used either drug in the prior year. Among high school seniors, 14% admitted to ever having used an opioid for a high, with almost 2% acknowledging the intake of heroin. For this younger population, figures for the prior 12 months were 9 and 1%, respectively.

The figures for most other countries are lower than those reported for the United States.[30,31] For example, a 1997 survey from Spain, of individuals aged 18 and older, revealed a lifetime prevalence for heroin of 0.6%, whereas in high school students in northern Mexico, the rate was about 0.5%. The lifetime prevalence of DSM-IV abuse and dependence of opioids in these countries is difficult to establish, but it is certainly much lower than for alcohol, stimulants, or cannabinoids.

6.1.3. Natural History

Despite large variations in course across individuals, some generalizations can be made. The usual heroin or other street drug user begins taking opioids occasionally, usually orally, but may progress to daily use, with tolerance and physical dependence rapidly following the transition to IV administration (which is often unplanned and frequently occurs through initiation by a friend).[32] This pattern is the one most likely to come to the attention of medical and mental health personnel as well as the police.

However, a number of individuals continue to take the drug only occasionally over an extended period of time, even when they use it by needle—i.e., subcutaneously (SQ) or intravenously. The exact number of people "chipping" these drugs is not known, but it is probable that they show a much higher level of life stability, having family, friends, and a job, than is true of the usual repeat user.

A related phenomenon is seen in individuals who are physically dependent, but who manage to hold jobs and to function fairly well socially. Another important observation grew out of Vietnam, where large numbers of soldiers with little or no prior experience with opioids found themselves in a situation of high stress and with drugs readily available.[33] Under such circumstances, as many as half of those given the opportunity did try opioids. Although many became physically dependent, those who had not used drugs before Vietnam tended to return to a drug-free status when back in their home communities.

The average street users tend to be young males, about half of whom demonstrate a prior history of delinquent behavior (the more severe the antisocial problems, the greater the chance of continued drug use).[34,35] Their average age of first use of *any* drug (which is usually marijuana) tends to be the mid-teens; the first use of heroin occurs at about 18; physical dependence emerges in the early 20s; and the first treatment in the mid-20s. Most users begin by experimenting with more readily available drugs, then try opioids orally or through smoking, and subsequently progress to IV use, although there is much variability in this pattern.[36–38] Those who are opioid dependent and also qualify for a diagnosis of the antisocial personality disorder, carry a worse prognosis for violent behavior and for continued drug and antisocial problems than the "average" street user.[35] Even here, however, there is likely to be a decrease in criminal activity with increasing age.[39]

The short-term prognosis for opioid-dependent men and women is relatively poor, with up to 90% returning to drugs within the first 6 months after treatment. However, this is followed by a trend toward an increasing percentage achieving abstinence over time.[34] Although the majority tend to show repeated exacerbations and remissions, long-term follow-ups (up to 30 years) have demonstrated that a third or more of people who are opioid dependent, even those impaired severely enough to be treated in a jail-hospital setting like the Federal facility in Lexington, Kentucky, are finally able to achieve abstinence.

The course for the remainder is far from benign, with at least a quarter dead at follow-up and one quarter still dependent.[40–43] The yearly mortality rate for opioid-dependent people is about 5–10 per thousand, with especially high levels of death from suicide, homicide, accidents, and diseases such as tuberculosis, AIDS, and other infections.

If remission occurs, it can be seen at any time, with a probable peak after age 40. When an opioid-dependent person remains abstinent for 3 years or longer, there is a good chance that he or she will not go back to drugs. Good prognostic signs include a history of relatively stable employment, being married, a history of few delinquent acts, little evidence of dependence on other substances, and few criminal activities unrelated to drugs.[33,38,44]

6.1.4. Concurrent Drug Use

Most opioid-dependent persons begin their substance problems with tobacco and alcohol, and then progress to marijuana and other drugs of abuse.[36,45] Because ethanol is legal, readily available, and does not always lead to dismissal from drug-treatment programs, people who are opioid dependent tend towards alcohol when their primary drug is not available, as alcohol can be used to boost the effects of other drugs.[45,46] Perhaps as many as 50% of men and 25% of women with opioid dependence meet the criteria for alcohol dependence within the first 5 years after active opioid involvement. The prevalence is higher in drug-treatment dropouts than it is in those who stay with therapy, and the progression to dependence is more likely in individuals who have a history of prior alcohol problems.

Several other drugs of abuse are also relatively closely associated with opioid dependence. First, perhaps to enhance the overall high or to diminish some of the side effects of intoxication, many opioid-dependent individuals inject cocaine at the same time in a mixture known as a "speedball".[8,46,47] Second, the combination of pentazocine (Talwin) along with the antihistamine tripelennamine (usually available in a blue colored pill under the street name of Ts and blues.)[7], is used by some individuals who are opioid dependent. A similar practice is seen when another opioid, codeine, is used in conjunction with the antihistamines and the ingredients of cough syrup.[48,49] Finally, the concomitant use of Bzs and opioids has become increasingly popular in some locales, and it is considered to be a special common problem among individuals on methadone maintenance.

6.1.5. Medical Abuse and Dependence

The misuse of opioids in medical settings has not been well studied, probably because it is not associated with an exceptionally high rate of death, serious crimes, or violence. Two groups of individuals stand out as being at high risk for this syndrome. First, it has been suggested that a substantial minority of people with pain syndromes misuse their prescribed drugs.[50,51] The second important subgroup, health-care professionals (especially physicians and nurses), may have the highest rate of analgesic drug abuse and dependence of any middle-class population.[52,53] Possible explanations include the stresses of caring for other people's problems, the manner in which their job interferes with their ability to relate to their families, the long hours of their jobs, and the ready availability of drugs.

6.1.6. Establishing the Diagnosis

Diagnosis requires an awareness of the possibility of opioid misuse in all patients. In addition, there are a number of physical symptoms, signs, and behavioral patterns to watch for, including the following:

1. Increased pigmentation over veins.
2. Evidence of clotted or thrombosed veins.
3. Other skin lesions and abscesses.
4. Clubbing of the fingers, possibly secondary to phlebitis.[54]
5. Constricted or small pupils (except with hydromorphone).
6. Swollen nasal mucosa (if the drug is "snorted").
7. Swollen lymph glands.
8. An enlarged liver.
9. Abnormal laboratory tests, including decreased globulins, evidence of AIDS, a positive latex fixation test [Venereal Disease Research Laboratory (VDRL) test], liver-function test abnormalities, and a relatively high white blood count.
10. Evidence of visiting many physicians (perhaps to get a supply of drugs), a complex medical history that is hard to follow, or a de novo visit with complaints of severe pain (e.g., kidney pain, back pain, headache, or abdominal pain), even with physical signs, as these signs are easy to produce at will (e.g., by placing a drop or two of blood in a urine sample).
11. Any health professional being seen for a syndrome for which analgesics might be prescribed.
12. Unexpected evidence of opioids on a blood or urine toxicological screen.

6.2. EMERGENCY PROBLEMS

The emergency difficulties most frequently seen with the opioids are toxic reactions (i.e., overdose) and medical problems.

6.2.1. Toxic Reactions or Overdose

See Sections 2.2.1 and 13.2.

6.2.1.1. Clinical Picture

6.2.1.1.1. History

The opioid overdose is usually an acute, life-threatening event that is most often accidental but that could represent a deliberate suicide attempt.[2,7,8,46,55–57] At least one overdose is likely to occur during the course of 50% of heroin users.[58] The patient is likely to be found in a semi-comatose condition with evidence of a recent IV injection (e.g., a needle in the arm or nearby). The risk for such deaths varies with a variety of factors, including an increasing risk with higher-quality heroin or use of a more potent opioid such as fentanyl (probably related to an overriding of any existing levels of tolerance), and a negative association with price, so the less the drug costs, the greater is the risk for death. Quinine, sometimes used to dilute the heroin, can itself create a major problem, as it can decrease the activity of the cardiac pacemaker, decrease cardiac electrical conductivity, and thereby induce a prolonged cardiac electrical refractory period that increases the risk for ventricular fibrillation.[59]

6.2.1.1.2. Physical Signs and Symptoms

Physical problems dominate the clinical picture. Specific symptoms depend on the opioid taken, how long ago it was ingested, and the patient's general condition. The range of symptomatology can include the following:

1. Decreased respiration.
2. Blue lips and pale or blue skin.
3. Pinpoint pupils (unless there is brain damage, in which case the pupils may be dilated).
4. Nasal mucosa hyperemia (for a patient snorting the drug).
5. Recent needle marks or a needle in the arm.
6. Pulmonary edema characterized by gasping, rattling respirations of unknown etiology (not related to heart failure), and a state of shock.[7]
7. Cardiac arrhythmias and/or convulsions, especially seen with codeine, propoxyphene (Darvon), or meperidine (Demerol).[2,7]
8. Death may result from a combination of respiratory depression and pulmonary and/or cerebral edema.[2,7] The pulmonary edema may be related to an idiosyncratic reaction to the opioid, shock, or may be an allergic response either to the drug or to one of the adulterants (such as quinine) in the injected substance. An alternate hypothesized mechanism is the possible development of cardiac arrhythmias, perhaps related to histamine release.

6.2.1.1.3. Psychological State

The patient is usually markedly lethargic or comatose.

6.2.1.1.4. Relevant Laboratory Tests

See Section 2.2.1.1.4.

It is necessary to rule out other causes of coma, such as head trauma (with a physical exam, a neurological evaluation, skull x-rays, etc.) and glucose or electrolyte abnormalities (as shown in Table 1.6). The level of cardiac functioning must be established with an EKG, and the level of brain impairment with an EEG if appropriate. A toxicological blood or urine screen may be helpful.

6.2.1.2. Treatment

See Section 2.2.1.2.

It has been suggested that the medical needs of the overdosed opioid-dependent person can be divided into emergency, acute, and subacute stages.[2,7] As outlined in Table 6.2, the general supports first address problems expected in any medical emergency. The general order in which the levels of care are listed are as follows:

1. Establish an adequate airway; intubate and place on a respirator if necessary, using compressed air at a rate of 10–12 breaths per minute unless pulmonary edema is present.

Table 6.2
Opioid Overdose: Signs, Symptoms, and Treatment

Symptoms
Unconscious and difficult to arouse
Blue lips and skin
Small pupils
Needle marks
Pulmonary and/or cerebral edema
Hypothermia
Decreased respiration
Treatment
Clear airway
Assist respiration
Treat hypotension with expanders or pressors
Treat arrhythmias
Positive-pressure oxygen if needed
Naloxone 0.4 mg (1 ml) IV; repeat Q 2–3 h as needed
Monitor 24+ h

2. Be sure there is a pulse; defibrillate, or administer intracardiac epinephrine if needed; also, give 50 ml of sodium bicarbonate by IV drip for serious cardiac depression.
3. Prevent aspiration either by positioning the patient on his side or by using a tracheal tube with an inflatable cuff.
4. Begin an IV (large-gauge needle), being prepared to replace fluids lost to urine plus 20 ml/h for insensible loss if the coma persists.
5. Deal with blood loss or hypotension with plasma expanders or pressor drugs as needed.
6. Treat pulmonary edema with positive-pressure oxygen, but beware of giving too much oxygen and thus, decreasing the respiratory drive.
7. Treat cardiac arrhythmias with the appropriate drug.
8. Administer a narcotic antagonist:
   a. Naloxone (Narcan) is the preferred initial drug, given in doses of 0.2–0.4 mg (1 ml) or 0.01 mg/kg IV, to be repeated in 3–10 min if no reaction occurs. Some authors suggest IV doses of 0.8 mg for each 70 kg of weight. Because this drug wears off in 2–3 h, it is important to monitor the patient's vital signs for at least 24 h for heroin and for 72 h for longer acting drugs such as methadone. Be prepared to deal with an opioid abstinence syndrome, precipitated by the narcotic antagonist (see Section 6.2.2.2).
   b. If naloxone is not available, use nalorphine (Nalline), 3–5 mg IV (1 cc = 5 mg), repeated as necessary.
9. Monitor arterial blood gases if there are respiratory problems.
10. Draw blood for baseline laboratory tests, including complete blood count (CBC) and the usual blood panel series, as well as a toxicological screen (10 cc). If hypoglycemia is involved, administer 50 cc of 50% glucose IV.
11. Establish vital signs every 15 min for 4 h, with continued careful monitoring for 24–72 h.
12. The more subacute and chronic care involve careful patient monitoring, dealing with withdrawal signs, and treating infections (over one half of individuals with pulmonary edema go on to develop pneumonia, but prophylactic antibiotics are not justified). Continue to monitor vital signs and laboratory tests, and consider tetanus immunization.
13. While treating an overdose, it is very important to beware of the possibility of mixed drug ingestion. Some clinicians suggest using 0.2 mg/min of flumazenil (Romazicon), up to 3 mg in an hour, as a precaution in case a benzodiazepine overdose might also exist (see Chapter 2). However, beware regarding problems described in Chapter 2, including depressant withdrawal and convulsions.

Table 6.3
Acute Opioid (Heroin) Withdrawal

Beginning in hours, peak in 36–72 h
Marked drive for the drug
Onset in 8–12 h, peak in 48–72 h
Tearing
Running nose
Yawning
Sweating
At 12–14 h, peaking in 48–72 h
Restless sleep
Beginning in 12 h, peaking in 48–72 h
Dilated pupils
Anorexia
Gooseflesh
Irritability
Tremor
At peak
Insomnia
Violent yawning
Weakness
Gastrointestinal (GI) upset
Chills
Flushing
Muscle spasm
Ejaculation
Abdominal pain

6.2.2. Opioid Withdrawal (292.0 in DSM-IV)

6.2.2.1. Opioid Withdrawal in the Adult

See Sections 2.2.2 and 4.2.2.

A withdrawal syndrome can be seen for all the opioid agonists discussed in this chapter including propoxyphene (Darvon), tramadol (Ultram), and buprenorphene (Buprenex).[60–63] Along with alcohol withdrawal, this was among the first of the well-described abstinence pictures. While somewhat arbitrary distinction between phases of withdrawal is outlined in Table 6.3, these phases overlap greatly.

6.2.2.1.1. Clinical Picture

6.2.2.1.1.1. Acute Withdrawal

1. *History:* Withdrawal usually begins at the time of the next habitual drug dose, ranging from 4 to 12 h for heroin, to 1–3 days or more for long-acting opioids such as methadone.[2,7] The acute abstinence

syndrome with heroin lasts 5 days or so, and withdrawal from methadone for at least several weeks. Acute withdrawal conditions are likely to be followed by months of decreasing symptoms as part of a protracted withdrawal.[64]

The prevalence and intensity of this picture increase directly with the dose and the duration of use, and inversely with the level of health, although there are large inter-individual differences.[2,7] The diagnosis may be fairly obvious when the patient demonstrates the physical signs and symptoms as well as the psychological state described, that follows and requests opioids, but frequently the clinician must have a suspicion that opioids may be a problem and probe for potential dependence and withdrawal.

The most usual withdrawal syndrome is a moderately intense mixture of emotional, behavioral, and physical symptoms.[2,7,65] This less severe picture may reflect the variability in the potency of heroin obtained on the street, ranging from 0 to 77% (with most around 5–10%). Adulterants, such as lidocaine, procaine, quinine, and lactose, make up most of the substances sold as street opioids.[2,7]

2. *Physical signs and symptoms:* Although variability can be expected, it is possible to make some generalizations for heroin and morphine.[2,7] Variations from the usual "heroin-like" picture outlined include methadone (a slower development of symptoms, a less intense clinical picture, persistence of acute problems for 3 weeks or more once they have developed), hydromorphone (Dilaudid) (small rather than large pupils during withdrawal, along with muscle twitching and only mild GI complaints), and codeine (tendency of symptoms to be relatively mild).[2,7] With these examples aside, the usual heroin or morphine withdrawal can be said to have the following characteristics:
   a. Within 6–12 h of the last dose, physical discomfort begins, characterized by tearing of the eyes, a runny nose, sweating, and yawning.
   b. Within 12–14 h, and peaking on the second or third day, the patient moves into a restless sleep (a "yen").
   c. Over the same time period, other symptoms begin to appear, including dilated pupils, loss of appetite, gooseflesh (hence the term "cold turkey"), back pain, and a tremor.
   d. This picture gives way to insomnia; incessant yawning; a flu-like syndrome consisting of weakness, GI upset, chills, and flushing; muscle spasm; ejaculation; and abdominal pain.
   e. The acute symptoms of withdrawal decrease in intensity by the fifth day, markedly improving in 1 week to 10 days.
3. *Psychological state:* As important as physical problems, these include a strong "craving" along with emotional *irritability*.

4. *Relevant laboratory tests:* For the usual moderate withdrawal, it is usually enough to carry out a good physical exam and to establish the baseline laboratory functions described in Table 1.6. Specific test results can include a decrease in carbon dioxide values secondary to increased respiratory rates, a possible increase in the WBC (e.g., 14,000 cells × 10^3 μ), and occasionally ketosis.[2,7] A toxicological screen may be helpful in establishing the most recent drugs used.

6.2.2.1.1.2. Protracted Abstinence

The acute abstinence phase is followed by a more protracted withdrawal, with two probable subphases.[8,64] The initial stage lasts from 4 to 10 weeks or longer, and consists of mild increases in blood pressure, temperature, respirations, and pupillary diameter. This is followed by a later phase lasting 30 weeks or more, consisting of mild decreases in the same signs with a lower respiratory response to carbon dioxide. The resulting vague discomfort may play an important role in driving the addict back to drug use.

6.2.2.1.2. Treatment

Also review Section 2.2.2.2.

Treatment of the opioid withdrawal syndrome in adults is briefly outlined in Table 6.4. However, detoxification alone is rarely sufficient for continued abstinence. Helping the patient achieve relative comfort and offering reassurance and good general supports during this period may be associated with a higher rate of retention of patients in rehabilitation.[66–69]

1. The first phase includes a good medical examination.
2. The caregiver must develop rapport to maximize cooperation.
3. After estimating the probable degree of physical dependence and thereby deciding whether pharmacological treatment is needed, it is

Table 6.4
Treatment of Short-Acting Opioid Withdrawal (e.g., Heroin)

General support:
Physical and laboratory exam
Rest
Nutrition
Reassurance
Appraisal of what symptoms are to be expected
Keep one doctor in charge
Example of opioid based treatment
Methadone 15–20 mg orally as a test
Determine dose on day 1 or 2
Give needed dose BID
Decrease by 20% per day or over 2 weeks

important to carefully explain the symptoms to expect, and that, while they cannot be totally eliminated, you will do everything you can to minimize his discomfort.

4. Establish a flow sheet of symptom severity and the treatments.
5. One treatment approach can begin with the re-administration of an opiate to greatly reduce symptoms on day 1, after which the drug dose is slowly decreased over a period of 5–14 days.[2,7] The focus should be on objective withdrawal signs, not subjective complaints.[70] Most jurisdictions in the US have restrictions on the prescription of opioids to dependent individuals. Unless the physician or clinic possesses a special license, treatment is usually limited to 72 h, and that too only in case of a medical emergency. Even if a permit is granted, detoxification is usually limited to a month or less. Therefore, I will first outline detoxification using opioids (the most "physiological" way to treat the syndrome), and then discuss alternate approaches.
   a. Any opioid can be used, but most authors recommend oral methadone.[2,7,8,71,72]
      i. Give a test of about 20 mg of methadone orally, repeating the dose if the symptoms are not alleviated, thus determining the minimum dose needed to control symptoms during the first 24–36 h. Note that 1 mg of methadone roughly equals 1.5 mg of oxycodone,[2,7] 2 mg of heroin, or 20 mg of meperidine (Demerol). This may require giving an opioid every 4 h until the symptoms significantly improve or the respiratory rate decreases to no less than 16 breaths per minute.[70]
      ii. Most people in withdrawal respond to 20–40 mg of methadone the first day. The necessary drug is then divided into twice- to four-times-daily doses, with daily decreases of 10–20% of the first day's dose, depending on the development of symptomatology.
   b. Similar approaches are used if another opioid is used. In general, a dose that markedly decreases withdrawal symptoms is established on the first day, after which the drug used for detoxification is decreased over about a 5-day period for dependencies on shorter-acting drugs like heroin, or over a 2–3 week period for detoxification from longer-acting opioids such as methadone, or a long-acting oxycodone form (OxyContin). In the past, protocols have been proposed using propoxyphene (Darvon), diphenoxylate (the opioid contained in the antidiarrheal medication Lomotil) and others.

      Some recent studies have focused on using the mixed opioid agonist–antagonist, buprenorphine (Buprenex). For detoxification, or as part of opioid maintenance, buprenorphine is sold as Subutex (2 and 8 mg sublingual—SL-tablets), or in a 4:1 ratio with the opioid antagonist naloxone as Suboxone (with the 2 and 8 mg tablets combined with 0.5 and 2 mg of naloxone, respectively). The combined drug is thought to be less likely to be misused for a high. A typical detox protocol would begin about 6 h following the last heroin dose, giving 2–4 mg SL in the morning, and 0–4 mg in the afternoon, depending upon the emergence of the symptoms. On day 2, the original day's dose (roughly 4–8 mg) should be decreased by 2 mg if the patient is showing signs of intoxication with the buprenorphine, but might be increased to as high as 16 mg total in 24 h, if moderately severe withdrawal symptoms remain. Doses are subsequently decreased from 2 to 4 mg of the prior day's dose, with the goal of stopping the drug by day 5–8.[73,74] Some physicians have recommended a longer period of taper (up to a month), but a shorter period should suffice for the average detoxification. Buprenorphine is also used for opioid maintenance treatment for a year or longer, as discussed in detail in Chapter 14.

c. A special case occurs when an individual has been taking part in a methadone-maintenance program. If they decide to stop the methadone, the withdrawal symptoms might be less intense but more long lasting than heroin detoxification, although not all studies agree.[75] Under these circumstances, it is advisable to decrease the methadone slowly to minimize the chance of development of symptoms. This usually means a diminution of approximately 3 mg from the daily dose each week, but even at this rate, some symptoms will be seen.

6. The most common detoxification approach for opioid-dependent patients was developed in response to the legal restrictions against prescribing opioids to dependent individuals for problems other than physical pain. This combination of medications addresses the symptoms of opioid withdrawal, recognizing that, in contrast to problems seen during depressant-drug withdrawal (see Chapter 2), opioid withdrawal is rarely, if ever, lethal and is not associated with convulsions or states of agitated confusion (delirium). At the core of the treatment are efforts to diminish autonomic nervous system overactivity through the use of alpha adrenergic agonists.[76] The most commonly used drug is clonidine (Catapres) at about 0.1–0.3 mg given two times per day.[2,7,8,77,78] The dose is titrated up to as much as 0.3 mg TID depending on the patient's withdrawal symptoms while monitoring vital signs to avoid hypotension or excessive sedation. Clonidine can also be administered as a transdermal skin patch combined with oral medications on day 1, along with one or two Catapres TTS-1 (0.1 mg dose) transdermal patches for the average 150-pound person, using oral doses of clonidine in addition if

needed. These elements of treatment (along with the others mentioned below) should be decreased in dose over approximately 5–7 days for a heroin-dependent individual, and over several weeks or more for patients withdrawing from longer-acting drugs such as methadone.

Additional symptomatic treatment is offered during the withdrawal period. These include the "as needed" use of loperamide (Imodium) for abdominal pain and diarrhea, non-opioid analgesics for the control of pain (e.g., 500 mg of naproxen) (e.g., Aleve) twice a day, nasal decongestants as needed, and the judicious use of benzodiazepines for relief of daytime anxiety (e.g., Diazepam or Valium 5–10 mg BID or TID) and for sleep [e.g., temazepam (Restoril) 15–30 mg HS].

7. An additional variation for the treatment of opioid withdrawal uses an opioid antagonist such as naltrexone (e.g., ReVia) to precipitate withdrawal in a highly sedated (sometime anesthetized) patient.[66,79,80] I do not recommend these approaches as the cost and dangers may not be justified. After a careful physical evaluation including an electrocardiogram, individuals can be treated with any of several procedures. One approach carried out in a hospital (sometimes using an intensive care unit) uses general anesthesia, intubation, and oxygen administration, giving IV naloxone 2 mg at 30 min intervals up to a total of 12 mg. IV clonidine can be used to diminish withdrawal symptoms, along with ajunctive medication (e.g., octreotide or Sandostatin IV) to diminish gastrointestinal symptoms. Following 4 h of anesthesia, the procedure is stopped and subjects allowed to wake up.[66] Other investigators have carried out ultra-rapid precipitated withdrawal using naltrexone (e.g., 50 mg prior to sedation), and some have used high levels of sedation without intubation.[81] While withdrawal can be precipitated effectively, it is not clear whether the potential physical dangers and high costs of these approaches offer any advantages over the usual treatment.

   A variation on this procedure (known as rapid detoxification) is usually carried out in an inpatient alcohol- and drug-treatment setting. Here, withdrawal is usually precipitated with naloxone (0.2–1.2 mg/day) or naltrexone (e.g., 1–10 mg every 4 h during the first several days, building up to a 50 mg dose on day 3–5). Patients are treated with clonidine and other symptomatic treatments described above, with one study using an opioid agonist (e.g., buprenorphine) to also help alleviate withdrawal symptoms.[81,82] While not as costly as ultra-rapid detoxification, this approach is still potentially dangerous, and it is not clear if it has any advantages regarding longer-term outcome.

8. Additional potential treatments include acupuncture, hypnosis, transcranial electrical stimulation, and additional approaches that possibly increase the body's own opiates, the endorphins.[7,83] However, few, if any, controlled data are available.
9. During detoxification, it is very important to institute plans for rehabilitation. Some patients enter detoxification primarily to decrease their need for high drug doses or in response to immediate life problems, and may not want to participate in a rehabilitation program. However, for those who might consider rehabilitation, the detoxification period is an excellent time to introduce the need for permanent abstinence, and counseling should be offered to everyone.

6.2.2.2. Opioid Withdrawal in the Neonate

A special case of opioid withdrawal is seen in the newborn, made passively dependent through the mother's dependence during the latter part of pregnancy.[2,7,63,84,85] However, physical dependence of the infant is only one part of the wide span of severe problems likely to accompany the use of opioids by pregnant women.[83] Difficulties also include elevated rates of intrauterine death, low-birth-weight infants, premature delivery, and up to a 5% or higher risk for neonatal mortality. In one series, only 31% of children delivered to women who were heroin dependent were free of potentially serious complications.

6.2.2.2.1. Clinical Picture

The syndrome consists of a high-pitched cry (seen in 90%), irritability, a tremor (in 80%), increased reflexes, increased respiratory rate, diarrhea, hyperactivity (seen in 60%), sweating (in 50%), vomiting (seen in 40%), and sneezing/yawning/hiccuping (in 30%).[83,86,87] The child usually has a low birth weight but may be otherwise unremarkable until the first or second day, when the symptoms usually begin. For children of women who are methadone dependent, symptoms might not appear until day 3 or 4 or even later, and, if the dose of methadone taken by the mother has been stable, the infant's withdrawal might be less severe.[2,7,86,87]

6.2.2.2.2. Treatment

1. A first step should be prevention. For pregnant dependent women on methadone maintenance, it is important that the drug be reduced to as low as possible during the last 6 weeks of pregnancy. If this cannot be done, efforts should be made to be sure that the dose is stable and to help the mother avoid the use of heroin.
2. Symptoms in the infant may indicate other disorders as well, and the clinician must carefully rule out hypoglycemia, hypocalcemia,

infections, CNS trauma, or anoxia and must aggressively treat any such syndromes that are uncovered.

3. Treatment of neonatal withdrawal consists of general support and observation, including keeping the child in a warm, quiet environment and monitoring electrolytes, glucose, and other physiological parameters.
4. In addition, the child with moderate to severe symptoms can be treated with paregoric, a total of 4 drops/kg/day, which translates to about 0.2 ml orally every 3–4 h as needed to control symptoms.[2,7] Doses can be increased up to a total of about 2 ml/kg/day in divided doses if needed.[88] Other approaches include a daily total of methadone, 0.1–0.5 or more mg/kg; or phenobarbital, 8 mg/kg; or diazepam, 2–5 mg, with any of these drugs being given in divided doses three or four times a day. Medications should be given for 10–20 days, the amounts being decreased toward the end of that period. Remember that, as is true throughout this text, the medications and doses noted here are very general guidelines that must be adjusted for the specific situation.
5. It is also possible to treat the physically dependent infants of mothers on methadone maintenance by having them breast-feed while they continue to take their methadone. Additional drugs can be given to the child as needed.

6.2.3. Delirium, Dementia, and Other Cognitive Disorders (292.81 in DSM-IV)

See Section 1.7.3

States of confusion are unusual with opioids except as part of an obvious overdose. One possible exception is the state of agitated confusion that can be seen with meperidine, perhaps related to its effects on acetylcholine[89] and possible neuropsychological impairments following long-term high-dose opioid use.[90] Finally, confusion can be seen when high doses of an antihistamine is taken with an opioid (e.g., Ts and blues).

6.2.4. Psychosis (292.81, 292.11, and 292.12 in DSM-IV)

See Section 1.7.4.

Unlike stimulants and depressants, the opioids are not likely to produce a substance-induced psychoses that resembles schizophrenia.[7] The exceptions are seen with individuals who ingest multiple drugs, including cocaine and heroin in a "speedball," where the stimulant is responsible for the psychotic symptoms.[46]

6.2.5. Flashbacks

The sedating nature and relatively short half-lives of most of these drugs, as well as their rapid disappearance make flashbacks unlikely.

6.2.6. Anxiety and Depression (292.84 and 292.9 in DSM-IV)

As is true with all sedating drugs of abuse, intoxicated individuals tend to be slowed down rather than panicked. Thus, severe states of anxiety are usually limited to those associated with drug-seeking behavior during withdrawal.

The major psychiatric symptom likely to be noted in people who are opioid dependent is sadness (rather than intense, long lasting, persistent major depressive episodes, such as those reported for alcohol).[9,91] However, at the time of entrance into treatment, between one third and two third of those with opioid dependence are likely to report some depressive symptoms.[92] Perhaps 20% may meet the criteria for major depressive disorders at intake, but these figures decrease to 10% showing major depressions at 3- to 6-month follow-ups, with only 2% of the sample demonstrating significant depression at both the points.[92,93] Some of the depression associated with opioid misuse may be pharmacologically and/or situationally induced, and symptoms tend to disappear within a relatively short time even without active antidepressant treatment. Such pictures are perhaps twice as likely to be seen in women as in men at treatment intake, but follow-ups show no differences in persisting depressions between the sexes. It should be remembered, however, that if depressions persist for more than 4 weeks and still meet the criteria for major depressive episodes, the judicious use of antidepressants should be considered (see Section 3.1.2.3 on alcohol-related depressions).

6.2.7. Medical Problems

When opioids are taken in their pure form (i.e., without adulterants) in moderate doses, even their long-term use is not necessarily associated with severe medical problems.[2,7,8] However, people with opioid dependence, especially those taking street drugs, frequently present for care in a medical crisis. This may be an overdose or other serious medical problem as a consequence of the adulterants in drug mixtures or the use of non-sterile needles.[46,94–97]

The most common deadly medical complication associated with IV drug use (with most of the individuals demonstrating dependence on heroin) is human immunodeficiency virus (HIV) infection.[7,98,99] Among IV drug users, the rate of positive tests for this infection is as high as 60%, depending on the city and the subpopulation evaluated. For individuals who do not enter formal treatment, the rate of new HIV infection (or seroconversion) may be greater than 22% over an 18-month period.[100] For those who actively participate in methadone maintenance, the conversion rate over the 18-month period was 3.5%.[100] While most HIV infections in this population result from sharing contaminated needles, many men and women who were infected by heterosexual activity acquired their disease through sex partners who were IV users. More than 70% of children infected with HIV had mothers who either were IV drug users or had had heterosexual contact with such individuals.

Efforts to stem the tide of this epidemic have focused on expanded numbers of treatment programs, education, needle exchange programs, and better access to methadone maintenance. These appear to help.

Another major relevant health problem, one that affects at least 4 million Americans is chronic hepatitis C virus (HCV) infection.[101,102] It has been estimated that the majority of newly acquired infections result from IV drug users who share needles, with an estimate that two thirds of such individuals eventually become HCV positive. This form of hepatitis frequently remains as a chronic infection with subsequent significantly elevated risks for both cirrhosis and liver cancer. The treatment includes interferon, and, reflecting the demanding nature of the regimen and the high levels of side effects, most programs recommend that drug-dependent individuals receive treatment for their dependence so that abstinence can be achieved and maintained for a period of time before the institution of antiviral treatments. Continuation of drug use or heavy drinking in the context of interferon not only diminishes the chance of a successful response, but is likely to add to the risk for side effects including depression and anxiety.

Additional problems associated with opioid dependence, especially in the context of IV drug use, include the following:

1. Abscesses and other infections of the skin and muscle, including *Clostridium botulinum*.[94]
2. Possible fetal damage, perhaps in part reflecting gene changes induced by the drug.[103]
3. Hepatitis and other liver abnormalities (60–80% of IV users test positive for hepatitis B antibodies).[7,104]
4. Meningitis.
5. Gastric ulcers.
6. Heart arrhythmias.
7. Endocarditis.
8. Anemias.
9. Electrolyte abnormalities, especially hyperkalemia.
10. Bone and joint infections.
11. Eyeground abnormalities, as they reflect emboli from the adulterant added to the street drug.
12. Kidney failure secondary to infections or adulterants.
13. Muscle destruction.
14. Pneumonia.
15. Lung abscesses.
16. Tuberculosis.
17. Bronchospasm and wheezing, especially likely after inhalation of opioid fumes (chasing the dragon).

18. Sexual functioning abnormalities, which may partially reflect the transiently low testosterone level seen during chronic administration and lasting at least a month after the opiate is stopped.[71,105]

These highlight the importance of a careful medical evaluation for all opioid-dependent patients.

6.3. REHABILITATION

After identification and acute treatment, all opioid-dependent individuals should be advised of the need for rehabilitation to help them abstain from street drugs. Such treatment is usually done through methadone-maintenance clinics, drug-free residential programs, or a variety of outpatient approaches. In keeping with my emphasis on acute drug problems, rehabilitation is discussed separately in Section 14.3.

REFERENCES

1. Simon, E. J. Opiates: Neurobiology. In J. H. Lowinson, P. Ruiz, R. B. Millman, & J. G. Langrod (Eds.), *Substance Abuse: A Comprehensive Textbook* (4th ed.). Baltimore, MD: Williams & Wilkins, 2004, pp. 164–179.
2. Knapp, C. M., Ciraulo, D. A., & Jaffe, J. Opiates: Clinical aspects. In J. H. Lowinson, P. Ruiz, R. B. Millman, & J. G. Langrod (Eds.), *Substance Abuse: A Comprehensive Textbook* (4th ed.). Baltimore, MD: Williams & Wilkins, 2004, pp. 180–194.
3. Gutstein, H. B., & Akil, H. Opioid analgesics. In J. G. Hardman, L. E. Limbird, & A. G. Goodman (Eds.), *The Pharmacological Basis of Therapeutics* (10th ed.). New York, NY: McGraw-Hill, 2001, pp. 569–620.
4. Springer, A. Heroin control: A historical overview. *European Addiction Research 2:*177–184, 1996.
5. Jun, J. H., Thorndike, E. B., & Schindler, C. W. Abuse liability and stimulant properties of dextromethorphan and diphenhydramine combinations in rats. *Psychopharmacology 172:*277–282, 2004.
6. Kirages, T. J., Sule, H. P., & Mycyk, M. B. Severe manifestations of coricidin intoxication. *American Journal of Emergency Medicine 21:*473–475, 2003.
7. Jaffe, J. H. Opioid-related disorders. In B. J. Sadock & V. A. Sadock (Eds.), *Comprehensive Textbook of Psychiatry* (7th ed.). Baltimore, MD: Williams & Wilkins, 2000, pp. 1038–1062.
8. Schuckit, M. A., & Segal, D. S. Opioid drug abuse and dependence. In D. L. Kasper, E. Brauwald, A. S. Fauci, *et al.* (Eds.), *Harrison's Principles of Internal Medicine* (16th ed.). New York: McGraw-Hill, 2004, pp. 2567–2569.
9. Zubieta, J.-K., Ketter, T. A., Bueller, J. A., Xu, Y., Kilbourn, M. R., Young, E. A., & Koeppe, R. A. Regulation of human affective responses by anterior cingulate and limbic μ-opioid neurotransmission. *Archives of General Psychiatry 60:*1145–1153, 2003.
10. Sora, I., Elmer, G., Funada, M., Pieper, J., Li, X-F., Hall, F. S., & Uhl, G. R. μ-Opiate receptor gene dose effects on different morphine actions: Evidence for differential *in vivo* μ-receptor reserve. *Neuropsychopharmacology 25:*41–54, 2001.
11. Hjelmstad, G. O., & Fields, H. L. Kappa opioid receptor activation in the nucleus accumbens inhibits glutamate and GABA release through different mechanisms. *Journal of Neurophysiology 89:*2389–2395, 2003.
12. Margolis, E. B., Hjelmstad, G. O., Bonci, A., & Fields, H. L. Kappa opioid agonists directly inhibit midbrain dopaminergic neurons. *Journal of Neuroscience*, in press.

13. Schlaepfer, T. E., Strain, E. C., Greenberg, B. D., Preston, K. L., Lancaster, E., Bigelow, G. E., Barta, P. E., & Pearlson, G. D. Site of opioid action in the human brain: Mu and kappa agonists' subjective and cerebral blood flow effects. *American Journal of Psychiatry 155:*4, 1998.
14. De Vries, T. J., Schoffelmeer, A. N. M., Binnekade, R., Raaso, H., & Vanderschuren, L. J. M. J. Relapse to cocaine- and heroin-seeking behavior mediated by dopamine D2 receptors is time-dependent and associated with behavioral sensitization. *Neuropsychopharmacology 26:*18–26, 2002.
15. Koob, G. F., & LaMoal, M. Drug addiction, dysregulation of reward, and allostasis. *Neuropsychopharmacology 24:*97–129, 2001.
16. Nestler, E. J., & Malenka, R. C. The addicted brain. *Scientific American 290:*78–85, 2004.
17. Kalivas, P. W. Neurocircuitry of addiction, In *Neuropsychopharmacology: The Fifth Generation of Progress* (Chap. 95) 1357–1366, 2002.
18. Goldstein, R. Z., & Volkow, N. D. Drug addiction and its underlying neurobiological basis: Neuroimaging evidence for the involvement of the frontal cortex. *American Journal of Psychiatry 159:*1642–1652, 2002.
19. Basile, A. S., Fedorova, I., Zapata, A., Liu, X., Shippenberg, T., Duttaroy, A., Yamada, M., & Wess, J. Deletion of the M_5 muscarinic acetylcholine receptor attenuates morphine reinforcement and withdrawal but not morphine analgesia. *PNAS 99:*11452–11457, 2002.
20. Steingart, R. A., Abu-Roumi, M., Newman, M. E., Silverman, W. F., Slotkin, T. A., & Yanai, J. Neurobehavioral damage to cholinergic systems caused by prenatal exposure to heroin or phenobarbital: Cellular mechanisms and the reversal of deficits by neural grafts. *Developmental Brain Research 122:*125–133, 2000.
21. Jones, K. L., Zhu, H., Jenab, S., Du, T., Inturrisi, C. E., & Barr, G. A. Attenuation of acute morphine withdrawal in the neonatal rat by the competitive NMDA receptor antagonist LY235959. *Neuropsychopharmacology 26:*301–310, 2002.
22. Porras, G., DiMatteo, V., Fracasso, C., Lucas, G., DeDeurwaerdere, P., Caccia, S., Esposito, E., & Spampinato, U. $5\text{-}HT_{2A}$ and $5\text{-}_{HtsC/2B}$ receptor subtypes modulate dopamine release induced in vivo by amphetamine and morphine in both the rat nucleus accumbens and striatum. *Neuropsychopharmacology 26:*311–324, 2002.
23. Vigano, D., Cascio, M. G., Rubino, T., Fezza, F., Vaccani, A., DiMarzo, V., & Parolaro, D. Chronic morphine modulates the contents of the endocannabinoid, 2-arachidonoyl glycerol, in rat brain. *Neuropsychopharmacology 23:*1160–1167, 2003.
24. Darke, S., Sims, J., McDonald, S., & Wickes, W. Cognitive impairment among methadone maintenance patients. *Addiction 95:*687–695, 2000.
25. Senne, I., Zourelidis, C., Irnich, D., Kurz, M., Hummel, T., & Zwissler, B. Central anticholinergic syndrome and apnea after general anesthesia. A rare manifestation of the central anticholinergic syndrome. *Anaethesist 52:*608–611, 2003.
26. American Psychiatric Association. *The diagnostic and statistical manual of mental disorders* (text rev.). Washington, DC: American Psychiatric Press, 2000.
27. Strang, J., Griffiths, P., & Gossop, M. Heroin in the United Kingdom: Different forms, different origins and the relationship to different routes of administration. *Drug and Alcohol Review 16:*329–337, 1997.
28. Strang, J., Griffiths, P., & Gossop, M. Heroin smoking by 'chasing the dragon': Origins and history. *Addiction 92:*673–683, 1997.
29. Johnston, L. D., O'Malley, P. M., & Bachman, J. G. *Monitoring the Future National Survey Results on Drug Use, 1975–2003. Vol. I: Secondary School Students* (NIH Publication No. 04-5507). Bethesda, MD: National Institute on Drug Abuse, 2004.
30. Royo-Bordonada, M. A., Cid-Ruzafa, J., Martin-Moreno, J. M., & Guallar, E. Drug and alcohol use in Spain: Consumption habits, attitudes and opinions. *Public Health 111:*277–284, 1997.
31. Mora, M. E., Villatoro, J., & Rojas, E. Drug use among students in Mexico's northern border states. In Department of Health and Human Services (Ed.), *Epidemiologic Trends in Drug Abuse*. Washington, DC: U.S. Government Printing Office, 1996, pp. 367–375.

32. Crofts, N., Louie, R., Rosenthal, D., & Jolley, D. The first hit: Circumstances surrounding initiation into injecting. *Addiction 91:*1187–1196, 1996.
33. Robins, L. N. Vietnam veterans' rapid recovery from heroin addiction: A fluke or normal expectation? *Addiction 88:*1041–1054, 1993.
34. Hser, Y. I., Hoffman, V., Grella, C. E., & Anglin, M. D. A 33-year follow-up of narcotics addicts. *Archives of General Psychiatry 58:*503–508, 2001.
35. Myers, M. G., Stewart, D. G., & Brown, S. A. Progression from conduct disorder to antisocial personality disorder following treatment for adolescent substance abuse. *American Journal of Psychiatry 155:*479–485, 1998.
36. Labouvie, E., & White, H. R. Drug sequences, age of onset, and use trajectories as predictors of drug abuse/dependence in young adulthood. In D. B. Kandel (Ed.), *Stages and Pathways of Drug Involvement: Examining the Gateway Hypothesis.* Cambridge, MA: Cambridge University Press, 2002, pp. 19–41.
37. Lynskey, M. T., Heath, A. C., Bucholz, K. K., Slutske, W. S., Madden, P. A. F., Nelson, E. C., Statham, D. J., & Martin, N. G. Escalation of drug use in early-onset cannabis users vs co-twin controls. *Journal of the American Medical Association 289:*427–433, 2003.
38. Strang, J., Griffiths, P., Powis, B., & Gossop, M. First use of heroin: Changes in route of administration over time. *British Medical Journal 304:*1222–1223, 1992.
39. Hanlon, T. E., Nurco, D. N., Kinlock, T. W., & Duszynski, K. R. Trends in criminal activity and drug use over an addiction career. *American Journal of Drug and Alcohol Abuse 16:*223–238, 1990.
40. Hulse, G. K., English, D. R., Milne, E., & Holman, C. D. J. The quantification of mortality resulting from the regular use of illicit opiates. *Addiction 94:*221–229, 1999.
41. Frischer, M., Goldberg, D., Rahman, M., & Berney, L. Mortality and survival among a cohort of drug injectors in Glasgow, 1982–1994. *Addiction 92:*412–427, 1997.
42. Gossop, M., Stewart, D., Treacy, S., & Marsden, J. A prospective study of mortality among drug misusers during a 4-year period after seeking treatment. *Addiction 97:*39–47, 2002.
43. Quaglio, G., Talamini, G., Lechi, A., Venturini, L., Lugoboni, F., Gruppo Intersert di Collaborazione Scientifica (GICS), & Mezzelani, P. Study of 2708 heroin-related deaths in north-eastern Italy 1985–98 to establish the main causes of death. *Addiction 96:*1127–1137, 2001.
44. Epstein, D. H., & Preston, K. L. Does cannabis use predict poor outcomes for heroin-dependent patients on maintenance treatment? Past findings and more evidence against. *Addiction 98:*269–279, 2003.
45. Kandel, D. B., & Davies, M. High school students who use crack and other drugs. *Archives of General Psychiatry 53:*71–80, 1996.
46. Coffin, P. O., Galea, S., Ahern, J., Leon, A. C., Vlahov, D., & Tardiff, K. Opiates, cocaine and alcohol combinations in accidental drug overdose deaths in New York City, 1990–98. *Addiction 98:*739–747, 2003.
47. Mello, N. K., & Negus, S. S. Effects of indatraline and buprenorphine on self-administration of speedball combinations of cocaine and heroin by Rhesus monkeys. *Neuropsychopharmacology 25:*104–117, 2001.
48. Mattoo, S. K., Basu, D., Sharma, A., Balaji, M., & Malhotra, A. Abuse of codeine-containing cough syrups: A report from India. *Addiction 92:*1783–1787, 1997.
49. Elwood, W. N. Sticky business: Patterns of procurement and misuse of prescription cough syrup in Houston. *Journal of Psychoactive Drugs 33:*121–133, 2001.
50. Trafton, J. A., Oliva, E. M., Horst, D. A., Minkel, D., & Humphreys, K. Treatment needs associated with pain in substance use disorder patients: Implications for concurrent treatment. *Drug and Alcohol Dependence 73:*23–31, 2004.
51. Stack, K., Cortina, J., Samples, C., Zapata, M., & Arcand, L. F. Race, age, and back pain as factors in completion of residential substance abuse treatment by veterans. *Psychiatric Services 51:*1157–1161, 2000.

52. Hughes, P. H., Storr, C. L., Brandenburg, N. A., Baldwin, D. C., Anthony, J. C., & Sheehan, D. V. Physician substance use by medical specialty. *Journal of Addictive Diseases 18:*23–37, 1999.
53. de Wet, C. J., Reed, L. J., & Bearn, J. The rise of buprenorphine prescribing in England: Analysis of NHS regional data, 2001-2003. *Addiction 100:*495-499, 2005.
54. Chotkowski, L. A., Clubbing of the fingers in heroin addiction. *New England Journal of Medicine 311:*262, 1984.
55. Powis, B., Strang, J., Griffiths, P., Taylor, C., Williamson, S., Fountain, J., & Gossop, M. Self-reported overdose among injecting drug users in London: Extent and nature of the problem. *Addiction 94:*471–478, 1999.
56. Darke, S., & Ross, J. Suicide among heroin users: Rates, risk factors and methods. *Addiction 97:*1383–1394, 2002.
57. Warner-Smith, M., Darke, S., & Day, C. Morbidity associated with non-fatal heroin overdose. *Addiction 97:*963–967, 2002.
58. McGregor, C., Darke, S., Ali, R., & Christie, P. Experience of non-fatal overdose among heroin users in Adelaide, Australia: Circumstances and risk perceptions. *Addiction 93:*701–711, 1998.
59. Ruttenbar, A. J., & Luke, J. L. Heroin-related deaths: New epidemiologic insights. *Science 226:*14–20, 1984.
60. Obadia, Y., Perrin, V., Feroni, I., Vlahov, D., & Moatti, J. P. Injecting misuse of buprenorphine among French drug users. *Addiction 96:*267–272, 2001.
61. Jenkinson, R. A., Clark, N. C., Fry, C. L., & Dobbin, M. Buprenorphine diversion and injection in Melbourne, Australia: An emerging issue. *Addiction 100:*197-205, 2005.
62. Woody, G. E., Senay, E. C., Geller, A., Adams, E. H., Inciardi, J. A., Schnoll, S., Muñoz, A., & Cicero, T. J. An independent assessment of MEDWatch reporting for abuse/dependence and withdrawal from Ultram (tramadol hydrochloride). *Drug and Alcohol Dependence 72:*163–168, 2003.
63. Kayemba-Kay, S., & Laclyde, J. P. Buprenorphine withdrawal syndrome in newborns: A report of 13 cases. *Addiction 98:*1599–1604, 2003.
64. Harris, G. C., & Aston-Jones, G. Altered motivation and learning following opiate withdrawal: Evidence for prolonged dysregulation of reward processing. *Neuropsychopharmacology 28:*865–871, 2003.
65. Chang, G., & Kosten, T. R. Detoxification. In J. H. Lowinson, P. Ruiz, R. B. Millman, & J. G. Langrod (Eds.), *Substance Abuse: A Comprehensive Textbook* (4th ed.). Baltimore, MD: Williams & Wilkins, 2004, pp. 579–586.
66. Ali, R., Thomas, P., White, J., McGregor, C., Danz, C., Gowing, L., Stegink, A., & Athanasos, P. Antagonist-precipitated heroin withdrawal under anesthetic prior to maintenance naltrexone treatment: Determinants of withdrawal severity. *Drug and Alcohol Review 22:*425–431, 2003.
67. Amato, L., Davoli, M., Ferri, M., Gowing, L., & Perucci, C. A. Effectiveness of interventions on opiate withdrawal treatment: An overview of systematic reviews. *Drug and Alcohol Dependence 73:*219–226, 2004.
68. Ling, W., Huber, A., & Rawson, R. A. New trends in opiate pharmacotherapy. *Drug and Alcohol Review 20:*79–94, 2001.
69. Chutuape, M. A., Jasinski, D. R., Fingerhood, M. I., & Stitzer, M. L. One-, three-, and six-month outcomes after brief inpatient opioid detoxification. *American Journal of Drug and Alcohol Abuse 27:*199–44, 2001.
70. Fishbain, D. A., Rosomoff, H. L., Cutler, R., & Rosomoff, R. S. Opiate detoxification protocols. *Annals of Clinical Psychiatry 5:*53–65, 1993.
71. Schuckit, M. A. *Educating Yourself About Alcohol and Drugs.* New York: Plenum Publishing Co., 1998.
72. Oliver, P., Horspool, M., & Keen J. Fatal opiate overdose following regimen changes in naltrexone treatment. *Addiction 100:*560-563, 2005.

73. Lintzeris, N. Buprenorphine dosing regime in the management of out-patient heroin withdrawal. *Drug and Alcohol Review 21:*39–45, 2002.
74. Kosten, T. R. Buprenorphine for opioid detoxification. A brief review. *Addictive Disorders & Their Treatment 2:*107–112, 2003.
75. Gossop, M., & Strang, J. A comparison of the withdrawal responses of heroin and methadone addicts during detoxification. *British Journal of Psychiatry 158:*697–699, 1991.
76. Gowing, L. R., Farrell, M., Ali, R. L., & White, J. M. α_2-Adrenergic agonists in opioid withdrawal. *Addiction 97:*49–58, 2002.
77. O'Connor, P. G., Carroll, K. M., Shi, J. M., Schottenfeld, R. S., Kosten, T. R., & Rounsaville, B. J. Three methods of opioid detoxification in a primary care setting: A randomized trial. *Annals of Internal Medicine 127:*526–530, 1997.
78. McCann, M. J., Miotto, K., Rawson, R. A., Huber, A., Shoptaw, S., & Ling, W. Outpatient non-opioid detoxification for opioid withdrawal: Who is likely to benefit? *American Journal of Addiction 6:*218–223, 1997.
79. De Jong, C. A. J., Laheij, R. J. F., & Krabbe, P. F. M. General anaesthesia does not improve outcome in opioid antagonist detoxification treatment: A randomized controlled trial. *Addiction 100:*206-215, 2005.
80. Roozen, H. G., de Kan, R., van den Brink, W., Kerkhof, A. J. F. M., & Geerlings, P. J. Dangers involved in rapid opioid detoxification while using opioid antagonists: Dehydration and renal failure. *Addiction 97:*1071–1073, 2002.
81. O'Connor, P. G., & Kosten, T. R. Rapid and ultrarapid opioid detoxification techniques. *Journal of the American Medical Association 279:*229–234, 1998.
82. Hall, W., Mattick, R. P., Saunders, J. B., & Wodak, A. Rapid opiate detoxification treatment. *Drug and Alcohol Review 16:*325–327, 1997.
83. Han, J.-S., Trachtenberg, A. I., & Lowinson, J. H. Acupuncture. In J. H. Lowinson, P. Ruiz, R. B. Millman, & J. G. Langrod (Eds.), *Substance Abuse: A Comprehensive Textbook* (4th ed.). Baltimore, MD: Williams & Wilkins, 2004, pp. 743–762.
84. Finnegan, L. P., & Kandall, S. R. Maternal and neonatal effects of alcohol and drugs. In J. H. Lowinson, P. Ruiz, R. B. Millman, & J. G. Langrod (Eds.), *Substance Abuse: A Comprehensive Textbook* (4th ed.). Baltimore, MD: Williams & Wilkins, 2004, pp. 805–839.
85. Schindler, S. D., Eder, H., Ortner, R., Rohrmeister, K., Langer, M., & Fischer, G. Neonatal outcome following buprenorphine maintenance during conception and throughout pregnancy. *Addiction 98:*103–110, 2003.
86. Hulse, G. K., Milne, E., English, D. R., & Holman, C. D. The relationship between maternal use of heroin and methadone and infarct birth weight. *Addiction 92:*1571–1579, 1997.
87. Hulse, G. K., Milne, E., English, D. R., & Holman, C. D. Assessing the relationship between maternal opiate use and neonatal mortality. *Addiction 93:*1033–1042, 1998.
88. Finnegan, L. P. Neonatal abstinence syndrome: Assessment and pharmacotherapy. In F. F. Rubaltelli & B. Granati (Eds.), *Neonatal Therapy: An Update*. New York: Elsevier, 1986, pp. 122–146.
89. Mintzer, M. Z., Copersino, M. L., & Stitzer, M. L. Opioid abuse and cognitive performance. *Drug and Alcohol Dependence 78:*225–230, 2005.
90. Rogers, R. D., Everitt, B. J., Baldacchino, A., Blackshaw, A. J., Swainson, R., Wynne, K., Baker, N. B., Hunter, J., Carthy, T., Booker, E., London, M., Deakin, J. F., Sahakian, B. J., & Robbins, T. W. Dissociable deficits in the decision-making cognition of chronic amphetamine abusers, opiate abusers, patients with focal damage to prefrontal cortex, and tryptophan-depleted normal volunteers: Evidence for monoaminergic mechanisms. *Neuropsychopharmacology 20:*322–339, 1999.
91. Marsden, J., Gossop, M., Stewart, D., Rolfe, A., & Farrell, M. Psychiatric symptoms among clients seeking treatment for drug dependence: Intake data from the National Treatment Outcome Research Study. *British Journal of Psychiatry 176:*285–289, 2000.
92. Handelsman, L., Aronson, M. J., Ness, R., Cochrane, K. J., & Kanof, P. D. The dysphoria of heroin addiction. *American Journal of Drug and Alcohol Abuse 18:*275–287, 1992.

93. Teesson, M., Havard, A., Fairbairn, S., Ross, J., Lynskey, M., & Darke, S. Depression among entrants to treatment for heroin dependence in the Australian Treatment Outcome Study (ATOS): Prevalence, correlates and treatment seeking. *Drug and Alcohol Dependence 78:*309-315, 2005.
94. Passaro, D. J., Werner, S. B., McGee, J., MacKenzie, W. R., & Vugia, D. J. Wound botulism associated with black tar heroin among injecting drug users. *Journal of the American Medical Association 279:*859–863, 1998.
95. Dinwiddie, S. H., Reich, T., & Cloninger, C. R. Lifetime complications of drug use in intravenous drug users. *Journal of Substance Abuse 4:*13–18, 1992.
96. Warner-Smith, M., Darke, S., Lynskey, M., & Hall, W. Heroin overdose: Causes and consequences. *Addiction 96:*1113–1125, 2001.
97. Burnam, M. A., Bing, E. G., Morton, S. C., Sherbourne, C., Fleishman, J. A., London, A. S., Vitiello, B., Stein, M., Bozzette, S. A., & Shapiro, M. F. Use of mental health and substance abuse treatment services among adults with HIV in the United States. *Archives of General Psychiatry 58:*729–736, 2001.
98. Gostin, L. O., Lazzarini, Z., Jones, T. S., & Flaherty, K. Prevention of HIV/AIDS and other blood-borne diseases among injection drug users. *Journal of the American Medical Association 277:*53–62, 1997.
99. Nguyen, T. A., Hoang, L. T., Pham, V. Q., & Detels, R. Risk factors for HIV-I seropositivity in drug users under 30 years old in Haiphong, Vietnam. *Addiction 96:*405–413, 2001.
100. Metzger, D. S., Woody, G. E., McLellan, A. T., O'Brien, C. P., Druley, P., Navaline, H., DePhilippis, D., Stolley, P., & Abrutyn, E. Human immunodeficiency virus seroconversion among intravenous drug users in- and out-of-treatment: An 18-month prospective follow-up. *Journal of Acquired Immunodeficiency 6:*1049–1056, 1993.
101. Davis, G. L., & Rodriguez, J. R. Treatment of chronic hepatitis C in active drug users. *New England Journal of Medicine 345:*215–217, 2001.
102. Dolan, K. A., Shearer, J., White, B., Zhou, J., Kaldor, J., & Wodak, A. D. Four-year follow-up of imprisoned male heroin users and methadone treatment: Mortality, re-incarceration, and hepatitis C infection. *Addiction 100:*560-563, 2005.
103. Shafer, D. A., Falek, A., Donahoe, R. M., & Madden, J. J. Biogenetic effects of opiates. *International Journal of Addiction 25:*1–18, 1991.
104. Lettau, L. A., McCarthy, J. G., Smith, M. J., Hadler, S. C., Morse, L. J., Ukena, T., Bessette, R., Gurwitz, A., Irvine, W. G., Fields, H. A. Outbreak of severe hepatitis due to delta and hepatitis B viruses in parental drug abusers and their contacts. *New England Journal of Medicine 317:*1256–1262, 1987.
105. Mendelson, J. H., Teoh, K. S., Mello, N. K., & Ellingbone, J. Buprenorphine attenuates the effects of cocaine on adrenocorticotropin (ACTH) secretion and mood states in man. *Neuropsychopharmacology 7:*157–162, 1992.

CHAPTER 7

Cannabinols

7.1. INTRODUCTION

Cannabis, or marijuana, and related substances are ancient drugs that are among the most widely used of those described in this text.[1] Their history dates back to at least 2700 BC in China and elsewhere, and marijuana was introduced to Europe in the nineteenth century by French soldiers who had served in Egypt.[2–4] Cannabinoids have been used in many cultures, including those in the Middle East, the Orient, and in Western countries.

The marijuana based drugs are available in multiple forms, named in relation to their source and potency.[5] Until recent years, most of the marijuana tobacco available in the United States has had relatively low potency, being harvested from the tops of uncultivated marijuana plants.[4] This form of the drug is also known as bang in India and elsewhere, and generally has a 1–10% THC content, which in past decades resulted in about 10–25 mg per cigarette (reefer). The next most potent form, harvested from the flowering tops and leaves of plants cultivated for their THC content, is known as ganja. Charas, also known as hashish, is a more potent form of cannabis harvested from the resin at the top of more mature plants, and has more than 10% THC content. A recent more potent form of marijuana with a 7% active ingredient or more and as much as 150 mg per reefer is known as sinsemilla.[3–5] Finally, there is a highly concentrated hashish oil with a THC potency of between 15 and 30%.[3] The freshness of any form of marijuana has an impact on potency, with a reported decrease of 5% a month when the cannabinoid product is stored at room temperature.[3]

In North America, THC is usually sold as marijuana or as hashish, and is marketed under any of the variety of names listed in Table 1.4. Pure THC is not available "on the streets," and samples so labeled are usually PCP or other substances that are relatively inexpensive or easy to produce (see Chapter 8). At low to moderate doses, THC produces fewer dramatic physiological and psychological alterations than do most other classes of drugs, including alcohol. However, the cannabinoids do have potent effects in the nervous and hormonal systems and impacts on driving ability. The peak age of use occurs in late adolescence when the brain and sexual systems are still developing, making these problems a focus of legitimate concern.

Cannabinols are taken through a variety of mechanisms including oral ingestion (often in brownies) with a slower and less complete absorption, smoking in a pipe, the use of a "bucket" where ignited cannabinol leaf or resin is inhaled from a plastic bottle, as a cigarette occasionally mixed with embalming fluid, and through a cigar-like delivery device known as a blunt.[5–7] Because the active ingredient, delta-9-tetrahydrocannabinol (THC) is insoluble in water, IV use is inefficient and rarely used. A medicinal cannabinol containing THC mixed with sesame oil is available as dronabinol (Merinol).

Diagnosing abuse or dependence of marijuana follows the same guidelines as other drugs.[8,9] Although marijuana is illegal, its relatively high acceptance by the general population and the high prevalence of users make it important to differentiate among use, misuse (implying temporary problems that may disappear), and abuse or dependence (implying a high potential for future problems). Legal proscriptions against use of this drug have a long history including the Marijuana Tax Act of 1937 in the United States, the World Health Organization (WHO) designation of this as a drug of dependence, and the classification by the U.S. Drug Enforcement Agency of cannabinols as a Class I, or highly restricted, drug.

7.1.1. Pharmacology

THC comes from the marijuana plant, *Cannabis sativa*, a relative of the source of rope or hemp, and grows readily in warm climates. There are more than 60 cannabinoids (or cannabinol-like products) plus other chemicals in marijuana smoke, the most important of which regarding intoxication is THC.[2,4,5]

7.1.1.1. General Characteristics

Although this drug is sometimes called a hallucinogen, at the doses most frequently taken the predominant effects are euphoria, giddiness, a change in time sense, increased appetite, an enhanced perception of sensory input, and a change in the level of consciousness without frank hallucinations. Marijuana can be administered primarily through smoking and eating. Oral ingestion results in an estimated 12% absorption of the active drug, while smoking results in about 50%. When smoked, peak plasma level is reached in about 10–20 min.[2,5] While prominent intoxication usually lasts between 2 and 4 h depending on the dose, the elimination half-life is almost 7 days, and some active drug can be found in body tissues for several weeks. When the plant is eaten, the onset is seen in 0.5–1 h, a peak blood level is reached in 2–3 h, and the effects last up to 8 h, with less intense residual actions for about 24 h. In the United States, the major legally prescribed cannabinoid is dronabinol, which is used to treat vomiting (i.e., antiemetic) and as an appetite stimulant during chemotherapy or in the context of AIDS.[2,5]

The relationship between THC blood levels and clinical effects is complex.[2] Once ingested, the drug tends to disappear rapidly from the plasma, becoming absorbed in tissues, especially those with high levels of fat, such as the brain and the testes.[2] Also contributing to the long half-life is the fact that cannabinols are also reabsorbed into the blood from the intestine. These substances are metabolized, mostly in the liver, to an 11-hydroxylated derivative with some psychoactivity, which is then excreted, mostly in the feces, but also in the urine. The remaining metabolites probably do not affect cognitive functioning.

In recent decades there have been important advances in knowledge regarding the mechanism of action of cannabinols.[5,10,11] These began with the discovery of a neuronal cannabinoid receptor (CB1) which is distributed in the cortex, limbic system, basal ganglia, cerebellum, thalamus, and peripheral nervous system, as well as a CB2 receptor that affects immune cells and might affect pain perception.[5,12,13] The existence of these receptors led to the discovery of endogenously produced cannabinoids, which are classified as an anandamides and include arachidonic acid, 2-arachidonoyl glycerol, and possibly virodhamine.[5,14,15] Activation of CB1 receptors produces a cascade of effects in the second messenger system within the cells, with an impact on dopamine-rich areas (e.g., the nucleus accumbens) as well as opioid, gamma aminobutyric acid (GABA) and glutamate systems.[5,10,16]

Recent efforts have produced cannabinoid antagonists.[17–19] Studies in mice and rats have identified effects of cannabinoid receptor blockade on behaviors, pain perception, appetite, as well as on patterns of alcohol, nicotine, and opioid consumption.[19–22]

Before leaving the topic of pharmacology, it is important to emphasize that cannabinols have been listed in pharmacopias for many years.[2–4] They have prominent effects on promoting appetite, diminishing nausea and vomiting, decreasing symptoms of muscle spasticity, and perhaps even antitumor activity and may provide beneficial effects in pain and some neurological disorders.[23–27]

7.1.1.2. Predominant Effects (Cannabis Intoxication, 292.89 in DSM-IV)

The greatest effects of THC are on the brain, the heart or cardiovascular system, and the lungs. Most changes, if not all, occur acutely and are reversible.

The altered mood seen with THC depends on the amount ingested and also on the setting in which the substance is taken and, as with any more "mild" drug, what one expects to happen.[2] In addition to giddiness and euphoria, the individual usually experiences an enhancement of sensory stimuli such as colors; a feeling of relaxation or "mellowness"; sleepiness; problems keeping accurate track of time; hunger; a dry mouth; and less social interaction.[2–5] The user has problems with attention and short-term memory, has enhanced impulsiveness, and may demonstrate an impairment of the ability to carry out multistep tasks.[2,3,5,28] A combination of effects that jeopardize the ability to drive safely include decreased coordination and an increased reaction time. These problems can last longer than obvious intoxication and, thus, most people have little insight into the level of driving impairment.[2,3]

Intoxication may also be associated with mild levels of suspiciousness or paranoia, along with some loss of insight.[2–4] This could relate to findings that users might enhance their risk for subsequent schizophrenia, especially if they have a family history of that disorder.[29] Frank hallucinations, usually visual, and sometimes accompanied by paranoid delusions, can be seen at very high doses, producing a temporary cannabinol-induced psychotic disorder with auditory hallucinations and paranoid delusions.[5,30] Severe intoxication can also be associated with confusion, disorientation, and feelings of panic.[2,5,31]

A variety of physiological changes can accompany moderate intoxication.[2,3,5] These include fine shakes or tremors, a slight decrease in skin temperature, a decrease in muscle strength and balance, increased pulse rate, decreased motor coordination, dry mouth, and bloodshot eyes (injected conjunctivae).[2,3] Some individuals experience nausea, headache, nystagmus, and mildly lowered blood pressure (perhaps from vasodilation).

THC may also precipitate seizures in people with epilepsy. Additional relevant EEG changes include a diffuse slowing and decreased percentage of alpha waves and interference with sleep stages, especially a decrease in Rapid Eye Movement (REM) sleep.

Along with an increased breathing rate, the respiratory effects of acute administration of THC include an increase in the diameter of the bronchial tubes, an action of potential significance in treating asthma. However, chronic use results in a decrease rather than an increase in the diameter and a worsening of breathing problems.[2,4]

7.1.1.3. Tolerance and Dependence

7.1.1.3.1. Tolerance

Modest toleration of increasing doses of the drug develops through both metabolic and pharmacodynamic mechanisms. These include adaptations of some physiological effects such as heart rate, some EEG changes, and feelings of intoxication. In addition, a mild level of cross-tolerance to alcohol has been demonstrated.[2–4]

7.1.1.3.2. Dependence (304.30 in DSM-IV) and Abuse (305.20 in DSM-IV)

Most of the dependence criterion items listed in DSM-IV can apply to the cannabinols.[32] These include spending a great deal of time using the substance, giving up important events to consume marijuana products, a persistent desire to use, taking more than intended, tolerance, and additional difficulties.

There has been a debate about whether there is a clinically relevant marijuana withdrawal syndrome, and, while DSM-IV does not list cannabis withdrawal, the majority of patients report subjective perceptions they describe as withdrawal-like.[32–34] A condition consistent with a rebound or withdrawal phenomenon has been described in animals, in case reports, and following laboratory experiments where participants consumed very high doses of marijuana for days or weeks at a time. Upon cessation of such use, a number of symptoms can develop, including anxiety, fatigue, problems concentrating, insomnia, a loss of appetite, tremor of the hands, sweating, and increased reflexes.[35,36]

Before leaving the topic of dependence, it is of interest to note that there are data to support the probability that between 30 and 60% of the predisposition toward dependence on these drugs might be explained by genetic mechanisms.[37–41] Dependence appears to run in families, and the risk for this syndrome is higher in identical twins of individuals with cannabinol dependence than it is for fraternal twin pairs. While there is crossover between a predisposition toward dependence on cannabinols and other drugs, perhaps through mechanisms such as high levels of disinhibition or impulsivity (see also Chapter 3 regarding genetics of alcoholism), a substantial proportion of the genetic influence may be specific for cannabinoids themselves.[42,43] More drug-specific predisposition might, at least theoretically, relate to genetic influences on CB receptors or cannabinol-metabolizing enzymes, among other possibilities.

The description of the signs and symptoms of intoxication given above also support the clinical relevance of a diagnosis of cannabis abuse.[8] The lack of mental drive and focus along with the cognitive impairments associated with cannabinoids can interfere with job or school performance, impair coordination and judgment important for driving or riding a bike, or contribute to legal problems, and many users continue intake despite social and interpersonal problems.

7.1.2. Epidemiology or Patterns of Use

Cannabinoids are the most commonly used illicit drug, and are named by 75% of recent drug users, with 55% of this group reporting only having used marijuana products in recent months.[44] The highest rates of recent use are seen for 18- to 25-year-olds (17%), with 8% of those age 12–17 reporting use in the prior 30 days.[44] The Monitoring the Future Study and other investigations noted that in 2003, 46% of high school seniors, 51% of college students, and 57% of young adults admitted to ever having used cannabinoids, including about a third who consumed these drugs over the prior year, and about 20% over the prior month.[1,45] The rates were about equal in men and women, fairly equitably distributed across the United States (with slightly lower figures in the north central and southern states), with lifetime use for young adults (aged 19–30) ranging from 46% in rural regions to 61% in large cities.[1] In these young adults, 4.4% ever met criteria for abuse or dependence on cannabinoids, with at least a twofold higher rate among men than women.[46] In 2002, almost 1 million men and women (about 0.4% of the population) had received treatment for marijuana use disorders over the prior year.[44]

The relatively high prevalence of use of cannabinoids extends to other western countries. For example, in the United Kingdom, 60% of university students ever used cannabinoids,[5] a similar figure was noted for 20-year-olds in the general population in Australia,[32] and 70% had ever used marijuana by age 21 in New Zealand.[47] In Australia, in the prior year 1.5% of the population aged 18 and over had met criteria for cannabinoid dependence, and 0.7% for abuse.[48]

7.1.3. The Clinical Course or Natural History

The first use of cannabinoids usually occurs in the mid-teens to early 20s, with most users taking the drug a few times a month or less.[9,32] The probability of cannabinoid intake increases when peers also use the drug, report histories of delinquency, smoke tobacco, or use alcohol.[9,49] Heavier use of cannabinols is seen in individuals who administer other drugs, and among persons with an earlier onset of use higher levels of sensation-seeking, conduct problems, other drug use or antisocial personality disorder.[9,38,50] Repetitive intake of cannabinoid drugs is associated with an enhanced probability of impaired school performance and dropout, even after additional risk factors are controlled.[51–54] Not surprisingly, use of these substances is associated with an enhanced risk for motor vehicle accidents.

The relationship between more frequent marijuana use and intake of other drugs has led to speculation about the possible role of cannabinoids as a "gateway" to subsequent experience with other illicit substances. In one Australian survey, a history of having used cannabinoids before the age of 17 was associated with a significant increase in the future risk for abuse or dependence on other substances, even among pairs of identical twins.[40] A 21-year longitudinal study in New Zealand reported that heavier use of marijuana (e.g., 50 or more times per year) was associated with an almost 60-fold increase in the risk for use of other illicit drugs.[47] Some authors believe that such progression might reflect the preexisting personality and values of the person who repeatedly uses marijuana, as well as additional characteristics such as the pattern of drug use among peers. Others have speculated that cannabinoid-induced changes in the brain, including alterations in dopamine and stress-related hormones, might contribute to disruptions in the brain reward system that increases the probability of both experimentation with and continued use of other agents.[55,56] Thus, while there are indications that the use of cannabinoids is associated with a higher prevalence of experience with other illicit drugs, the mechanisms explaining this relationship are likely to be varied and complex.

Finally regarding the usual course of cannabinoid use, it is interesting to note a report from Australia that indicates the possibility that, similar to studies done with alcohol,[57] the quality of the initial response to cannabinoids may have an impact on the chances that a person will continue to take the substance.[58] In this instance, the important characteristics seem to be a report of more positive feelings associated with early use, including feeling especially "high," happy, and relaxed.

7.1.4. Establishing the Diagnosis

Recognizing whether social, psychiatric, and medical problems are associated with marijuana and with hashish use requires knowledge of the drug and an adequate history from the patient. Although THC is thought to exacerbate depression and to intensify preexisting psychoses,[5,30,59] there are no known definitive physical signs and available laboratory tests. Urinary toxicology screens can be positive for 1–3 weeks after heavier use, but a negative test cannot definitely rule out a role for this drug in causing temporary psychiatric symptoms or in exacerbating a prior mental condition. Similar to other drugs, the key to a diagnosis is to be familiar with the signs and symptoms associated with cannabinols, and to have a high index of suspicion that this highly prevalent drug might have caused life problems, contributed to difficulties at school or work, contributed to an accident, induced medical problems such as bronchitis, exacerbated a preexisting condition, or precipitated a temporary substance-induced disorder.

7.2. EMERGENCY PROBLEMS

7.2.1. Toxic Reactions

See Section 1.7.1.

7.2.1.1. Clinical Picture

Toxic, or overdose, reactions are relatively mild, characterized by temporary anxiety, a rapid pulse, delirium, and/or paranoia. Life-threatening overdose is rare.

7.2.1.2. Treatment

The treatment parallels steps outlined for anxiety symptoms in Section 7.2.6.2. The approach involves offering good general support and reassurance and allowing the passage of time in a room with no excessive external stimuli. It is best to treat this disorder symptomatically, avoiding the administration of other drugs.

7.2.2. Withdrawal (292.9 in DSM-IV)

It is not certain whether a clinically relevant withdrawal syndromes occurs with marijuana and with hashish.[33] Cannabis withdrawal is not recognized in DSM-IV, although it is listed for ICD-10.[8,60] However, the subjective report of some withdrawal symptoms may be expressed by almost three quarters of cannabinoid-dependent persons[32,34,61], and rebound symptoms have been noted in animal models.[10] In humans the most frequent symptoms are decreased appetite, impaired sleep, and craving, along with restlessness and irritability which will last for several days.[62]

Treatment is supportive.

7.2.3. Delirium, Dementia, and Other Cognitive Disorders (292.81 in DSM-IV)

See Sections 1.7.3 and 14.4.

7.2.3.1. Clinical Picture

Animal and human studies support the impact that acute cannabinoid intoxication has on cognitive functioning.[63,64] These include problems tracking time, interference with short-term memory, higher impulsivity, and difficulties carrying out multiple-step procedures. Such problems are likely to impair driving and ability.[5] In light of the long half-life of THC and its release from fat stores for days or weeks following abstinence, these cognitive problems can persist for days or weeks.[65] However, there are few convincing data that deficits last for months or longer following abstinence.[66,67] These results might reflect the ability of the brain to recover after drug use, even following long-term substance intake. It is also possible that relatively subtle problems remain but are hard to document.

Anecdotal reports indicate the development of apathy, decreased self-awareness, impaired social judgment, and decreased goal-directed drives in some chronic cannabinoid users.[52,65,66] Thus, it is possible that an *amotivational syndrome* exists in which the person loses interest in tasks and in accomplishments. Such symptoms probably reflect the actions of THC that remains in the body for weeks after heavy intake, and should disappear within weeks or a month or so of abstinence. It is also possible that individuals who are becoming apathetic and withdrawing from competition and from society in general also find the chronic use of marijuana attractive.

7.2.3.2. Treatment

The temporary nature of the clinical picture of any state of confusion and the relatively mild level of impairment make the focus of treatment careful observation and reassurance. Treatment involves supportive measures and reassurance, allowing time for the problems to dissipate.

7.2.4. Psychosis (292.11 and 292.12 in DSM-IV)

See Sections 5.2.4, 1.7.4, and 8.2.4.

A *temporary* psychotic state, characterized by paranoia and hallucinations without confusion, can be seen with marijuana, but, as with most drugs, there is little evidence that it results in permanent mental impairment. Cannabinoids may also intensify preexisting psychotic symptoms in individuals with schizophrenia, and they might precipitate a long-term psychosis in people predisposed to such problems.[5,29,68]

7.2.4.1. Clinical Picture

The temporary paranoid state accompanied by visual hallucinations is usually a reaction to excessive doses of the drug.[69,70] In countries with easy access to potent forms of cannabinols, heavy users can also demonstrate auditory hallucinations and paranoid delusions that resemble schizophrenia but that disappear in several weeks to a month of abstinence. This is virtually identical to the stimulant-induced psychosis described in Chapter 5. If a frankly psychotic state does not clear within a month, the patient is likely to have a preexisting psychiatric disorder made worse by the cannabinol.

A possible connection between heavy cannabinol use and the future development of schizophrenia has also been reported.[29,71] Interesting data come from a cohort of Swedish army conscripts where any use of marijuana-type drugs was associated with a twofold increased risk for schizophrenia during the follow-up period, and 50 or more ingestions with a sixfold increase. However, of the almost 300 men who did develop schizophrenia, only 21 were in the high-marijuana-use group, and 50 men with schizophrenia had never used marijuana. These findings indicate that the association between marijuana use and the future development of schizophrenia is relatively weak and might relate to preexisting factors found in individuals before the onset of their use of cannabinoids and psychotic problems.[72]

7.2.4.2. Treatment

It is imperative that a history of prior psychiatric problems be obtained for all individuals who present with what appears to be a marijuana-related psychotic problem. Any underlying prior psychiatric diagnosis (e.g., major depressive disorder or schizophrenia) is an important factor to be addressed in treatment.

1. If the individual is out of contact with reality (i.e., psychotic), a short-term hospitalization can keep him out of trouble until the psychosis clears.
2. The patient should be told that his problem is temporary, and attempts should be made to help him with reality testing (e.g., by offering insight into his hallucinations and delusions).
3. Short-term antipsychotic medication can be initiated for a psychosis if behavior control is absolutely necessary. You might use haloperidol (Haldol) at approximately 5 mg/day in divided doses (rarely up to 20 mg daily), chlorpromazine (Thorazine) at 25–50 mg IM or 50–150 mg by mouth, or comparable doses of risperidone (Risperdal) for several days to several weeks.
4. Anyone demonstrating a grossly psychotic condition that lasts more than a month should be carefully reevaluated for other major psychiatric disorders, especially schizophrenia.

7.2.5. Flashbacks (292.9 in DSM-IV)

See Sections 1.7.5 and 8.2.5.

7.2.5.1. Clinical Picture

Flashbacks involve the unexpected recurrence of feelings and perceptions experienced in the past in the intoxicated state.[2,5] They are seen for marijuana and the hallucinogens, and while not officially listed in DSM-IV, this condition might be referred to as a cannabis persisting perception disorder.

The clinical picture involves a feeling of intoxication, including a change in time sense or a feeling of slowed thinking, generally at a lower level of intensity than that experienced when the user was high. The flashbacks tend to be time-limited (usually lasting only minutes), and the major difficulty is that the individual may fear a loss of control. It has been reported that marijuana may precipitate flashbacks in individuals who have taken hallucinogens in the past. In rare instances, the symptoms may be more persistent, but all are likely to disappear with time.

7.2.5.2. Treatment

The treatment involves education and reassurance, following all the steps outlined for the treatment of the depressive and anxiety states in Section 7.2.6.

7.2.6. Anxiety and Depression (292.89 or 292.9 in DSM-IV)

See Sections 1.7.6, 5.2.6, 8.2.6, and 13.7.

7.2.6.1. Clinical Picture

Acutely, the cannabinoids can produce a feeling of panic, labeled in DSM-IV as a cannabis-induced anxiety disorder with an onset during intoxication. The clinical picture includes an exaggeration of the usual marijuana effects, which can be perceived by the person as threatening and as part of losing control or going crazy. This can be seen in individuals with no preexisting psychopathology.[5,73,74]

A growing literature has evaluated whether there is an association between cannabinol use and major depressive syndromes.[59,75–78] While the causal implications of a relationship are unclear, heavy users of cannabinoids may have an increased risk for depressive symptoms, and, perhaps, full-blown depressive episodes. On the other hand, adolescents with interpersonal and emotional problems may be more likely to use cannabinoids. More research will be required to determine if a relationship exists, and whether earlier use or cannabinoids enhances the risk for later development of depressive episodes.

7.2.6.2. Treatment

Treatment is predicated on carefully establishing a diagnosis, determining whether depressive or anxiety symptoms relate to an independent or preexisting psychiatric condition. If, on the other hand, a substance-induced condition is present, the optimal approach may involve reassurance along with cognitive-behavioral therapy.

1. A physical examination is necessary to rule out signs of other drugs of intoxication and preexisting medical disorders. It is advisable to draw blood (10 cc) or collect urine (50 ml) for a toxicological screen for cannabinols and for other drugs.
2. A history should establish the dose taken and the individual's prior experience with the drug.
3. The individual should be reassured that his problems are likely to improve within a few hours to a few weeks of abstinence.
4. It helps to place the patient in a quiet room, constantly reassure him, and allow friends to help "talk him down."
5. For anxiety, the level of intoxication may fluctuate over the next 5 h or so, as the active drug is released from the tissues.
6. No specific drug should be used to treat every anxiety syndrome. If, however, the anxiety cannot be controlled in any other manner, the drugs of choice are benzodiazepines, such as chlordiazepoxide (Librium), 10–25 mg orally, which may be repeated in an hour, if needed.

7. Because of the persistence of THC in the body, patients should be warned that they may experience some mild feelings of drug intoxication over the next 2–4 days.

7.2.7. Medical Problems

The risk of medical consequences grows with increasing amount, frequency of intake, and years of exposure to these drugs.[79–81] Some of the more important areas of possible damage are presented below, primarily to help you in answering questions from patients and from their relatives.

7.2.7.1. Lungs

1. Marijuana reefers contain 3–5 times the content of tar and carcinogens as tobacco cigarettes.[5] These and other inhaled compounds are irritating, and can produce a bronchitis and an enhanced risk for emphysema for which 3 reefers are estimated to have the same risk as 20 tobacco cigarettes.[5]
2. Although the acute administration of marijuana causes dilation of the bronchial tree, chronic use is thought to cause constriction, with a resulting asthma-like syndrome.
3. The chronic use of any substance that irritates the lungs can cause temporary or permanent destruction of lung architecture, and there is evidence of a decreased vital lung capacity in chronic smokers—even healthy young men.[80]
4. Although it is difficult to definitively document, heavy marijuana smokers appear to have increased rates of lung cancer, both as a result of carcinogens in the smoke and immunosuppression.[5,82] Animal experiments have corroborated a possible increased rate of cancer after many years of heavy marijuana intake.

7.2.7.2. Nose and Throat

A chronic inflammation of the sinuses (sinusitis), as well as pharyngitis, has been reported in heavy smokers of marijuana.[82] There is also the possibility that heavy marijuana smokers have the same increased risk of cancers of the head and neck as heavy tobacco smokers.

7.2.7.3. Cardiovascular System

Marijuana acutely produces an increased heart rate, vasodilatation, and a decreased strength of heart contractions.[2,5] This reaction can be dangerous for heart patients, as there is an associated decrease in oxygen delivery to the heart muscle and a decrease in the amount of exercise an individual on cannabinoids can tolerate before the onset of heart pain or angina.

7.2.7.4. Immune System

White blood cell function and other aspects of the immune system are sensitive to THC, with decreases in the ability to carry out immune responses.[12,13,15] This may increase the risk for infections as well as cancers.

7.2.7.5. Reproductive System

Cannabinoid use may impair sperm production in heavy users, and has been associated with an increased risk for chromosomal breakage.[5] Chronic marijuana use may decrease the size of the prostate and the testes in males and block ovulation in females, although these changes are reversible. In mice, chronic exposure to these drugs decreases the reproductive functioning of adult males.[83]

Because cannabinoids cross the placenta and are also found in breast milk, it is also likely that THC can have an effect on the developing fetus. Smoking by pregnant mothers is likely to produce problems with oxygenation of the baby, and can be associated with decreased growth as well as altered behavior and learning in newborns.[83–86] The clinical importance of these findings has not yet been demonstrated, and the purported teratogenic action of the cannabinols has also been questioned.

7.2.7.6. Endocrine System

Decreased levels of several hormones, including leutenizing hormone and testosterone, have been demonstrated in heavy marijuana smokers,[87] but these abnormalities appear to be temporary. It is also possible that growth-hormone production and prolactin levels may be altered in heavy marijuana smokers, but the clinical significance to humans has not been established.[88]

7.2.7.7. Interactions with Other Drugs

THC and other constituents of marijuana are metabolized by liver enzymes. Therefore, the destruction of other drugs that use the same enzyme systems can occur at a slower rate, and the presence of these additional drugs can decrease the rate of metabolism of the cannabinoids. These drug interactions can be seen with alcohol, with barbituates, and with theophylline (Theo-Dur).

7.2.8. Other Emergency Problems

7.2.8.1. Accidents

One prominent danger of marijuana is a heightened risk for accidents as a consequence of the decreased judgment, the impaired ability to estimate time and distance, and the decreased motor performance that follow use.[2–5] These effects are similar to those of alcohol, and it appears that the two substances may potentiate each other. Marijuana significantly decreases automobile-driving ability for up to 8 hours after smoking, and almost 20% of drivers in fatal auto accidents test positive for cannabinols.[89,90]

REFERENCES

1. Johnston, L. D., O'Malley, P. M., & Bachman, J. G. *Monitoring the Future National Survey Results on Drug Use, 1975–2003, Vol. II: College Students and Adults Ages 19–40* (NIH Publication No. 04-5506). Bethesda, MD: National Institute on Drug Abuse, 2004.
2. O'Brien, C. P. Drug addiction and drug abuse. In J. G. Hardman, L. E. Limbird, & A. G. Goodman (Eds.), *The Pharmacological Basis of Therapeutics* (10th ed.). New York: McGraw-Hill, 2001, pp. 621–642.
3. Edwards, G. *Matters of Substance: Drugs and Why Everyone's a User*. London: Penguin Books, 2004.
4. Grinspoon, L., Bakalar, J. B., & Russo, E. Marihuana: Clinical aspects. In J. H. Lowinson, P. Ruiz, R. B. Millman, & J. G. Langrod (Eds.), *Substance Abuse: A Comprehensive Textbook* (4th ed.). Baltimore, MD: Williams & Wilkins, 2004, pp. 263–276.
5. Ashton, C. H. Pharmacology and effects of cannabis: A brief review. *The British Journal of Psychiatry 178:*101–106, 2001.
6. Soldz, S., Huyser, D. J., & Dorsey, E. The cigar as a drug delivery device: Youth use of blunts. *Addiction 98:*1379–1386, 2003.
7. Elwood, W. N. TCADA research brief: "Fry": A study of adolescents' use of embalming fluid with marijuana and tobacco. Texas Commission on Alcohol and Drug Abuse Research Brief, pp. 1–19, 2001.
8. American Psychiatric Association. *The Diagnostic and Statistical Manual of Mental Disorders* (4th ed., text revision, DSM-IVTR). Washington, DC: American Psychiatric Press, 2000.
9. Coffey, C., Lynskey, M., Wolfe, R., & Patton, G. C. Initiation and progression of cannabis use in a population-based Australian adolescent longitudinal study. *Addiction 95:*1679–1690, 2000.
10. Howlett, A. C., Breivogel, C. S., Childers, S. R., Deadwyler, S. A., Hampson, R. E., & Porrino, L. J. Cannabinoid psychology and pharmacology: 30 years of progress. *Neuropharmacology 47:*345–358, 2004.
11. Crippa, J. A. S., Zuardi, A. W., Garrido, G. E. J., Wichert-Ana, L., Guarnieri, R., Ferrari, L., Azevedo-Marques, P. M., Hallak, J. E. C., McGuire, P. K., & Busatto, G. F. Effects of cannabidiol (CBD) on regional cerebral blood flow. *Neuropsychopharmacology 29:*417–436, 2004.
12. Ibrahim, M. M., Deng, H., Zvonok, A., Cockayne, D. A., Kwan, J., Mata, H. P., Vanderah, T. W., Lai, J., Porreca, F., Makriyannis, A., & Malan, T. P., Jr. Activation of CB2 cannabinoid receptors by AM1241 inhibits experimental neuropathic pain: Pain inhibition by receptors not present in the CNS. *PNAS 100:*10529–10533, 2003.
13. Quartilho, A., Mata, H. P., Ibrahim, M., Vanderah, T. W., Porreca, F., Makriyannis, A., & Malan, T. P., Jr. Inhibition of inflammatory hyperalgesia by activation of peripheral CB2 cannabinoid receptors. *Anesthesiology 99:*955–960, 2003.
14. Felder, C. C., Sauer, J.-M., Knierman, M. D., Berna, M. J., Nomikos, G. G., Bymaster, F. P., Leese, A. B., Bensinger, J., Li, J., & Porter, A. C. Characterization of a novel endocannabinoid, Virodhamine. *Poster Presentation, ANCP Meeting*, San Juan, Puerto Rico, December 2002.
15. Vigano, D., Cascio M. G., Rubino, T., Fezza, F., Vaccani, A., DiMarzo, V., & Parolaro, D. Chronic morphine modulates the contents of the endocannabinoid, 2-arachidonoyl glycerol, in rat brain. *Neuropsychopharmacology 23:*1160–1167, 2003.

16. Houchi, H., Babovic, D., Pierrefiche, O., Ledent, C., Daoust, M., & Naassila, M. CB1 receptor knockout mice display reduced ethanol-induced conditioned place preference and increased striatal dopamine D2 receptors. *Neuropsychopharmacology 30:*339-349, 2005
17. Huestis, M. A., Gorelick, D. A., Heishman, S. J., Preston, K. L., Nelson, R. A., Moolchan, E. T., & Frank, R. A. Blockade of effects of smoked marijuana by the CB1-selective cannabinoid receptor antagonist SR141716. *Archives of General Psychiatry 58:*322–328, 2001.
18. Griebel, G., Stemmelin, J., & Scatton, B. Effects of the cannabinoid CB1 receptor antagonist rimonabant in models of emotional reactivity in rodents. *Biological Psychiatry 57:*261-267, 2005.
19. Le Foll, B., & Golberg, S. R. Rimonabant, a CB_1 antagonist, blocks nicotine-conditioned place preferences. *NeuroReport 15:*2139–2143, 2004.
20. Ortiz, S., Oliva, J. M., Pérez-Rial, S., Palomo, T., & Manzanares, J. Chronic ethanol consumption regulates cannabinoid CB_1 receptor gene expression in selected regions of rat brain. *Alcohol & Alcoholism 39:*88–92, 2004.
21. Wang, L., Liu, J., Harvey-White, J., Zimmer, A., & Kunos, G. Endocannabinoid signaling via cannabinoid receptor 1 is involved in ethanol preference and its age-dependent decline in mice. *PNAS 100:*1393–1398, 2003.
22. Monteleone, P., Matias, I., Martiadis, V., De Petrocellis, L., Maj, M., & Di Marzo, V. Blood levels of the endocannabinoid anandamide are increased in anorexia nervosa and in binge-eating disorder, but not in bulimia nervosa. *Neuropsychopharmacology 30:*1216-1221, 2005.
23. Darmani, N. A. Tetrahydrocannabinol and synthetic cannabinoids prevent emesis produced by the cannabinoid CB1 receptor antagonist/inverse agonist SR 141716A. *Neuropsychopharmacology 24:*198–203, 2001.
24. Galve-Roperh, I., Sànchez, C., Cortés, M. L., Gomez del Pulgar, T., Izquierdo, M., & Guzmán, M. Anti-tumoral action of cannabinoids: Involvement of sustained ceramide accumulation and extracellular signal-regulated kinase activation. *Nature Medicine 6:*313–319, 2000.
25. Robson, P. Therapeutic aspects of cannabis and cannabinoids. *The British Journal of Psychiatry 178:*107–115, 2001.
26. Zajicek, J., Fox, P., Sanders, H., Wright, D., Vickery, J., Nunn, A., & Thompson, A., on behalf of UK MS Research Group. Cannabinoids for treatment of spasticity and other symptoms related to multiple sclerosis (CAMS study): Multicentre randomised placebo-controlled trial. *The Lancet 362:*1517–1526, 2003.
27. Berman, J. S., Symonds, C., & Birch, R. Efficacy of two cannabis based medicinal extracts for relief of central neuropathic pain from brachial plexus avulsion: Results of a randomized controlled trial. *Pain 112:*299-306, 2004.
28. Lane, S. D., Cherek, D. R., Tcheremissine, O. V., Lieving, L. M., & Pietras, C. J. Acute marijuana effects on human risk taking. *Neuropsychopharmacology 30:*800-809, 2005.
29. Smith, F., Bolier, L., & Cuijpers, P. Cannabis use and the risk of later schizophrenia: A review. *Addiction 99:*425–430, 2004.
30. Grace, R. F., Shenfield, G., & Tennant, C. Cannabis and psychosis in acute psychiatric admissions. *Drug and Alcohol Review 19:*287–290, 2000.
31. Solowij, N., & Grenyer, B. F. S. Are the adverse consequences of cannabis use age-dependent? *Addiction 97:*1083–1086, 2002.
32. Vandrey, R., Budney, A. J., Kamon, J. L., & Stanger, C. Cannabis withdrawal in adolescent treatment seekers. *Drug and Alcohol Dependence 78:*205-210, 2005.
33. Budney, A. J., Hughes, J. R., Moore, B. A., & Vandrey, R. Review of the validity and significance of cannabis withdrawal syndrome. *American Journal of Psychiatry 161:*1967–1977, 2004.
34. Haney, M., Hart, C. L., Vosburg, S. K., Nasser, J., Bennett, A., Zubaran, C., & Foltin, R. W. Marijuana withdrawal in humans: Effects of oral THC or divalproex. *Neuropsychopharmacology 29:*158–170, 2004.

35. Wiesbeck, G. A., Schuckit, M. A., Kalmijn, J. A., Tipp, J. E., Bucholz, K. K., & Smith, T. L. An evaluation of the history of a marijuana withdrawal syndrome in a large population. *Addiction 91:*1469–1478, 1996.
36. Crowley, T. J., Macdonald, B. S., Whitmore, E. A., & Mikulich, S. K. Cannabis dependence, withdrawal, and reinforcing effects among adolescents with conduct symptoms and substance use disorders. *Drug and Alcohol Dependence 50:*27–37, 1998.
37. Kendler, K. S., Karkowski, L. J., Neale, M. C., & Prescott, C. A. Illicit psychoactive substance use, heavy use, abuse, and dependence in a U.S. population-based sample of male twins. *Archives of General Psychiatry 57:*261–269, 2000.
38. Lynskey, M. T., Heath, A. C., Nelson, E. C., Bucholz, K. K., Madden, P. A., Slutske, W. S., Statham, D. J., & Martin, N. G. Genetic and environmental contributions to cannabis dependence in a national young adult twin sample. *Psychological Medicine 32:*195–207, 2002.
39. Miles, L. D. R., Van Den Bree, N. B. M., Gupman, A. E., Newlin, D. B., Glantz, M. D., Pickens, R. W. A twin study on sensation seeking, risk taking behavior and marijuana use. *Drug and Alcohol Dependence 62:*57–68, 2001.
40. Lynskey, M. T., Heath, A. C., Bucholz, K. K., Slutske, W. S., Madden, P. A., Nelson, E. C., Statham, D. J., & Martin, N. G. Escalation of drug use in early-onset cannabis users vs. co-twin controls *Journal of the American Medical Association 289:*427–433, 2003.
41. Olsson, C. A., Coffey, C., Toumbourou, J. W., Bond, L., Thomas, L., & Patton, G. Family risk factors for cannabis use: A population-based survey of Australian secondary school students. *Drug and Alcohol Review 22:*143–152, 2003.
42. Kendler, K. S., Jacobson, K. C., Prescott, C. A., & Neale, M. C. Specificity of genetic and environmental risk factors for use and abuse/dependence of cannabis, cocaine, hallucinogens, sedatives, stimulants, and opiates in male twins. *American Journal of Psychiatry 160:*687–695, 2003.
43. Hoofer, C. J., Stallings, M. C., Hewitt, J. K., & Crowley, T. J. Family transmission of marijuana use, abuse and dependence. *Journal of the American Academy of Child and Adolescent Psychiatry 42:*834–841, 2003.
44. Substance Abuse and Mental Health Services Administration. *Results from the 2002 National Survey on Drug Use and Health: National Findings* (Office of Applied Studies, NHSDA Series H-22, DHHS Publication No. SMA 03-3836). Rockville, MD, 2003.
45. Gledhill-Hoyt, J., Lee, H., Strote, J., & Wechsler, H. Increased use of marijuana and other illicit drugs at U.S. colleges in the 1990's: Results of three national surveys. *Addiction 95:* 1655–1667, 2000.
46. Compton, W. M., Grant, B. F., Colliver, J. D., Glantz, M. D., & Stinson, F. S. Prevalence of marijuana use disorders in the United States: 1991–1992 and 2001–2002. *Journal of the American Medical Association 291:*2114–2121, 2004.
47. Fergusson, D. M., & Horwood, L. J. Does cannabis use encourage other forms of illicit drug use? *Addiction 95:*505–520, 2000.
48. Swift, W., Hall, W., & Teesson, M. Cannabis use and dependence among Australian adults: Results from the National Survey of Mental Health and Wellbeing. *Addiction 96:*737–748, 2001.
49. Kandel, D. B., & Chen, K. Types of marijuana users by longitudinal course. *Journal of Studies on Alcohol 61:*367–378, 2000.
50. van den Bree, M. B. M. & Pickworth, W. M. Risk factors predicting changes in marijuana involvement in teenagers. *Archives of General Psychiatry 62:*311–319, 2005.
51. Fergusson, D. M., Horwood, L. J., & Beautrais, A. L. Cannabis and educational achievement. *Addiction 98:*1681–1692, 2003.
52. Chen, C.-Y., O'Brien, M. S., & Anthony, J. C. Who becomes cannabis dependent soon after onset of use? Epidemiological evidence from the United States, 2000-2001. *Drug and Alcohol Dependence 79:*11-22, 2005.
53. Ramaekers, J. G., Berghaus, G., van Laar, M., & Drummer, O. H. Dose related risk of motor vehicle crashes after cannabis use. *Drug and Alcohol Dependence 73:*109–119, 2004.

54. Lynskey, M. T., Coffey, C., Degenhardt, L., Carlin, J. B., & Patton, G. A longitudinal study of the effects of adolescent cannabis use on high school completion. *Addiction 98:*685–692, 2003.
55. Anggadiredja, K., Nakamichi, M., Hiranita, T., Tanaka, H., Shoyama, Y., Watanabe, S., & Yamamoto, T. Endocannabinoid system modulates relapse to methamphetamine seeking: Possible mediation by the arachidonic acid cascade. *Neuropsychopharmacology 29:*1470–1478, 2004.
56. Pistis, M., Perra, S., Pillolla, G., Melis, M., Muntoni, A. L., & Gessa, G. L. Adolescent exposure to cannabinoids induces long-lasting changes in the response to drugs of abuse of rat midbrain dopamine neurons. *Biological Psychiatry 56:*86–94, 2004.
57. Schuckit, M. A. Vulnerability factors for alcoholism, In K. Davis (Ed.), *Neuropsychopharmacology: The Fifth Generation of Progress.* Baltimore, MD: Lippincott, Williams & Wilkins, 2002, pp. 1399–1411.
58. Fergusson, D. M., Horwood, J., Lynskey, M. T., & Madden, P. A. F. Early reactions to cannabis predict later dependence. *Archives of General Psychiatry 60:*1033–1039, 2003.
59. Degenhardt, L., Hall, W., & Lynskey, M. Exploring the association between cannabis use and depression. *Addiction 98:*1493–1504, 2003.
60. World Health Organization. *The ICD-10 Classification of Mental and Behavioural Disorders.* Geneva: World Health Organization, 1992.
61. Moore, B. A., Budney, A. J., Vandrey, R. G., & Hughes, J. R. The time course and significance of cannabis withdrawal. *Journal of Abnormal Psychology 112:*393–402, 2003.
62. Budney, A. J., Hughes, J. R., Moore, B. A., & Novy, P. L. Marijuana abstinence effects in marijuana smokers maintained in their home environment. *Archives of General Psychiatry 58:*917–924, 2001.
63. Verrico, C. D., Jentsch, J. D., Roth, R. H., & Taylor, J. R. Repeated, intermittent 9-tetrahydro-cannabinol administration to rats impairs acquisition and performance of a test of visuospatial divided attention. *Neuropsychopharmacology 29:*552–529, 2004.
64. Hart, C. L., van Gorp, W., Haney, M., Foltin, R. W., & Fischman, M. W. Effects of acute smoked marijuana on complex cognitive performance. *Neuropsychopharmacology 25:*757–765, 2001.
65. Solowij, N., Stephens, R. S., Roffman, R. A., Babor, T., Kadden, R., Miller, M., Christiansen, K., McRee, B., & Vendetti, J., for the Marijuana Treatment Project Research Group. Cognitive functioning of long-term heavy cannabis users seeking treatment. *Journal of the American Medical Association 287:*1123–1131, 2002.
66. Pope, H. G., Jr., Gruber, A. J., Hudson, J. I., Huestis, M. A., & Yurgelun-Todd, D. Neuropsychological performance in long-term cannabis users. *Archives of General Psychiatry 58:*909–915, 2001.
67. Fletcher, J. M., Page, J. B., Francis, D. J., Copeland, K., Naus, M. J., Davis, C. M., Morris, R., Krautzkopf, D., & Satz, P. Cognitive correlates of long-term cannabis use in Costa Rica men. *Archives of General Psychiatry 53:*1051–1057, 1996.
68. Degenhardt, L., Hall, W., & Lynskey, M. Testing hypotheses about the relationship between cannabis use and psychosis. *Drug and Alcohol Dependence 71:*37–48, 2003.
69. D'Souza, D. C., Perry, E., MacDougall, L., Ammerman, Y., Cooper, T., Wu, Y.-T, Braley, G., Gueorguieva, R., & Krystal, J. H. The psychomimetic effects of intravenous delta-9-tetrahydrocannabinol in healthy individuals: Implications for psychosis. *Neuropsychopharmacology 29:*1558–1572, 2004.
70. Stefanis, N. C., Delespaul, P., Henquet, C., Bakoula, C., Stefanis, C. N., & Van Os, J. Early adolescent cannabis exposure and positive and negative dimensions of psychosis. *Addiction 99:*1333–1341, 2004.
71. Ferguson, D. M., Horwood, L. J., & Ridder, E. M. Tests of causal linkages between cannabis use and psychotic symptoms. *Addiction 100:*354–366, 2005.
72. D'Souza, D. C., Abi-Saab, W. M., Madonick, S., Forselius-Bielen, K., Doersch, A., Braley, G., Gueorguieva, R., Cooper, T. B., & Krystal, J. H. Delta-9-tetrahydrocannabinol effects in

schizophrenia: Implications for cognition, psychosis, and addiction. *Biological Psychiatry 57:*594-608, 2005.

73. Agosti, V., Nunes, E., & Levin, F. Rates of psychiatric comorbidity among U.S. residents with lifetime cannabis dependence. *The American Journal of Drug and Alcohol Abuse 28:*643–652, 2002.
74. Johns, A. Psychiatric effects of cannabis. *The British Journal of Psychiatry 178:*116–122, 2001.
75. Milich, R., Lynam, D., Zimmerman, R., Logan, T., Mattin, C., Leukefield, C., Portis, C., Miller, J., & Clayton, R. Differences in young adult psychopathology among drug abstainers, experimenters, and frequent users. *Journal of Substance Abuse 22:*69–88, 2000.
76. Bovasso, G. B. Cannabis abuse as a risk factor for depressive symptoms. *American Journal of Psychiatr*y 158:2033–2037, 2001.
77. Strakowski, S. M., DelBello, M. P., Fleck, D. W., & Arndt, S. The impact of substance abuse on the course of bipolar disorder. *Biological Psychiatry 48:*477–485, 2000.
78. Fergusson, D. M., Horwood, L. J., & Swain-Campbell, N. Cannabis use and psychosocial adjustment in adolescence and young adulthood. *Addiction 97:*1123–1135, 2002.
79. Taylor, D. R., Fergusson, D. M., Milne, B. J., Horwood, L. J., Moffitt, T. E., Sears, M. R., & Poulton, R. A longitudinal study of the effects of tobacco and cannabis exposure on lung function in young adults. *Addiction 97:*1055–1061, 2002.
80. Cunningham, J. A., Bondy, S. J., & Walsh, G. W. The risks of cannabis use: Evidence of a dose–response relationship. *Drug and Alcohol Review 19:*1137–142, 2000.
81. deWit, D. J., Hance, J., Offord, D. R., & Ogborne, A. The influence of early and frequent use of marijuana on the risk of persistance and of progression to marijuana-related harm. *Preventive Medicine 31:*455–464, 2000.
82. Hall, W. The respiratory risks of cannabis smoking. *Addiction 93:*1461–1463, 1998.
83. Smith, A. M., Fried, P. A., Hogan, M. J., & Cameron, I. Effects of prenatal marijuana on response inhibition: An fMRI study of young adults. *Neurotoxicology and Teratology 26:*533-542, 2004.
84. Robins, L. N., & Mus, J. L. Effects of in utero exposure to street drugs. *American Journal of Public Health*, Supplement to Volume 83, 1993.
85. Wang, X., Dow-Edwards, D., Anderson, V., Minkoff, H., & Hurd, Y. L. In utero marijuana exposure associated with abnormal amygdale dopamine D2 gene expression in the human fetus. *Biological Psychiatry 56:*909-915, 2004.
86. Goldschmidt, L., Richardson, G. A., Cornelius, M. D., & Day, N. L. Prenatal marijuana and alcohol exposure and academic achievement at age 10. *Neurotoxicology and Teratology 26:*521-532, 2004.
87. Block, R. I., Farinpour, R., & Schlechte, J. A. Effects of chronic marijuana use on testosterone, luteinizing hormone, follicle stimulating hormone, prolactin, and cortisol in men and women. *Drug and Alcohol Dependence 28:*121–128, 1991.
88. Murphy, L. L., Muñoz, R. M., Adrian, B. A., & Villanúa, M. A. Function of cannabinoid receptors in the neuroendocrine regulation of hormone secretion. *Neurobiology of Disease 5:*432–446, 1998.
89. Kurzthaler, I., Hummer, M., Miller, C., Sperner-Unterweger, B., Gunther, V., Wechdorn, H., Battista, H. J., & Fleischhacker, W. W. Effect of cannabis use on cognitive functions and driving ability. *Journal of Clinical Psychiatry 60:*395–399, 1999.
90. Liguori, A., Gatto, C. P., & Robinson, J. H. Effects of marijuana on equilibrium, psychomotor performance, and simulated driving. *Behavioural Pharmacology 9:*599–609, 1998.

CHAPTER 8

Hallucinogens and Related Drugs

8.1. INTRODUCTION TO HALLUCINOGENS

This chapter covers the variety of substances listed in Table 8.1, each of which can enhance sensory perceptions such as colors and sounds. I also include in this chapter phencyclidine (PCP) and associated drugs [e.g., ketamine (Ketalar)] (see Section 8.3.1), reflecting their overlap with classical hallucinogens in some clinical effects and the manner in which they are used "on the streets." The hallucinogens rarely produce schizophrenia-like auditory hallucinations on paranoid ("crazy") thoughts in the context of a clear sensorium and, thus, are not really "psychotomimetic."[1–3] However, high doses of these drugs can produce visual hallucinations, most often involving lights, colors, or geometric shapes, but the user is likely to understand (or have insight) that these were caused by the substance of abuse.

Drugs that enhance sensory perceptions and attention have been used for more than 3500 years.[2–5] Hallucinogen-like substances, probably derived from mushrooms, were called "soma" in Sanskrit, and referred to as "mushroom stones" in preliterate cultures in Guatemala. The Aztecs recognized the potential sensory enhancement properties of Psilocbe mushrooms, peyote, and morning glory seeds.

One of the most often used hallucinogens in modern times, lysergic acid diethylamide (LSD), resembles a component of an ergot fungus that infects grains, such as rye. In the middle ages, epidemics of intoxication with this ergot caused visual hallucinations, delirium, and muscle contractions in a potentially fatal disorder referred to as St Anthony's fire.

The modern age of hallucinogen use began in 1938 when Albert Hofman synthesized LSD, subsequently experiencing an accidental intoxication. He then voluntarily subjected himself to an oral administration of a large dose, which resulted in an anxiety-laden "bad trip." LSD was commercially marketed in the early 1940s as Delysid, supposedly to enhance psycho-

Table 8.1
Some Hallucinogenic Drugs[1–3]

Drug name	Usual source	Usual dose
Indolealkylamines (serotonin-like)		
Lysergic acid diethylamide (LSD)[a]	Synthetic	100–200 μg
N,N-Dimethyltryptamine (DMT)	Synthetic	50–100 mg
Diethyltryptamine (DET)	Synthetic	50–75 mg
Psilocybin and psilocin	Mushrooms	10–200 mushrooms
Bufotenine	Toad skin	5–10 mg
Phenylethylamines (amphetamine-like)		
Mescaline	Peyote cactus	6–12 catcus buttons or 200–500 mg
Dimethoxy methamphetamine (DOM or STP)	Synthetic	5 mg
Methylene dioxyamphetamine (MDA)	Synthetic	75–200 mg
Methylene dioxymethamphetamine (MDMA)	Synthetic	60–200 mg

[a]As a point of interest, the abbreviation LSD comes from the original German: *Lyserg Säure Diethylamid.*

logical insight in psychotherapy, but no careful studies have supported its use in this manner.[6] Consequently, the potential benefits of hallucinogen intoxication have been touted by numerous individuals including Aldous Huxley, Alan Ginsberg, and Timothy Leary. Concern regarding the burgeoning use of LSD and similar substances resulted in a 1965 proscription against sales, and a subsequent placement of these drugs on Schedule I, indicating substances with no medical usefulness, but high potential for misuse.

Cannabinols are known to produce some physiological and psychological changes that overlap with the hallucinogens. However, because the mechanisms of action of the hallucinogens are quite different, reflecting the lack of cross-tolerance between cannabinols and hallucinogens, as well as in light of differences in the associated symptoms of intoxication, the cannabinoids are described in a separate chapter. Some more closely related (yet still distinct) substances such as nutmeg, morning glory seeds, catnip, loco weed, betel nut, nitrous oxide, and nitrate inhalants are described below.

8.1.1. Pharmacology

The most widely accepted classification scheme distinguishes between the amphetamine-like substances called phenethylamines, and the serotonin-like drugs diethylamine (DMT), diethyltryptamine (DET), psilocybin, and bufotenin.[1–3] The more stimulating, amphetamine-like phenethylamines include mescaline, dimethoxy methylamphetamine (DOM, also known as Serenity, Tranquility, and Peace (STP), as well as methylene dioxyamphetamine (MDA or Eve), and its close cousin methylene dioxymethamphetamine (MDMA or Ecstasy).

Drugs of both major hallucinogen subclasses function as postsynaptic agonists at a variety of serotonin receptors, most prominently the 5-HT_2 and the 5-HT_{2C}.[1,2,7,8] Relatively close correlations have been observed between the binding affinity to these receptors and the hallucinogen potency of the drugs. Additional shared properties are their oral absorption (except for DMT which must be smoked, snorted, or taken IV) and their metabolism in the liver, usually via hydroxylation and conjugation.[2]

On a milligram basis, LSD has 100 times the potency of the "magic mushroom" constituents of psilocybin and psilocin, and is 4,000 times more potent than mescaline, but is weaker than STP or DOM. These relative potencies are of limited clinical importance because users adjust the dose to get desired effects. The drugs also demonstrate some different side-effect profiles, (e.g., there is a greater likelihood of vomiting with mescaline at even low doses) and different ratios between feelings of euphoria and self-awareness and actual hallucinations (e.g., DOM and DET tend to show more euphoria at lower doses, and may require higher levels of intake before visual hallucinations are observed). Overall, however, about 100–200 µg of LSD produces a fairly typical enhanced perception of sensory stimuli. Thus, the generalizations given for LSD at this dose can be assumed to hold for most other drugs, unless specifically noted.

The hallucinogens also differ in their length of action, with the "high" from LSD and mescaline having an onset after 30–60 min, peaking at 2–4 h, and lasting as long as 6–12 h.[1–3,9] Most other hallucinogens have clinically relevant actions that last for between 2 and 8 h.[1–3] These differences tend to reflect rates of metabolism.

8.1.1.1. Predominant Effects and Intoxication (292.89 in DSM-IV)

The earliest effects, seen an hour or so after consuming LSD, are likely to involve stimulant-like physical changes such as pupillary dilation, along with increases in heart rate, blood pressure, and body temperature.[2,3] Some investigators have reported the likelihood of tremors and paresthesias at this stage, along with an increase in both blood sugar and several hormones (e.g., cortisol, ACTH, and prolactin).[3,10]

Accompanying these physiological changes are prominent alterations in perceptions. This usually involves an increased awareness of sensory stimuli including vivid colors and a sharpened sense of hearing, along with problems distinguishing between sensory modalities such as sight versus smell.[1,2] Mood changes are prominent, sometimes alternating between enhanced feelings of self-confidence or euphoria versus feelings of depression and anxiety.[2] Users also describe a subjective feeling of enhanced mental activity, a perception of usual environmental stimuli as novel events, altered body images, an inward turning of thoughts, and a decreased ability to tell the difference between oneself and one's surroundings.

Some clinicians have felt that these experiences, especially as they relate to LSD or MDMA (ecstasy), might serve to increase mental insights and feelings of empathy.[6] Because of this, it was hoped that use of these agents might enhance psychotherapy, but there is *no evidence* that such benefits occur. In addition to the possibility that the drugs will increase feelings of anxiety and sadness, some hallucinogens are also said to alter gene expression in the brain[11] and produce a "knight's move" pattern of jumping in logical sequences and nonlinear thinking—making it harder to reason one's way through problems.

8.1.1.2. Tolerance, Abuse and Dependence

8.1.1.2.1. Tolerance

The modest increased need for higher doses to maintain effects reflects both behavioral and pharmacological mechanisms of tolerance. This develops after as little as 3 or 4 days at one dose per day, and disappears within 4 days to a week after stopping use.[1–3] These changes might parallel decreases in the amount of 5-HT_2 binding sites.[2] Cross-tolerance exists among most of the hallucinogens, including LSD, mescaline, and psilocybin, but this does not appear to extend to marijuana, PCP, or stimulants.[3]

8.1.1.2.2. Dependence and Abuse (304.50 and 305.30 in DSM-IV)

Regular users of hallucinogens can demonstrate most of the seven DSM-IV dependence criteria.[12] These include tolerance, persistent but unsuccessful efforts to control use, spending a great deal of time taking the drug or recovering from effects, giving up important activities in order to get high, and so on. However, there is no known clinically significant abstinence syndrome for the hallucinogens.[2,3]

Frequent users of hallucinogens who are not dependent on these drugs can demonstrate syndromes consistent with DSM-IV abuse. These include recurrent problems with fulfilling work or family obligations, repeatedly taking hallucinogens while engaging in hazardous activities such as driving a car, as well as repetitive legal or social problems.

8.1.1.3. Specific Drugs

Most of the drugs described in prior chapters of this text are readily available on the street and are usually (but not always) what the seller advertises them to be (a notable exception being the virtual nonexistence of pure THC). This, however, is often *not* the case for the hallucinogens. As many as 95% of mescaline or peyote units contain either no drug, or are actually PCP or LSD, and the figures are probably similar for the other hallucinogens. In addition, even those samples that actually have the alleged substance usually also contain an adulterant, often amphetamines. Thus, it is *not* safe to assume that one can predict the reaction just by knowing what substance the individual *thinks* he or she has taken.

8.1.1.3.1. Lysergic Acid Diethylamide (LSD)

This is a potent drug that produces some physiological and psychological changes at doses as low as 20–35 μg, with the usual street dose ranging from 100–300 μg.[1,2] At 0.5–2.0 μg/kg, the individual experiences dizziness, weakness, and a series of physiological changes that are replaced by euphoria and occasionally visual hallucinations lasting from 4 to 12 h. The actual "high" depends on the dose, the individual's emotional set, the environment, prior drug experiences, and the psychiatric history.

LSD can be purchased as a powder, a liquid, a capsule, or a pill. The colorless, tasteless substance is also sold dissolved on sugar cubes or pieces of blotter paper. Although the drug is usually taken orally, it has been known to be administered transcutaneously or intravenously. LSD can be placed on tobacco and smoked, but the intoxication obtained by this method is usually mild.

8.1.1.3.2. 3,4-Methylene Dioxymethamphetamine (MDMA or Ecstasy)

Reflecting the structural similarity that this drug and its cousin methylene dioxyamphetamine (MDA or Eve) have to the amphetamines, it would have been possible to place MDMA in the chapter on stimulants. However, MDMA is primarily used on the streets as a hallucinogen-like drug, and the other phenethylamine hallucinogens bear a striking structural similarity to the amphetamines as well. Thus, in this text and in most others, these drugs are presented as hallucinogens.[1–3]

MDMA may have become one of the two or three most commonly used hallucinogens in recent years, especially on college campuses.[1,13] This drug was first synthesized in Germany in 1912, patented in 1914, and was originally evaluated for potential use as an appetite suppressant. Known on the street by a variety of names including ecstasy, XTC, and E, this drug is most often taken orally as a tablet or capsule containing between 60 and 250 mg (an average of 120 mg). MDMA powder can also be snorted (intranasally), taken as a suppository (causing a much slower onset with a longer lasting high), or injected IV or subcutaneously. Taken orally, the effects have an onset within minutes to a half-hour, a "high" that often lasts 5 h, and with residual effects that can remain for several days.[2,14] The intoxication includes euphoria, a feeling of spirituality and closeness to others, as well as increases in blood pressure, pulse rate, changes in hormones, and sweating.[15] Reflecting its stimulant-like properties, ecstasy can produce anxiety, panic attacks, muscle contractions, dry mouth, and a labile mood.[1]

This substance came into vogue in the mid to late 1980s, and it has been estimated that between 13 and 15% of late teenagers and young adults have had at least one use of this drug.[16] MDMA shares all of the major complications associated with the other hallucinogens, but carries the added potential danger of possible longer term, even permanent, alterations in functioning of serotonin-rich nerve cells.[17–19]

Pharmacological effects of MDMA include dopamine release, but the most prominent actions appear to be on serotonin neurons.[20] There is impressive evidence from animal studies that even modest doses of this drug are associated with the destruction of these nerve cells and their axons. However, reflecting methodological difficulties, the prevalence of this phenomenon in humans has been more difficult to document. Nonetheless, cognitive changes are observed during intoxication, and a day or so after taking the drug, users are still likely to demonstrate problems with mental arithmetic, immediate and delayed recall, and impairments in delayed memory. MDMA users are also likely to complain of moodiness and sleep problems. Both animal and human studies suggest problems with memory for days post MDMA use, and lethal effects have been reported, especially in the presence of additional drugs.[21,22]

8.1.1.3.3. Mescaline or Peyote

The hard, dried brown buttons of the peyote or mescal cactus (*Lophophoria williamsii* and *Anhalonium lewinii*) contain mescaline, one of the more widely used hallucinogens.[3] Taken as a powder and softened with saliva, mescaline has a slower onset than LSD, and is more likely to produce unpleasant side effects such as nausea and vomiting. The hallucinations, usually involving lights and colors, commonly last 1–2 h, up to 6–10 h after a usual dose[3] between 200 and 500 mg.

8.1.1.3.4. Psilocybin or Psilocyn

Psilocybin is obtained from "magic" mushrooms (*Psilocybe mexicana*), many of which grow wild in the United States and Mexico.[3] The resulting effects are similar to those noted for LSD and mescaline. This drug is usually taken by mouth and has a rapid onset: effects are demonstrated within 15 min after a dose of 4–8 mg. Reactions peak at about 90 min and begin to wane at 2–3 h, but they do not disappear for 5–6 h. Higher doses tend to produce longer periods of intoxication.

8.1.1.3.5. 2,5-Dimethoxy-4-methylamphetamine (DOM or STP)

This is a synthetic hallucinogen bearing a structural resemblance to both amphetamine and mescaline, and resembling LSD in its effects. The usual dose is 5 mg or more; thus, the drug is between 50 and 100 times less potent than LSD.[3] The onset of action is usually within 1 h, and peak effects occur at 3–5 h, disappearing by 7 or 8 h. The physiological changes are adrenaline-like, including increases in pulse, blood pressure, and pupillary size, paralleling those of LSD.

8.1.1.3.6. *N,N,*-Dimethyltryptamine (DMT)

This synthetic indoleamine hallucinogen is often taken in doses of between 50 and 100 mg.[3] Although intoxication is reported to be similar to that observed with LSD, this substance is relatively unique among the hallucinogens because it is not well absorbed orally. Most users take DMT through snorting, smoking, or IV injection. Regarding the latter, the onset of effects is almost immediate, and intoxication lasts approximately one-half hour. Because of the short period of intoxication, this drug has also been referred to as the "businessman's LSD," inferring that it can be taken during the lunch hour, after which an individual might be able to return to work.[3]

8.1.2. Epidemiology and Patterns of Use

The hallucinogens were, along with marijuana, among the first of the "middle-class" street drugs to cause public concern in the 1960s. Although it is impossible to be certain of the extent of abuse or dependence, studies of students, the street culture, as well as emergency room admissions, indicate a peak prevalence in 1966–1967, with a subsequent leveling off and decline until another modest increase in the mid-1990s.[16]

Recent data on the extent of the use of these substances is available from several sources. First, the National Survey on Drug Use and Health (formerly known as National Household Survey on Drug Abuse) has reported information regarding the use of illicit substances for individuals in the US of age 12 and over. These include a lifetime prevalence of hallucinogen use of about 6% for youth age 12–17, and 24% for those aged 18–25. Overall, about 1% of the US population had used a hallucinogen in the prior month.[23] Reflecting the importance of the pattern of use in youth, the 2003 Monitoring the Future Study reported a lifetime prevalence of hallucinogen use of 11% in 12th graders, 7% in 10th graders, and 4% in 8th graders.[16] Lifetime rates are 14% in college students and 20% in young adults. Looking at PCP, lifetime rates were about 3% in young adults and in 12th grade students, with less than 1% having used in the past year. The 1-year prevalence rates were 2% for 10th and 12th graders, 1% in 8th, and about 1% in college students and other young adults.

Use patterns are generally similar across the races, but there is a trend for a higher prevalence of abuse among Caucasians.[3,16] The rate of experimentation with specific hallucinogens (e.g., MDMA) varies across different locales. As is true for most drugs, rates outside the United States are lower.[24]

8.2. EMERGENCY PROBLEMS ASSOCIATED WITH HALLUCINOGENS

The most common hallucinogen-related difficulties seen in emergency rooms are anxiety, flashbacks, and toxic reactions.

8.2.1. Toxic Reactions

See Sections 1.7.1, 2.2.1, 5.2.1, 6.2.1, and 13.2.

8.2.1.1. Clinical Picture

8.2.1.1.1. History

The usual toxic reaction consists of the rapid onset (over minutes to hours) of confusion and the physical symptoms described below. Although death following higher doses of hallucinogens appears to be quite rare for most drugs, ingestion of high levels of MDA and probably of MDMA might carry higher risk.[2,3]

8.2.1.1.2. Physical Signs and Symptoms

Although the psychological state dominates the picture, vital sign abnormalities consistent with anxiety and panic are also observed. These include palpitations, increases in blood pressure and body temperature, sweating, and blurred vision. With intense overdoses, often with MDA or MDMA, symptoms can include body temperatures greater than 103°F orally, cardiovascular collapse, and convulsions. MDMA-like drugs can also result in rapid muscle destruction (rhabdomyelysis), and subsequent kidney and liver failure.[3]

8.2.1.1.3. Psychological State

This usually resembles an intense panic reaction. The individual has taken a higher than usual dose of the drug, with resulting anxiety along with visual hallucinations, depersonalization, paranoia, and confusion. The clinical picture diminishes as the drug is metabolized, but the symptoms tend to wax and wane over the subsequent 8–24 h.

8.2.1.1.4. Relevant Laboratory Tests

There are no specific laboratory tests except for the possible use of a toxicological screen (10 cc of blood or 50 ml of urine). It is important to monitor the vital signs, especially the blood pressure and the body temperature. If confusion is present, it is necessary to rule out head trauma.

8.2.1.2. Treatment

See Sections 2.2.1.2, 5.2.1.2, and 6.2.1.2.

1. The patient may present with convulsions or hyperthermia. The treatments usually involved for any life-threatening drug emergency must be instituted.[9]
   a. Closely observe vital signs.
   b. Establish an airway.
   c. Treat convulsions with anticonvulsants or a slow injection of diazepam (5–20 mg IV) if needed (see Section 5.2.1.2).
   d. Use ice baths or a hypothermic blanket for hyperthermia.
   e. Support blood pressure with medications, if needed (see Sections 6.2.1.2 and 13.2.3.1).
2. A thorough physical examination, including a neurological evaluation, should be carried out. The vital signs should be monitored for at least 24 h.
3. It is important to gain the patient's confidence with an empathic but firm approach. Consistent verbal contact and reality-orienting cues must be given, generally for up to 24 h.[2,3]
4. Reflecting the rapid absorption of most of these drugs, gastric lavage is not likely to be of use and may frighten the patient. However, some authors suggest lavage with activated charcoal (e.g., 1g/kg) when pills (e.g., MDMA) are used.[2,9]
5. I prefer to avoid all medications. However, when necessary, I usually fall back on:
   a. Diazepam (Valium), 5–30 mg orally, repeating 5–20 mg every 4 h as needed.[2]
   b. Chlordiazepoxide (Librium), 10–50 mg orally, followed by up to 25–50 mg every 4 h as needed.
   c. It may be best to avoid chlorpromazine (Thorazine) or other typical antipsychotics that have anticholinergic properties. There are few data, but clinically relevant doses of atypical neuroleptic drugs with prominent serotonin antagonism such as risperidone (Risperdal) might be useful.
6. If the clinical problem does not improve within 24 h, suspect that the drug ingested might be STP (which might last for several days to 2 weeks) or PCP, as discussed in Section 8.3. Treatment in this situation is similar to that outlined above.

8.2.2. Withdrawal

No clinically significant withdrawal picture is known for the hallucinogens.

8.2.3. Delirium, Dementia, and Other Cognitive Disorders (292.81 in DSM-IV)

See Sections 1.7.3, 2.2.3, 4.2.3, and 13.4.

8.2.3.1. Clinical Picture

Symptoms of confusion with hallucinogens usually develop in the midst of a toxic reaction (an overdose). The treatment of these syndromes was outlined in Section 8.2.1.2.

Some clinicians are concerned that prolonged exposure to hallucinogens may cause permanent decreased intellectual functioning or a long-term dementia, but there are few solid data to support this contention. Chronic use of these drugs may be associated with unfocused or "magical thinking," or problems with abstract thinking.[3,25] It is difficult to establish a "cause-and-effect" relationship for these pictures, as people likely to use these drugs might previously have tended toward more global thought patterns, might have had some level of brain impairment before drug use, and often have a history of multiple substance use. Another possible indication of brain damage comes from reports of visual afterimages (palinopsia), even years after achieving abstinence.[26]

8.2.3.2. Treatment

The individual suffering a delirium or dementia possibly associated with hallucinogen intoxication should be treated symptomatically. The approach should include a recommendation of abstinence from drugs and all other medications (including alcohol), a reevaluation of the degree of impairment over time, and vocational or educational rehabilitation, if appropriate.

8.2.4. Psychosis (292.1 and 292.2 in DSM-IV)

See Sections 1.7.4, 4.2.4, 5.2.4, 7.2.4, and 13.5.

8.2.4.1. Clinical Picture

True hallucinations or delusions that occur without insight (i.e., the person believes they are real) are much rarer with hallucinogens than with stimulants. When a hallucinogen-related psychosis occurs, it is most often marked by visual hallucinations (a state different from that likely to be seen in schizophrenia), and the symptoms usually disappear within hours to days. In the past, there have been case reports of potential paranoid delusions and/or hallucinations,[27,28] but few such case descriptions have been published in recent years. Because the condition is so rare, it is difficult to gather accurate data on potential causes. Perhaps the clinical picture represents an overdose with associated changes in vital signs, along with delusions or hallucinations, especially in the context of symptoms of confusion.

8.2.4.2. Treatment

The treatment depends on the clinical picture.

1. If the clinical picture is limited to intense anxiety or signs of a toxic reaction, the treatment is as described in Section 8.2.1.2.
2. In an individual with preexisting major depressive episodes or obvious preexisting schizophrenia, emergency treatment for a psychotic reaction resembles that outlined in Section 8.2.1.2, but with an emphasis on therapy aimed at the specific psychiatric disorder.
3. A drug-induced psychosis occurring in an individual without a preexisting psychiatric disorder is treated with reassurance, education, and cognitive approaches similar to steps outlined in Section 8.2.1.2. Hospitalization may be required if the loss of contact with reality is severe.
4. Appropriate short-term medications to control symptoms can include haloperidol at 2–4 mg IM Q2–4 h, or chlordiazepoxide (Librium, 25 mg PO Q4 h as needed).[29] The atypical antipsychotic drugs, such as rispiridone (Risperidal) have prominent effects on serotonin and are worth considering here, although there are a few data addressing their use.
5. If the psychosis does not clear within several days to several weeks, and no prior psychiatric disorder is apparent, the clinician should note the unusual nature of the syndrome. As with any atypical picture, other clinical conditions (e.g., an intracranial lesion, or concomitant stimulant dependence) must be considered. Treatment is symptomatic, requiring careful observation, good history taking, and constant reevaluation for a possible underlying pathological diagnoses.

8.2.5. Flashbacks (292.89 in DSM-IV, Listed as Hallucinogen Persisting Perception Disorder)

See Sections 1.7.5, 7.2.5, and 13.6.

8.2.5.1. Clinical Picture

This relatively benign condition usually comes to the attention of the health-care practitioner because an individual is concerned that the recurrence of drug effects might represent permanent brain damage.[2,3,29] Symptoms of *flashbacks* include simple visual images, lines or tracing of objects, and complex emotional experiences similar but not identical to the prior drug experience.[1] The patient may demonstrate sadness, anxiety, or even paranoia, which may recur periodically for days to weeks after taking the drug. This recurrence of hallucinogen effects may be set off by stress, fatigue, anxiety, taking another drug such as marijuana, or even the use of a clinically prescribed drug that enhances serotonin activity, such as a selective serotonin reuptake inhibitor (SSRI).[1,3]

The prevalence of flashbacks depends on the definition used and the study methods invoked. The rate of these problems seems to increase with the number of times an individual has taken the hallucinogen, but does not appear to be clearly related to the doses taken.[3] It is probable that between 15 and 30% of users have had a flashback of some sort.[1,3]

The person usually notes a feeling of euphoria and detachment, which is frequently associated with visual illusions (actual sensory inputs that are misinterpreted by the individual) lasting several minutes to hours.[1–3] The hallucinations usually involve lights or geometric figures seen out of the corner of the eye, often when entering darkness or just before falling asleep, or a trail of light following a moving object. Only rarely do they interfere with an individual's ability to function. Other types of flashbacks, including feelings of depersonalization or a recurrence of distressing emotional reactions experienced while under the drug effects, can also occur.

8.2.5.2. Treatment

Therapy for the self-limited picture is relatively simple.[3]

1. Care is based on reassurance that the syndrome will gradually decrease in intensity and disappear.
2. The patient should be educated about the course and the probable causes (e.g., residual drug) of the flashback.
3. It is important that other substances, especially marijuana and stimulants, as well as nonessential medications such as SSRIs and antihistamines be avoided.
4. If medication is needed (I usually choose to use no medication), consider diazepam (Valium) in doses of 10–20 mg orally, repeated at 5-mg doses if the flashback recurs, or comparable oral doses of chlordiazepoxide (e.g., 10–30 mg). One study suggested the usefulness of clonidine (Catapres) 0.25 mg PO TID.[30]
5. As is true in any drug-related problem, in an emergency situation it is important to consider the possibility that it is the result of a preexisting psychiatric disorder and not a flashback. Therefore, a careful history of prior psychiatric problems and a family history of psychiatric illness (which may indicate a propensity toward illness for this individual) must be taken.

8.2.6. Anxiety and Depression (292.89 and 292.84 Pictures in DSM-IV)

See Sections 1.7.6, 5.2.6, 7.2.6, and 13.7.

8.2.6.1. Clinical Pictures

Because these drugs cause both stimulation and altered feeling states at relatively low doses, it is not surprising that the most common problem connected with hallucinogens seen in emergency room settings is the high level of anxiety and fear.[1,3,31] Regarding anxiety, the individual is highly stimulated, frightened, may be hallucinating, and is usually fearful of losing his or her mind. This is one example of a "bad trip," the other being the toxic reaction seen in individuals who have taken higher doses (see Section 8.2.1).

These temporary anxiety reactions are most likely to be found in people with limited prior exposure to hallucinogens. The emotional discomfort tends to last for the length of action of the drug, for example, up to 8–12 h for LSD and closer to 2–4 h for mescaline and peyote.

Hallucinogens are also likely to create temporary mood disturbances.[32] The depression and sleep disturbances are likely to improve over a matter of days to weeks.

8.2.6.2. Treatment

1. Therapy is based on education through explaining the causes and course of the anxiety or depression reaction to the individual, and offering reassurance that he will totally recover.
2. Care should be given in the presence of friends or family members if possible.
3. It is important to establish a supportive, nonthreatening environment in which constant verbal contact can be maintained.[1]
4. Hospitalization is not usually needed if a temporary quiet, safe atmosphere can be arranged.
5. Medications are usually *not* needed. However, if it is impossible to control the patient otherwise, most authors suggest the use of an antianxiety drug such as:
   a. Diazepam (Valium), 10–30 mg orally, repeated in 1–2 h as needed.[1]
   b. Chlordiazepoxide (Librium) in doses of 10–50 mg orally, which may be repeated in 1–2 h.
   c. Be careful regarding the use of chlorpromazine (Thorazine) or other antipsychotic drugs because of the possibility that they might increase anticholinergic effects of adulterants or of the ingested drug.
6. It is important to obtain a clear history of other drug abuse or dependence and prior psychiatric disorders, and to establish a differential diagnosis, particularly ruling out mania and schizophrenia.
7. It is suggested that a follow-up visit be arranged to help the individual deal with his drug-taking problems, and to rule out any major coexisting psychiatric disorder.
8. Refer the patient for treatment of the substance use disorder.

8.2.7. Medical Problems

It has been difficult to prove persisting unique physiological impairments directly related to these drugs.[25] One area of concern has been the possibility of chromosomal damage.[11] Although broken chromosomes have been demonstrated with LSD-type drugs, and birth abnormalities have been seen in the offspring of mothers using hallucinogens (especially LSD in the first trimester), the causal nature of the relationship has not been established. Many substances (including aspirin) cause chromosomal breakage but have not been demonstrated to have definitely affected the fetus. Nonetheless, these substances are very potent. They may pose a danger of fetal abnormalities when they are used by pregnant women, and they may be associated with a significant increase in spontaneous abortions.[33]

Additional potential medical problems relate to the toxicity associated with MDA and MDMA.[17,19,21,34,35] The evidence of long-term and permanent damage to serotonin-rich neurons in animals, and the potential implications of these results to humans, were presented in Section 8.1.1.3.2. In addition, high doses of these hallucinogens have been reported to produce a variety of rare, but dangerous, medical problems including widespread muscle destruction with associated kidney failure, coagulation difficulties, and a syndrome of high body temperature, convulsions, and muscle contractions similar to the complication of antipsychotic medications known as the "neuroleptic malignant syndrome."

8.3. RELATED DRUGS (e,g., PCP) AND EMERGENCY PROBLEMS ASSOCIATED WITH THEIR USE

These are drugs that produce effects similar to hallucinogens but whose structures or additional actions contributed to the decision to list them separately. Thus, most commonly used substances in this category are PCP and related compounds. The more exotic (and usually less potent) drugs worthy of mention include *nutmeg*, *morning glory seeds*, *catnip*, *betel nut*, *nitrous oxide*, and *amyl* or *butyl nitrite*. The active ingredients of most "hallucinogen-like" plants and mushrooms are usually LSD-like or atropine-like substances.[36]

8.3.1. PCP and Related Drugs

Analogues of PCP were first introduced as general anesthetics in the 1950s (PCP as Sernyl or Sernylan, and ketamine as Ketalar, Ketaject, and Ketavet). In more recent years, this group has also included experimental drugs such as dizocilpine and cyclohexamine.[37–39] PCP-like drugs have the benefit of allowing anesthesia (lack of pain) through a dissociative state in which the subject is not in a deep "coma," thus producing relatively little depression of blood pressure, respiration, and other vital signs.[1,38] However, by 1965, PCP itself was no longer used for anesthesia in humans because approximately 20% of patients developed agitation, often with hallucinations, during the immediate postoperative period.[37,38] Currently, less potent analogues of PCP (e.g., ketamine) are still used in anesthesia.

PCP has become widely misused as an adulterant of other, sometimes more expensive street drugs.[40] In its own right, the drug has become widely misused as a "hallucinogen," known on the street by a variety of names (indicated in Table 1.4). It is taken as a pill, used as a powder that can be snorted or taken orally, or as a dried blot on a paper.[37,38] It can also be injected IV or sprayed on other drugs, such as marijuana, which is smoked.[37]

8.3.1.1. Pharmacology

PCP, a white solid substance, is a member of the arylcycloalkylamine group of drugs, all of which share similar types of actions in the brain.[41] These substances readily dissolve in fats, with a resulting accumulation in fatty tissues and an easy access to the brain, where drug levels can be sixfold to ninefold higher than in blood.[37,38] Taken orally, the PCP-like drugs are rapidly absorbed, and are then reabsorbed from the intestine and recirculated in the blood, resulting in longer lasting or recurrent effects.

The usual half-life of PCP is approximately 20 h, but storage in fats can result in very long-lasting effects in some individuals. PCP and related substances are metabolized primarily in the liver, mostly by hydroxylation, with metabolites and small amounts of the active drug excreted directly in the urine.[37,38]

When used for anesthesia, the PCP analogue, ketamine, is often given from 1.0 to 4.5 mg/kg, infused IV over a minute, or 6.5–13 mg/kg when given IM.[41] For PCP itself (which is no longer used clinically) 50 μg/kg can cause intense emotional withdrawal and disordered thinking, as demonstrated by bizarre responses on psychological testing.[1] The usual oral street dose is often between 5 and 10 mg, with the lower amount resulting in blood levels of between 0.01 and 0.1 μM.[37] The average marijuana cigarette laced with PCP is estimated to have higher doses (often greater than 20 mg) per "joint."[38] The usual blood levels on the street are not too far away from the estimated 1.0 μM levels that are capable of producing coma and respiratory distress.[38]

Four neurochemical actions of the PCP-like drugs are felt to contribute to the clinical effects. The most prominent involves a brain protein, or receptor, that is relatively specific for PCP-like drugs, and which is located as part of a complex that is named as the NMDA receptor.[42–44] The protein is activated by glutamate, the most prominent of the stimulatory, or excitatory, neurotransmitters in the brain.[39] The second neurochemical system prominently affected by PCP-like drugs involves dopamine.[45] Similar to the actions of stimulants, PCP appears to facilitate dopamine release and inhibit the dopamine transporter, with a resulting diminished reuptake of dopamine into synaptosomes and higher level in the synapse. These actions are thought to contribute to the stimulatory and hallucination-inducing effects of the PCP-like drugs, and might also explain why PCP might sometimes be substituted for amphetamines or cocaine in drug samples sold on the street. The third relevant neurochemical system involves serotonin.[46] The PCP-like drugs appear to inhibit the reuptake of serotonin into synaptosomes, decrease the rate of turnover of this neurotramsitter, and might also decrease the rate of firing of some serotonin neurons. Finally, the PCP-like substances have direct actions on both nicotinic and muscarinic cholinergic receptors, might impact on opiate receptors, and produce either direct or indirect actions on additional neurotransmitters including norepinephrine and GABA.[37,38,41]

8.3.1.2. Intoxication, Tolerance, Abuse, and Dependence (292.89, 304.90, and 305.90 in DSM-IV)

The intoxicating effects of PCP-like drugs are dose-related, with 1–5 mg producing incoordination, a floating feeling of euphoria, and heightened emotions, along with increases in heart rate, sweating, and tearing of the eyes. The usual intoxication lasts 4–6 h, though some additional time must pass before a person returns to normal.[38] At doses between 5 and 10 mg, the individual is likely to experience disorganized thinking, changes in body image, misperceptions of sensory input, feelings of unreality, a decreased ability to concentrate, and increased talkativeness. At this dose, physiological signs can include nystagmus (lateral, horizontal, or rotary), modest elevations in blood pressure, and a high heart rate.[37,38] At doses of about 15 mg, the signs and symptoms progress to vertigo, nausea and vomiting, weakness, a prominent decrease in movement, an increased reaction time, analgesia, and a sadness that can last up to 14 h.[37] Greater than 15 mg can produce deepening analgesia, anesthesia, and convulsions.

Tolerance for the PCP-like drugs has been noted in animals.[1,37,38] People have been reported to take as much as 1000 mg of PCP-like drugs per day without coma, reports that are consistent with prominent tolerance.[38]

Aspects of *dependence* have also been noted with regular PCP use. In animals, PCP is reinforcing, and monkeys have been reported to give up other activities in order to bar press for this drug.[1,37] Animals have also been noted to demonstrate a "withdrawal-like" syndrome when they precipitously stop taking PCP after repeated exposure, with symptoms including somnolence, tremor, diarrhea, vocalizations, bruxism, and piloerection.[1,37,47] However, few, if any, definitive cases of PCP withdrawal have been reported in humans. The remaining aspects of DSM-IV dependence can all be observed with repeated use of this drug (e.g., spending a great deal of time using, giving up important events, and so on).

8.3.1.3. Emergency Problems

8.3.1.3.1. Toxic Reactions

See Sections 1.7.1, 2.2.1, 6.2.1, and 13.2.

The toxic reaction, or overdose, consists of a combination of sympathetic (adrenaline-like) overactivity, the consequences of NMDA receptor actions, along with alterations in cholinergic functioning that can range from overactivity to anticholinergic effects.[37,38] Moderate doses (i.e., 10 mg and above) can result in catalepsy, mutism, and even a "light" level of coma. The vital signs and autonomic changes intensify at higher doses, and anything in excess of 15–50 mg is capable of producing an intense coma and/or convulsions. The patient is likely to demonstrate sweating and a fever; the blood pressure may be alarmingly high; the increase in deep tendon reflexes (DTRs) can progress to muscle rigidity and then convulsions; and the changes in heart and respiratory rate can progress to failure in both systems.

Although moderate to severe toxic reactions may develop rapidly, the clinical picture is likely to clear less quickly. One can expect a progression of recovery from severe intoxication (e.g., coma) through more moderate intoxication and on to light levels of impairment, with the entire picture taking from a few days to as long as 2–6 weeks to clear. The coma may progress to a severe delirium, with or without psychotic symptoms, which in turn slowly disappears. Therefore, a toxic reaction to PCP can be one of the longest lasting produced by drugs of abuse. The combination of a comalike state, open eyes, nystagmus, increased DTRs, decreased brain perceptions, and temporary periods of excitation should raise suspicion that a PCP toxic state is being observed.[36,37,47]

Regarding *treatment*, there are no specific antagonists to PCP intoxication.[36–38] The approach follows the common-sense rules of offering general support while avoiding the use of other medications unless necessary. When a medication is chosen to treat the PCP intoxication, the side effects must be kept in mind, and low doses should be used over as short a time as possible. The most important step is supporting the vital signs. Thus, it is worthwhile to review the material in Sections 2.2.1.2, 4.2.1.2, 6.2.1.2, and 13.2.3.1. Specific medications that might be helpful include physostigmine (Antilirium) at a dose of 2 mg every 20 min as needed if prominent anticholinergic symptoms are observed, diazepam (Valium) at 5–10 mg infused slowly IV for treatment of convulsions, and some recent data suggest that atypical antipsychotics or lamotrigine (Lamictal) may be beneficial for psychotic symptoms or severe agitation.[41,48,49]

8.3.1.3.2. Withdrawal

Reflecting the structure of PCP (which resembles depressants), a withdrawal syndrome after chronic administration is possible, and has been illustrated by studies of monkeys.[36] However, this has not been reported to be of clinical relevance in humans. A "rebound" can be expected after abrupt discontinuation of any medication (even aspirin), and patients may relate some level of discomfort, although there is no evidence that active treatment is required.[50]

8.3.1.3.3. Delirium, Dementia, and Other Cognitive Disorders (e.g., 292.89 or 292.81 in DSM-IV)

See Sections 1.7.3, 2.2.3, 4.2.3, and 13.4.

Antagonism of the NMDA glutamate receptor complex and/or changes in the cholinergic systems can produce prominent memory problems.[51–53] Thus, a state of confusion and/or decreased intellectual functioning is a usual component of the toxic reactions with PCP-like drugs, and has been reported in 25% of such patients.[36] The confusion may last for 4 weeks or longer and may be associated with violence. Some residual level of impairment of recent memory and ability to carefully think through problems has been reported to last in some individuals for months.[36,37]

8.3.1.3.4. Psychosis (e.g., 292.81 in DSM-IV)

See Sections 1.7.4, 5.2.4, and 13.5.

The ability of PCP-like drugs to induce psychotic pictures has been reported since the introduction of this drug as an dissociative anesthetic in the 1950s.[54] Psychotic symptoms have been documented in previously normal human subjects with doses of PCP of between 0.05 and 0.1 mg/kg IV, and with doses of ketamine of 0.77 mg/kg given IV over an hour.[55] The symptoms, likely to begin within minutes of the infusion of a bolus of a PCP-like drug, include social withdrawal, concrete thinking, and bizarre responses to proverbs and projective testing, even the absence of a delirium.[36,55] PCP-induced psychotic states often include significant elevations in blood pressure and/or nystagmus.[36] For the average patient, the psychotic symptoms last approximately 4 days, but can persist for 30 days or more in some individuals.[36] In addition, even at low doses, both PCP and ketamine are likely to intensify both positive and negative psychotic symptoms among schizophrenics.[37]

Regarding *treatment*, because the psychosis might be part of a continuum with the toxic reaction, the treatment parallels that outlined in Section 8.3.1.3.1. The best approach is to offer the patient a quiet, sheltered environment where his psychosis is not likely to lead to harm to himself or to those around him (e.g., a locked psychiatric ward). If possible, physical restraints should be avoided, and IM or oral antipsychotics or Bzs (e.g., diazepam in doses up to 60 mg or haloperidol up to 30 mg/day, if needed) can be used for the period of the psychosis, but should then be stopped as soon as possible. Of course, the adequate treatment of any psychotic state requires a careful evaluation to rule out any preexisting psychiatric disorders that may require long-term treatment (e.g., manic-depressive disease or schizophrenia).

8.3.1.3.5. Anxiety, Depression, and Violence (292.89 and 292.84 in DSM-IV)

See Sections 1.7.6, 5.2.6, and 8.2.6.

Any drug with sympathomimetic properties can produce prominent anxiety, and one third of patients presenting after using PCP report such problems. These hyperstimulated states are often associated with confusion and a decrease in behavioral controls. Thus, an important aspect of this type of anxiety can be violence. A history of physical or verbal aggressiveness, often impulsive, bizarre, and unprovoked, is reported in a third to 75% of chronic PCP users.[36] These follow a possible progression from anger and irritability to violence as PCP use is continued. Frank depressions resembling a major depressive disorder are not usually observed. Mood swings, however, are to be expected.[36]

The treatment of these conditions is aimed at the symptoms. As is true in most anxiety syndromes, it is best to avoid medications, offer reassurance, and decrease external stimuli by placing the person in a quiet, dimly lit room.[36] Depressive symptoms can be treated with education, reassurance, and cognitive therapy.

8.3.1.3.6. Medical Problems

PCP is not closely related to failure in any specific major organ system.[36] However, these drugs can cause physiological consequences, such as muscle rigidity and subsequent muscle destruction, as discussed above. In addition, animal studies indicate at least temporary vacuolization in some neurons when 5 mg/kg or more of PCP is ingested, with similar changes after high doses of other PCP-like drugs, such as ketamine and dizocilpine (e.g., 5 mg/kg).[1,35,37,55] At much higher doses, actual neuronal death can be observed within 48 h of the acute administration of these drugs. These changes might be related to ischemic neuronal death and/or might occur secondary to alterations in receptors associated with excitatory amino acids such as glutamate. Although few, if any, definitive cases of neuronal damage have been demonstrated in humans, this is a potential concern.

8.3.2. Nutmeg

The nutmeg plant, used since antiquity for the treatment of pain and diarrhea, can be ground up and either inhaled or ingested in large amounts to produce a change in consciousness.[56,57] The unpleasant side effects of high doses of these substances (including vomiting), and the long lag time (as much as 6 h) between ingestion and intoxication generally limit their use to places, such as prisons, where other drugs are not available.[57] The oral ingestion of two grated nutmeg pods will produce, after a latency of hours, a feeling of heaviness in the arms and legs, depersonalization (a feeling of not being oneself), derealization (a feeling of unreality), and apprehension.[57–59]

Along with this reaction come physiological changes such as dry mouth, thirst, increased heart rate, and flushing. Very high doses have been reported to cause abdominal pain and insomnia. One of the side effects of chronic use may be constipation.

The specific chemicals that contribute to the effects (probably myristicin and elemicin) have been suggested, but not proven. Also, details about the mechanisms of the action of nutmeg are not known, but part of the picture relates to its ability to inhibit prostagladin and affect serotonin systems.

Recovery from signs of intoxication usually occurs within 24–48 h. No specific treatment for the toxic reaction is needed. None of the other categories of drug abuse problems are known to occur with nutmeg.

8.3.3. Morning Glory Seeds

The seeds of the more common varieties of morning glory flowers contain LSD-related substances including ergine (*d*-lysergic acidlike) and isoergine. If ingested in high enough amounts, these can produce a mild hallucinatory state.[3] The usual effect of morning glory seeds, known on the streets as *heavenly blue* or *pearly gates*, is a change in self-awareness along with visual hallucinations that can lead to inappropriate behaviors.

The treatment of any panic, toxic, or potential psychotic reactions would follow that outlined for the hallucinogens in general in Section 8.2.

8.3.4. Catnip

Catnip is derived from the plant *Nepeta cataria* (a member of the mint family), and has a long history in folk-medicine as a prescription for abdominal irregularities.[60] The plant contains a variety of substances, including tannin and atropine-like drugs. It can be obtained in pet stores and has been given to cats to make them appear contented, and somewhat intoxicated. When catnip is used by humans, usually by smoking, the intoxication can be similar to that from marijuana. Visual hallucinations, euphoria, and fairly rapid changes in mood associated with headaches can occur, but these tend to clear rather quickly. There is no known treatment needed for the panic or toxic state that can be noted with the substance.

8.3.5. Locoweed

Another relevant substance is locoweed (*Astragalus* and *Oxytropis*), which is widely distributed in the western United States.[61] This plant is usually associated with accidental ingestion in animals, the result of which is a clinical picture of incoordination, depression, and difficulty in eating as well as an exaggerated reaction to stress. The active ingredients are indolizidine alkaloids, including swainsonine, which have some characteristics in common with the hallucinogens described in this section.[62,63]

8.3.6. Betel Nut

Betel nut is probably the most widely used drug in the Western Pacific and in parts of Africa and Asia, with an estimated use in up to 20% of the world's population.[64] This ancient substance, with use dating back to at least the year 600, was brought to Europe by Marco Polo in approximately AD 1300. Derived from the betel palm (*Areca catechu*), the substance is consumed as either fresh chunks or dried powder, which is chewed as a "quid" or mixture of peppermint and mustard along with leaves of the pepper plant (*Piper betel*).[65] These ingredients are subsequently mixed with slake lime from either limestone or the residue of burning seashells or coral stones in the presence of water. In addition to these basic ingredients, other substances such as tobacco, Asian spices, and dyes are also added, with different mixtures typical of different parts of the world. The combination of nut, mustard, lime, and additional ingredients is chewed; when mixed with saliva it produces a red color that stains the teeth.

The major active ingredient of this betel nut mixture is arecoline, present in concentrations estimated to be 0.25%. The quid also contains small amounts of pilocarpine and muscarine, natural plant products that affect the body in a manner similar to the brain neurochemical acetylcholine. There may also be indirect effects in catecholamine release and GABA inhibition.[65] Chewing produces symptoms similar to those of nicotine, and include euphoria, general arousal, and increased motor activity. Physical changes include sweating, an increase in saliva, tearing of the eyes (lacrimation), and an increased temperature, pulse, and breathing rate.[65] Individuals can also experience a decrease in appetite or diarrhea.

There are significant dangers to this acetylcholine-like substance. This is not surprising in light of the similar but more intense effects that are associated with reactions in some mushroom poisonings. High doses might precipitate convulsions, and regular use may enhance the risk for cirrhosis of the liver.[64,66] Chronic users can also develop psychological dependence, mood swings, and a feeling of tiredness when they stop using the drug. A more prevalent danger, however, is the result of the effect of the active ingredients and the lime on the lining of the mouth and throat. Regular consumption of betel nut is associated with a life-threatening cancer in those regions, squamous cell carcinoma, with rates projected to be as high as 5–10% among regular users.[67] The betel nut mixture also produces excessive fiber formation just beneath the gums, which can be responsible for a stiffness in the lining of the mouth that can become severe enough to interfere with eating.

8.3.7. Nitrous Oxide (N_2O)

This is a relatively weak general anesthetic that is either used as an adjunct to other agents or given on its own by dentists and obstetricians.[68–70] Possible mechanisms of action include interactions with the dopamine and opiate systems, and inhibitory effects on *N*-methyl-D-aspartate (NMDA) receptors.[70] This drug is reinforcing, and animals will self-administer it. Misuse of this inhalant tends to occur among professionals such as dentists, but it also occurs in as many as 10% of people from the general population who use the propellant from canned whipped cream and other sources.[71] Intake of the drug for a number of months on a daily basis can result in a temporary confused state, sometimes accompanied by paranoia. There are also dangers associated with lack of judgment, poor coordination, and possible orthostatic changes in blood pressure associated with intoxication.[72] These problems are likely to clear fairly rapidly when the drug use is stopped. More severe medical problems have also been noted including possible spinal cord degeneration.[71]

8.3.8. Amyl or Butyl Nitrite

These potent vasodilators appear to be widely used in homosexual men in an attempt to feel intoxicated and to postpone and enhance orgasm during sexual intercourse.[72] The substance is marketed under a variety of names, including Vaporole, and is sold in "adult" bookstores as Rush, Kick, Belt, and so on. These drugs dilate the blood vessels and have been used in the treatment of angina, although they now have limited medical usefulness.[73] Nitrites cause a slight euphoria and flushing of the skin, and may slow down time perception.

Approximately 17% of 18- to 25-year-olds and 60% of a sample of 150 homosexual men admitted using amyl nitrite, including almost 20% of the latter who took the substance at least once or twice a week. Heavier use is not likely in urban residents and, either directly or indirectly, with greater evidence of promiscuity, group sexual practices, and heavy intake of alcohol. Regarding the latter, approximately 48% of the heavier amyl nitrite users versus 23% of less intense users or nonusers reported being drunk at least weekly over the prior year.

The most common clinical problems of intoxication are toxic and anxiety reactions, which usually clear spontaneously with simple reassurance and abstinence. In addition, the drug can cause nausea, dizziness, and ataxia, as well as a drop in blood pressure.[74] The nitrites can also change the red-blood-cell pigment hemoglobin to methemoglobin and thereby impair the oxygen-carrying capacity of the blood. If severe, this can precipitate a coma which may respond to 1.5 mg/kg of a solution with methylene blue which reverses the process.[75] Amyl nitrite has also been reported to produce a potentially life-threatening hemolytic anemia.[76]

REFERENCES

1. O'Brien, C. P. Drug addiction and drug abuse. In J. G. Hardman, L. E. Limbird, & A. G. Goodman (Eds.), *The Pharmacological Basis of Therapeutics* (10th ed.). New York: McGraw-Hill, 2001, pp. 621–642.

2. Abraham, D. H. Hallucinogen-related disorders. In B. J. Sadock & V. A. Sadock (Eds), *Kaplan & Sadock's Comprehensive Textbook of Psychiatry* (8th ed.). Philadelphia, PA: Lippincott, Williams & Wilkins, 2004, pp. 1015–1024.
3. Pechnick, R. N., & Ungerleider, J. T. Hallucinogens. In J. H. Lowinson, P. Ruiz, R. B. Millman, & J. G. Langrod (Eds.), *Substance Abuse: A Comprehensive Textbook* (4th ed.). Baltimore: Williams & Wilkins, 2004, pp. 313–323.
4. Gouzoulis-Mayfrank, E., Thelen, B., Maier, S., Heekeren, K., Kovar, K.-A., Sass, H., & Spitzer, M. Effects of the hallucinogen psilocybin on covert orienting of visual attention in humans. *Neuropsychobiology 45:*205–212, 2002.
5. Edwards, G. *Matters of Subtance: Drugs and Why Everyone's a User*. London: Penguin Ltd., 2005.
6. Halpern, J. H. The use of hallucinogens in the treatment of addiction. *Addiction Research* (Vol. 4). Amsterdam: Harwood Academic Publishers, 1996, pp. 177–189.
7. Vollenweider, F. X., Vontobel, P., Hell, D., & Leenders, K. L. 5-HT modulation of dopamine release in basal ganglia in psilocybin-induced psychosis in man—a PET study with [^{11}C]raclopride. *Neuropsychopharmacology 20:*424–433, 1999.
8. Aghajanian, G. K., & Marek, G. J. Serotonin and hallucinogens, *Neuropsychopharmacology 21(Suppl):* 16S–23S, 1999.
9. Glaspy, J. N. Drugs of abuse. In O. J. Ma & D. M. Cline (Eds.) *Emergency Medicine Manual* (6th ed.). New York: McGraw-Hill Medical Publishing Division, 2004, pp. 499–504.
10. Strassman, R. J., Qualls, C. R., & Berg, L. M. Differential tolerance to biological and subjective effects of four closely spaced doses of *N,N*-dimethyltryptamine in humans. *Biological Psychiatry 39:*784–795, 1996.
11. Nichols, C. D., & Sanders-Bush, E. A single dose of lysergic acid diethylamide influences gene expression patterns within the mammalian brain. *Neuropsychopharmacology 26:*634–642, 2002.
12. American Psychiatric Association. *The Diagnostic and Statistical Manual of Mental Diseases* (4th ed., text revised). Washington, DC: American Psychiatric Press, 2000.
13. Grob, C. S., & Poland, R. E. MDMA. In J. H. Lowinson, P. Ruiz, R. B. Millman, & J. G. Langrod (Eds), *Substance Abuse: A Comprehensive Textbook* (4th ed.). Baltimore, MD: Williams & Wilkins, 2004, pp. 374–386.
14. Harris, D. S., Baggott, M., Mendelson, J. H., Mendelson, J. E., & Jones, R. T. Subjective and hormonal effects of 3,4-methylenedioxymethamphetamine (MDMA) in humans. *Psychopharmacology 162:*396–405, 2002.
15. Gouzoulis-Mayfrank, E., Becker, S., Pelz, S., Tuchtenhagen, F., & Daumann, J. Neuroendocrine abnormalities in recreational Ecstasy (MDMA) users: Is it Ecstasy or Cannabis? *Biological Psychiatry 51:*766–769, 2002.
16. Johnston, L. D., O'Malley, P. M., Bachman, J. G., & Schulenberg, J. E. (2004). *Monitoring the Future National Survey Results on Drug Use, 1975–2003, Vol. II: College Students and Adults Ages 19–40* (NIH Publication No. 04-5506). Bethesda, MD: National Institute on Drug Abuse.
17. Gowing L. R., Henry-Edwards, S. M., Irvine, R. J., & Ali, R. L. The health effects of ecstasy: A literature review. *Drug and Alcohol Review 21:*53–63, 2002.
18. Cowan, R. L., Lyoo, I. K., Sung, S. M., Ahn, K. H., Kim, M. J., Hwang, J., Haga, E., Vimal, R. L. P., Lukas, S. E., & Renshaw, P. F. Reduced cortical gray matter density in human MDMA (Ecstasy) users: A voxel-based morphometry study. *Drug and Alcohol Dependence 72:*225–235, 2003.
19. Gouzoulis-Mayfrank, E., Fischermann, T., Rezk, M., Thimm, B., Hensen, G., & Daumann, J. Memory performance in polyvalent MDMA (ecstasy) users who continue or discontinue MDMA use. *Drug and Alcohol Dependence 78:*317–323, 2005.
20. Buchert, R., Thomasius, R., Wilke, F., Petersen, K., Nebeling, B., Obrocki, J., Schulze, O., Schmidt, U., & Clausen, M. A voxl-based PET investigation of the long-term effects of "Ecstasy" consumption on brain serotonin transporters. *American Journal of Psychiatry 161:*1181–1189, 2004.

21. Vuori, E., Henry, J. A., Ojanpera, I., Nieminen, R., Savolainen, T., Wahlsten, P., & Jantti, M. Death following ingestion of MDMA (ecstasy) and moclobemide. *Addiction 98:*365–368, 2003.
22. Reneman, L., Lavalaye, J., Schmand, B., de Wolff, F. A., van den Brink, W., den Heeten, G. J., & Booij, J. Cortical serotonin transporter density and verbal memory in individuals who stopped using 3,4-methylenedioxymethamphetamine (MDMA or "Ecstasy"). Preliminary findings. *Archives of General Psychiatry 58:*901–906, 2001.
23. Substance Abuse and Mental Health Services Administration. *Overview of Findings from the 2002 National Survey on Drug Use and Health* (Office of Applied Studies, NHSDA Series H-21, DHHS Publication No. SMA 03-3774). Rockville, MD, 2003.
24. Cuomo, M. J., Dyment, P. G., & Gammino, V. M. Increasing use of "ecstasy" (MDMA) and other hallucinogens on a college campus. *Journal of American College of Health 42:*271–274, 1994.
25. Roiser, J. P., Cook, L. J., Cooper, J. D., Rubinsztein, D. C., Sahakian, B. J. Association of a functional polymorphism in the serotonin transporter gene with abnormal emotional processing in ecstasy users. *American Journal of Psychiatry 162:*609-612, 2005.
26. Kawasaki, A., & Purvin, V. Persistent palinopsia following ingestion of lysergic acid diethylamide (LSD). *Archives of Ophthalmology 114*:47–50, 1996.
27. Gouzoulis, E., Borchardt, D., & Hermle, L. A case of toxic psychosis induced by "Eve" (3,4-methylenedioxyethylamphetamine). *Archives of General Psychiatry 50*:75, 1993.
28. Hermle, L., Funfgeld, M., Oepen, G., Botsch, H., Borchardt, D., Gouzoulis, E., Fehrenbach, R. A., & Spitzer, M. Mescaline-induced psychopathological, neuropsychological, and neurometabolic effects in normal subjects: Experimental psychosis as a tool for psychiatric research. *Biological Psychiatry 32*:976–991, 1992.
29. Lerner, A. G., Finkel, B., Oyffe, I., Merenzon, I., & Sigal, M. Clonidine treatment for hallucinogen persisting perception disorder. *American Journal of Psychiatry 155*:1460, 1998.
30. McCann, U. D., & Ricaurte, G. A. MDMA "ecstasy" and panic disorder: Induction by a single dose. *Biological Psychiatry 32*:950–953, 1992.
31. Gouzoulis, E., Steiger, A., Ensslin, M., Kovar, A., & Hermle, L. Sleep EEG effects of 3, 4-methylenedioxyethamphetamine (MDE; "Eve") in healthy volunteers. *Biological Psychiatry 32*:1108–1117, 1992.
32. Abraham, H. D., & Aldridge, A. M. Adverse consequences of lysergic acid diethylamide. *Addiction 88*:1327–1334, 1993.
33. Croft, R. J., Klugman, A., Baldeweg, T., & Gruzelier, J. H. Electrophysiological evidence of serotonergic impairment in long-term MDMA ("Ecstasy") users. *American Journal of Psychiatry 158:*1687–1692, 2001.
34. McCann, U. D., Ricaurte, G. A., & Molliver, M. E. "Ecstasy" and serotonin neurotoxicity. *Archives of General Psychiatry 58:*907–908, 2001.
35. Riba, J., Rodríguez-Fornells, A., Urbano, G., Morte, A., Antonijoan, R., Montero, M., Callaway, J. C., & Barbanoj, M. J. Subjective effects and tolerability of the South American psychoactive beverage *Ayahuasca* in healthy volunteers. *Psychopharmacology 154:*85–95, 2001.
36. Zukin, S. R. Phencyclidine (or Phencyclidine-like) -related disorders, In B. J. Sadock & V. A. Sadock (Eds.), *Kaplan and Sadock's Comprehensive Textbook of Psychiatry* (8th ed.). Philadelphia, PA: Lippincott, Williams & Wilkins, 2004, pp. 1063–1070.
37. Zukin, S. R., Sloboda, Z., & Javitt, D. C. Phencyclidine (PCP). In J. H. Lowinson, P. Ruiz, R. B. Millman, & J. G. Langrod (Eds.), *Substance Abuse: A Comprehensive Textbook* (4th ed.). Baltimore: Williams & Wilkins, 2004, pp. 324–335.
38. Al-Amin, H. A., & Schwarzkopf, S. B. Effects of the PCP analog dizocilpine on sensory gating: Potential relevance to clinical subtypes of schizophrenia. *Biological Psychiatry 40*:744–754, 1996.
39. Holland, J. A., Nelson, L., Ravikumar, P. R., & Elwood, W. N. Embalming fluid-soaked marijuana: New high or new guise for PCP? *Journal of Psychoactive Drugs 30:*215–219, 1998.

40. Evers, A. S. & Crowder, C. M. General anesthetics. In J. G. Hardman, L. E. Limbird, & A. G. Goodman (Eds.), *The Pharmacological Basis of Therapeutics* (10th ed.). New York, NY: McGraw-Hill, 2001, pp. 337–366.
41. Anand, A., Charney, D. S., Oren, D. A., Berman, R. M., Hu, X. S., Cappiello, A., & Krystal, J. H. Attenuation of the neuropsychiatric effects of ketamine with lamotrigine. Support for hyperglutamatergic effects of *N*-methyl-D-aspartate receptor antagonists. *Archives of General Psychiatry 57:*270–276, 2000.
42. Krystal, J. H., Bennett, A., Abi-Saab, D., Belger, A., Karper, L. P., D'Souza, D. C., Lipschitz, D., Abi-Dargham, A., & Charney, D. S. Dissociation of ketamine effects on rule acquisition and rule implementation: Possible relevance to NMDA receptor contributions to executive cognitive functions. *Biological Psychiatry 47:*137–143, 2000.
43. Lindahl, J. S., & Keifer, J. Glutamate receptor subunits are altered in forebrain and cerebellum in rats chronically exposed to the NMDA receptor antagonist phencyclidine. *Neuropsychopharmacology 29:*2065–2075, 2004.
44. Balla, A., Sershen, H., Serra, M., Koneru, R., & Javitt, D. C. Subchronic continuous phencyclidine administration potentiates amphetamine-induced frontal cortex dopamine release. *Neuropsychopharmacology 28:*34–44, 2003.
45. Rabin, R. A., Doat, M., & Winter, J. C. Role of serotonergic 5-HT2a receptors in the psychotomimetic actions of phencyclidine. *International Journal of Neuropsychopharmacology 3:*333–338, 2000.
46. Spielewoy, C., & Markou, A. Withdrawal from chronic phencyclidine treatment induces long-lasting depression in brain reward function. *Neuropsychopharmacology 28:*1106–1116, 2003.
47. Winger, G.,Woods, J. H., & Hofmann, F. G. *A Handbook on Drug and Alcohol Abuse* (4th ed.). New York: Oxford University Press, 2004.
48. Malhotra, A. K., Adler, C. M., Kennison, S. D., Elman, I., Pickar, D., & Breier, A. Clozapine blunts *N*-methyl-D-asparate antagonist-induced psychosis: A study with ketamine. *Biological Psychiatry 42*:664–668, 1997.
49. Farber, N. B., Price, M. T., Labruyere, J., Nemnich, J., St Peter, H., Wozniak, D. F., & Olney, J. W. Antipsychotic drugs block phencyclidine receptor-mediated neurotoxicity. *Biological Psychiatry 34*:119–121, 1993.
50. Hurt, P. H., & Ritchie, E. C. A case of ketaminie dependence. *American Journal of Psychiatry 151*:5, 1994.
51. Curran, H. V., & Morgan, C. Cognitive, dissociative and psychotogenic effects of ketamine in recreational users on the night of drug use and 3 days later. *Addiction 95:*575–590, 2000.
52. Curran, H. V., & Monaghan, L. In and out of the K-hole: A comparison of the acute and residual effects of ketamine in frequent and infrequent ketamine users. *Addiction 96:*749–760, 2001.
53. Morgan, C. J. A., Monaghan, L., & Curran, H. V. Beyond the K-hole: A 3-year longitudinal investigation of the cognitive and subjective effects of ketamine in recreational users who have substantially reduced their use of the drug. *Addiction 99:*1450-1461, 2005.
54. Adler, C. M., Malhotra, A. K., Elman, I., Goldberg, T., Egan, M., Pickar, D., & Breier, A. Comparison of ketamine-induced thought disorder in healthy volunteers and thought disorder in schizophrenia. *American Journal of Psychiatry 156:*1646–1649, 1999.
55. Breier, A., Malhotra, A.K., Pinals, D.A., Weisenfeld, N. I., & Pickar, D. Association of ketamine-induced psychosis with focal activation of the prefrontal cortex in healthy volunteers. *American Journal of Psychiatry 154*:805–811, 1997.
56. Grover J. K., Khandkar S., Vats, V., Dhunnoo Y., & Das, D. Pharmacological studies on myristica fragrans—antidiarrheal, hypnotic, analgesic and hemodynamic (blood pressure) parameters. *Methods and Findings in Experimental and Clinical Pharmacology 24:*675–680, 2002.
57. Kelly, B. D., Gavin, B. E., Clarke, M., & Lane A. Nutmeg and psychosis. *Schizophrenia Research 60:*95–96, 2003.

58. Sangalli, B. C., & Chiang, W. Toxicology of nutmeg abuse. *Journal of Toxicology. Clinical Toxicology 38:*671–678, 2000.
59. Stein, U., Greyer, H., & Hentschel, H. Nutmeg (myristicin) poisoning—report on a fatal case and a series of cases recorded by a poison information centre. *Forensic Science International 118:*87–90, 2001.
60. Nostro A, Cannatelli, M. A., Crisafi, G., & Alonzo, V. The effect of Nepeta cataria extract on adherence and enzyme production of Staphylocccus aureus. *International Journal of Antimicrobial Agents 18:*583–585, 2001.
61. Pfister, J. A., Stegelmeier, B. L., Cheney, C. D., James, L. F., Molyneux, R. J. Operant analysis of chronic locoweed intoxication in sheep. *Journal of Animal Science 74*:2622–2632, 1996.
62. Gardner, D. R., Lee, S. T., Molyneux, R. J., & Edgar, J. A. Preparative isolation of swainsonine from locoweed: extraction and purification procedures. *Phytochemical Analysis 14:*259–266, 2003.
63. Rooprai, H. K., Kandanearatchi, A., Maidment, S. L., Christidou, M., Trillo-Pazos, G., Dexter, D. T., Rucklidge, G. J., Widmer, W., & Pilkington, G. J. Evaluation of the effects of swainsonine, captopril, tangeretin and nobiletin on the biological behaviour of brain tumour cells in vitro. *Neuropathology and Applied Neurobiology 27:*29–39, 2001.
64. Tsai, J. F., Jeng, J. E., Chuang, L. Y., Ho, M. S., Ko, Y. C., Lin, Z. Y., Hsieh, M. Y., Che, S. C., Chuang, W. L., Wang, L. Y., Yu, M. L., Dai, C. Y., & Ho, C. Habitual betel quid chewing as a risk factor for cirrhosis: a case-control study. *Medicine 82:*365–372, 2003.
65. Chu, N. S. Effects of Betel chewing on the central and autonomic nervous systems. *Journal of Biomedical Science 8:*229–236, 2001.
66. Huang, X., Xiao, B., Wang, X., Li, Y., & Deng, H. Betel nut indulgence as a cause of epilepsy. *Seizure 12:*406–408, 2003.
67. Liao, C. T., Chen, I. H., Chang, J. T., Wang, H. M., Hsieh, L. L., & Cheng, A. J. Lack of correlation of betel nut chewing, tobacco smoking, and alcohol consumption with telomerase activity and the severity of oral cancer. *Chang Gung Medical Journal 26:*637–645, 2003.
68. Alho, H., Methuen, T., Paloheimo, M., Strid, N., Seppa, K., Tiainen, J., Salaspuro, M., Roine, R. Long-term effects of and physiological responses to nitrous oxide gas treatment during alcohol withdrawal: Double blind, placebo-controlled trial. *Alcoholism: Clinical and Experimental Research 26:*1816–1822, 2002.
69. Zacny, J. P., Janiszewski, D., Sadeghi, P., & Black, M. L. Reinforcing, subjective, and psychomotor effects of sevoflurane and nitrous oxide in moderate-drinking healthy volunteers. *Addiction 94:*1817–1828, 1999.
70. Jevtovic-Todorovic, V., Beals, J., Benshoff, N., & Olney, J. W. Prolonged exposure to inhalational anesthetic nitrous oxide kill neurons in adult rat brain. *Neuroscience 122:*609–616, 2003.
71. Ng, J., O'Grady, G., Pettit, T., & Frith, R. Nitrous oxide use in first-year students at Auckland University. *Lancet 361:*1349–1350, 2003.
72. Culley, D. J., Baxter, M. G., Yukhananov, R., & Crosby, G. Long-term impairment of acquisition of a spatial memory task following isoflurane-nitrous oxide anesthesia in rats. *Anesthesiology 100:*309–314, 2004.
73. Haverkos, H. W., & Drotman, D. P. NIDA technical review: Nitrate inhalants. *Biomedicine & Pharmacotherapy 50*:228–230, 1996.
74. Kopelman, M. D., Reed, L. J., Marsden, P., Mayes, A. R., Jaldow, E., Laing, H., & Isaac, C. Amnesic syndrome and severe ataxia following the recreational use of 3,4-methylenedioxymethamphetamine (MDMA, 'ecstasy') and other substances. *Neurocase 7:*423–432, 2001.
75. Modarai, B., Kapadia, Y. K., Kerins, M., & Terris, J. Methylene blue: A treatment for severe methaemoglobinaemia secondary to misuse of amyl nitrite. *Emergency Medicine Journal 19:*270, 2002.
76. Graves, T. D., & Mitchell, S. Acute haemolytic anaemia after inhalation of amyl nitrite. *Journal of Royal Society of Medicine 96:*594–595, 2003.

CHAPTER 9

Glues, Inhalants, and Aerosols

9.1. INTRODUCTION

9.1.1. General Comments

This chapter describes a heterogeneous group of industrial substances that share the ability to produce generalized CNS depression and signs of confusion through disturbances in physiological functioning within neurons.[1–5] Although labeled as glues, solvents, and aerosols, in deference to the DSM-IV system, this chapter uses the more generic term of inhalants,[6] reflecting the ability of these substances to be administered through inhalation via the lungs. Some other drugs are also inhaled, including tobacco and several agents discussed with the hallucinogens (e.g., amyl and butyl nitrite and nitrous oxide), but the clinical and biological effects of these other drugs make it more appropriate that they be discussed in Chapters 8 and 11.

It is likely that inhalant use has existed since ancient times, in one form or another. The practice reached almost epidemic proportions by the late nineteenth and early twentieth centuries as substances like chloroform, gasoline, and other agents became generally available.[1] A marked expansion of the pattern of use of these drugs was also observed in World War II, and again in the early 1960s with the inhalation of model airplane glue. Despite the efforts of the hobby industry to modify its products by removing some of the more toxic substances and adding an irritating smell, problems have continued with inhalation of aerosol propellants and industrial solvents.

The more frequently misused agents and their contents (Table 9.1) include cleaning solvents (such as carbon tetrachloride), toluene, gasoline, lighter fluids, typewriter correction fluid, nail polish remover, and the fluorinated hydrocarbons used in aerosols. These products are popular because they induce euphoria and are readily available, cheap, legal, and easy to conceal. The onset of mental change occurs rapidly and disappears fairly quickly, and, with the exception of headache, serious hangovers are usually not seen.

Table 9.1
Groups of Inhalants[1,3,4]

I. Glues and adhesives	Toluene, hexane, ethyl acetate, benzene, methyl chloride, acetone, xylene, chloroform, and others
PVC cement	Trichloroethylene
II. Aerosol propellants (including thosefor paints, deodorants, analgesics, asthma treatments, etc.)[a]	Fluorinated hydrocarbons plus butane, toluene, propane, and others (depending on the source)
Fire extinguishers	Bromochlorodifluoromethane
III. Cleaning and dry cleaning solutions, and degreasers	Tetra- and trichloroethylene, trichloroethane, carbon tetrachloride, petroleum products, and others
IV. Paints, paint thinners, and nail polish removers	Toluene, acetone, methanol, ethylacetate, methylene chloride
Correction fluid	Trichloroethylene, trichloroethane
V. Fuels	
Gasoline	Gasoline, lead, other petroleum products
Lighter gas and fluids	Butane, isopropane

[a]Nitrous oxide is used as a propellant for whipping cream, and amyl or butyl nitrite are discussed in Chapter 8 on hallucinogens.

9.1.2. Pharmacology

9.1.2.1. General Characteristics

The inhalants are all fat-soluble organic substances that easily pass through the blood–brain barrier to produce a change in the state of consciousness similar to the more mild stages of anesthesia.[4] Because the inhalants easily dissolve in fats, they are likely to accumulate in fat-rich organs such as the liver and the brain.[1] The drugs in this category are all efficiently and rapidly absorbed through the lungs and are also taken into the body via the skin.

The substances are diverse in structure, and most commercial products contain a combination of these inhalants along with other chemicals. Some of their actions may reflect alterations in the lipid-rich neuroglial membranes in the CNS. There are also both direct and indirect changes, in the turnover and tissue levels of brain neurotransmitters, including dopamine, glutamate, and GABA.[7–9] The alterations in dopamine probably contribute to the reinforcing effects of these drugs. The metabolism of most solvents occurs in both the kidneys and the liver, but much of the substance is directly exhaled.[4,7]

This diverse group of inhalants can be roughly divided into the five subgroups given in Table 9.1.[1,4] The glues (including airplane hobby glue and rubber cement) contain prominent amounts of toluene, hexane, acetone, and other petroleum products. Another adhesive, PVC cement, contains trichloroethylene. The second category of inhalants involves the propellants used in aerosol containers, along with the major active ingredients in the commercial product itself, such as paints, analgesics, asthma treatments, or deodorants. Prominent in most of these containers are fluorinated hydrocarbons, and many of them also contain butane, toluene, and propane.

The third class of these drugs includes substances usually used as cleaning solutions, especially to get rid of grease. These include tetrachloroethylene, trichloroethylene, carbon tetrachloride, and other products. The fourth group, paint thinners and nail polish removers, also contain toluene and acetone, along with methanol and other chemicals, whereas a related substance, typewriter correction fluid, contains trichloroethylene and trichloroethane. Finally, the fifth subgroup of inhalants includes fuels such as gasoline and substances used in cigarette lighters. These contain many petroleum products, sometimes include lead, and are likely to incorporate butane and isopropane. Although this brief review is structured to help the reader categorize substances, it is always best to carefully read the list of ingredients whenever the original source of the inhalant intoxication is available.

It is worthwhile to briefly review some of the properties of several specific inhalants.

Toluene is considered unsafe when levels in the environment reach 100 parts per million (ppm), but inhalation of toluene containing glues or paint products can produce concentrations of 10,000 ppm.[1] Blood levels of toluene for patients hospitalized after exposure to this substance often range from about 1.0 to 8.0 μg per gram of blood.[1] Once inhaled, about 20% of the substance is excreted through the breath, with the rest metabolized in the liver to hippuric acid, which is then excreted in the urine.[1] Inhalation of toluene by a person who is also consuming alcohol results in higher blood levels of both substances as they compete for liver enzymes in their metabolism. Problems associated specifically with toluene include cognitive impairment, cerebellar dysfunction, renal toxicity, lung damage, and optic, but not peripheral, neuropathies.[3,4]

Trichloroethylene (also known as TCE) is prominent in PVC cement, cleaning solutions, typewriter correction fluid, and in dry-cleaning solutions. This inhalant can cause a relatively persistent (and slowly reversible) trigeminal neuropathy.

Benzene is prominent in many glues and adhesives. Whereas mild intoxication can cause euphoria, dizziness, and headache, severe intoxication can result in blurred vision, shallow respirations, heart arrhythmias, paralysis, and unconsciousness.[2] Long-term exposure to this toxic inhalant can cause aplastic anemia and might increase the risk for leukemia.

Hexane, found in glues and other inhalants, can cause a peripheral neuropathy, but it is less likely to induce confusion or other brain dysfunction, than some other inhalants, unless very high levels are used. *Methylene chloride* can produce carboxyhemoglobin with resulting decreased oxygen carrying capacity of the blood. *Gasoline*, often inhaled as a 1% vapor, produces a variety of temporary cognitive problems and can expose the user to lead intoxication, with severe cognitive impairment[10], although the latter problem has become less common as lead has been removed from most fuels.

Finally, *methanol*, used in carburetor cleaning fluids and in some paint products, can be severely toxic to both the brain and to peripheral nerves.[3] These and other medical problems are also discussed in Section 9.2.7.

9.1.2.2. Predominant Effects (Intoxication is 292.89 in DSM-IV)

When used for a high, inhalants are all taken through the lungs. Initial administration is either via sniffing through the nose, by huffing (sucking on a rag saturated with the inhalant), through bagging (where the substance is placed in a paper or plastic bag, sometimes heated, and inhaled through the mouth and nose—a method where increased carbon dioxide and decreased oxygen also contribute to intoxication), or by spraying an aerosol directly into the mouth.[4,10] Although aerosol propellants can be inhaled directly, most users attempt to remove particulate contents by straining through a cloth. Gasoline is sometimes inhaled directly from gas tanks.

The usual "high" begins within minutes (perhaps 15 inhalations) and lasts for a quarter to three quarters of an hour, during which time the individual feels giddy, dizzy, and light-headed.[1,2,4] Most users report a decrease in inhibitions along with a floating sensation, misperceptions or illusions, clouding of thoughts (with possible visual hallucinations), drowsiness, and occasionally a period of amnesia during the height of the inhalation episode.

Acute intoxication is accompanied by a variety of potentially disturbing physiological symptoms (Table 9.2), including headache, irritation of the eyes, sensitivity to light, double vision, nystagmus, ringing in the ears, irritation of the lining or mucous membranes of the nose and mouth, and a cough. The user may also complain of nausea, vomiting, and diarrhea. Some faint (especially with a fluorinated hydrocarbon aerosol), perhaps secondary to cardiac arrhythmias. Additional symptoms can include incoordination, shallow respiration, paralysis, and unconsciousness.[2] Intoxication is usually associated with a slowing of the brain waves to an 8–10 s^{-1} pattern on the EEG.

9.1.2.3. Tolerance and Dependence (304.60 and 305.90 in DSM-IV)

Most users begin to take the substance in the early to mid-teens, with inhalation often occurring in a sporadic and temporary manner.[4,5] Whereas for most people, the frequency and intensity of use of inhalants decreases with increasing age,[3] severe repetitive problems can develop and last into adulthood, especially for individuals with antisocial personality disorder and among IV drug users.[1] Adolescents who use inhalants are also more likely to use alcohol, nicotine, and other illicit substances.[5,11]

A host of different problems related to dependence can develop. Tolerance, or the need for larger amounts of the substance to get the usual

Table 9.2
Common Signs and Symptoms of Acute Inhalant Intoxication[1,2]

Sensory	Light sensitivity
	Eye irritation and injection
	Double vision
	Ringing ears
Respiratory	Sneezing
	Wheezing
	Runny nose
	Cough
	Perioral rash
Gastrointestinal	Nausea
	Salivation
	Vomiting
	Diarrhea
	Loss of appetite
Other	Chest pain
	Incoordination
	Ataxia
	Lethargy
	Decreased reflexes
	Abnormal heart rhythm
	Muscle and joint aches

effects, has been observed in both animals and in humans, but is difficult to quantify.[1,3,4,9] Some users will spend a great deal of time seeking out the substance and recovering from its effects, will give up important events in order to huff or bag, and will continue to take the inhalant despite obvious medical and psychological consequences.[8,9,12] Studies in animals have shown that repeated exposure to an inhalant such as trichloroethane can be associated with convulsions when the drug is stopped, a phenomenon that can be blocked by toluene, alcohol, or barbiturates.[1] However, there is no clear evidence from clinical case studies that a relevant withdrawal syndrome exists in humans.

9.1.3. Epidemiology and Patterns of Use

Inhalants are usually taken intermittently and often as part of a fad among adolescents in their early teens or among groups with limited access to drugs. Teenagers tend to abandon the use of inhalants after a year or two as they mature and move on to other substances, but a small percentage continue with solvents as their drug of choice for periods of 15 years or more.[13] Long-term intake is often associated with antisocial personality disorder, and it has been estimated that 30% or more of prison inmates have used inhalants at sometime in their lives.[3]

The temporary use of inhalants is estimated to be among the top two or three most prevalent substances of abuse in adolescent populations in many parts of the world[8,9,11,14] with populations in the United States reporting the highest prevalence rates. The 2003 National Monitoring the Future Study reported that almost 16% of 8th graders, 13% of 10th graders, and more than 11% of 12th graders had ever used inhalants for intoxication, including 9, 5, and 4% in the prior year, as well as 4, 2, and 2% in the prior 30 days. These figures are a bit lower than those reported in 1994, with the early 1990s being the highest prevalence rates in recent decades.[13] Regarding specific areas of the US, the lifetime risk in adolescents in Illinois was reported as 14%, but greater than 22% in Texas youth.[15,16] Among college students, the lifetime rate was 8%, prior year 2%, and last 30 days 1% for the use of inhalants, with figures in young adults in the general population of 12, 2, and <1%. These results are consistent with reports that the prevalence of use decreases rapidly with increasing age, and that the chances of ever having been intoxicated with an inhalant are higher for individuals with lower levels of education, as well as those having problems at school.[5,11,16] One survey of students in an alternative (i.e., nonacademic high school), reported a lifetime prevalence of 27%.[5]

A variety of other characteristics have been reported as likely to relate to a higher prevalence of inhalant misuse. Most studies report a greater probability of intake among males, although this is not reported in all samples, and use may be especially high among Native Americans and Aboriginals in Australia.[5,11,17,18] It has also been reported to be elevated among Hispanics living in socioeconomically deprived areas, but appears to be lower among African-Americans than the general population.[4,18,19] Regular users of inhalants are also more likely to report symptoms of depression, alienation from peers, and the use of additional substances, including nicotine and alcohol.[5,11]

9.2. EMERGENCY PROBLEMS

The most common emergency situations seen with the inhalants are toxic reactions, cognitive impairments, and medical complications.

9.2.1. Toxic Reactions

See Sections 1.7.1, 2.2.1, 4.2.1, 6.2.1, and 13.2.

9.2.1.1. Clinical Picture

9.2.1.1.1. History

The patient can experience an abrupt onset (within minutes) of severe physical distress while using an inhalant.[1,3,20] Death during intoxication can also occur through aspiration of vomitus, from suffocation as a result of using a plastic bag, cardiac arrhythmias, or accidents.[1,4,16,21]

9.2.1.1.2. Physical Signs and Symptoms

It has been estimated that inhalants lead to the death of 1–2% of children aged 10–19 years in the United Kingdom.[22] In the US, at least 240 inhalant-related deaths were reported between 1996 and 1999, and in one series, the victims were an average of 25 years old with the two most common agents being freon and chlorinated hydrocarbons.[4,16] A life-threatening toxic picture characterized by respiratory depression, cardiac arrhythmias, and possibly convulsions can follow the administration of inhalants at any age.[22–24]

9.2.1.1.3. Psychological State

The physically ill individual may present with anxiety and mental impairment that can range from confusion, sometimes with associated hallucinations or delusions, to coma.[24]

9.2.1.1.4. Relevant Laboratory Tests

Although these are rarely helpful in establishing the diagnosis, some inhalants, such as toluene, can be identified in the blood.[1] The major metabolite of this substance, hippuric acid, can also be found in urine, with ratios of 1 g or more of hippurate to 1 g of creatinine suggesting recent intoxication.[1]

For those with toxic reactions, it is advisable to monitor cardiac functioning through an EKG and to establish the RBC and WBC counts (see Table 1.6) as well as the levels of liver and kidney functions (see Section 9.2.7). Other tests that should be considered include arterial blood gases if breathing is compromised, creatinine, as well as a chest x-ray.[20]

9.2.1.2. Treatment

There are no specific antidotes for the inhalant overdose. The treatment consists of offering good supportive care, controlling arrhythmias, and aiding respiration (up to and including an endotrachial tube, if needed). If considerable hypotension is present, an IV crystalloid infusion should be considered, as adrenalin-like drugs might intensify arrhythmias. A beta blocker (e.g., propranolol or inderol) may be used for arrhythmias, if needed.[20] This approach is similar to the general life supports outlined for opioids in Section 6.2.1.2, except that naloxone (Narcan) has no use here. The severe confusion or psychotic symptoms can be treated with antipsychotic medications, and one report suggests possible benefits for carbamazepine (Tegretol).[24]

9.2.2. Withdrawal

No clinically relevant withdrawal syndrome from inhalants has been described in humans, although this is still under study. Some users have reported experiencing sleep problems, nausea, irritability, and a tremor following cessation of use,[4] but there are few convincing data that these reflect a true rebound or withdrawal syndrome.

9.2.3. Delirium, Dementia, and Other Cognitive Disorders (292.89, 292.81, and 292.82 in DSM-IV)

9.2.3.1. Clinical Picture

See Sections 1.7.1, 2.2.3, and 13.4.

Inhalant intoxication can include the rapid onset of confusion and disorientation. The patient may have a rash around the nose or the mouth from inhaling, may have the odor of the inhalant in his breath, and may have been found in a semiconscious state with inhalants near him.

A frequent neurological finding is an EEG pattern of diffuse encephalopathy with an otherwise basically normal clinical neurological examination. Protracted long-term use can result in temporary or even longer lasting brain damage as demonstrated by a coarse tremor, a staggering gait, and scanning speech, perhaps reflecting cerebellar impairment, along with memory impairment.[1,4] Motor-related symptoms (e.g., myoclonus, chorea, and hyperactive reflexes) are especially likely following long-term inhalation of leaded gasoline.[10] Some patients also show evidence of brain atrophy, especially loss of white matter, with chronic toluene use.[1,3] These findings may be accompanied by disorders of thought, such as tangentiality, but usually occur without evidence of gross delusions or hallucinations. Although long-term follow-ups have not been carried out, this clinical picture has been observed for 5 months or longer after abstinence, and may be permanent.[25]

9.2.3.2. Treatment

Acute cognitive deficits are usually short-lived, and clear within a matter of hours. As with any delirium state, treatment centers on reassurance, the elimination of ambiguous or misleading stimuli (i.e., shadows or whispers), protection of the patient from the consequences of hostile outbursts, and the provision of a generally supportive environment. Few data are available on the optimal care for longer term cognitive impairment.

9.2.4. Psychosis (292.82 in DSM-IV)

See Section 5.2.4.

The most likely mental status change with inhalants, is an agitated confusion, or delirium. While visual hallucinations may occur during the state of confusion, delusions and/or hallucinations in the absence of confusion (a clear sensorium) are rare. Of course, as is true of all drugs of abuse, these agents can exacerbate any preexisting psychopathology and might precipitate longer term psychotic syndromes in people who are predisposed.

The treatment of any substance-induced psychopathological state is aimed at controlling the patient's behavior until the syndrome clears. Efforts include reassurance and physical or pharmacological controls such as diazepam (Valium), 15–30 mg or more by mouth, or chlordiazepoxide, 25–50 mg or more, which can be repeated in 1 h, if needed. Some authors suggest the use of antipsychotic medications or carbamazepine (Tegretol), although there are no double-blind controlled data on this issue.[24] If psychotic symptoms do not clear within several days, the possibility of a concomitant or a preexisting psychiatric disorder must be considered. This requires that the clinical picture be reviewed and that information be obtained from additional informants.

9.2.5. Flashbacks (Persisting Perception Disorder in DSM-IV)

See Sections 1.7.5, 8.2.5, and 13.6.

With the exception of temporary residual cognitive deficits, flashbacks are not known to occur with these drugs.

9.2.6. Anxiety and Depression (292.89 and 292.84 in DSM-IV)

Because the period of intoxication is short (15–45 min), intense anxiety states usually abate before an individual seeks professional care. Temporary periods of panic attacks and enhanced feelings of general anxiety can be seen with deliberate intoxication as well as with inadvertent exposure to these substances at home or in the workplace. As is true of all panic episodes, education, reassurance, and supplying a comfortable and non-threatening atmosphere form the basis of treatment.

Intoxication and its aftereffects can also produce emotional lability with considerable mood swings. Treatment involves taking care to identify any independent major depressive syndromes and offering reassurance if the symptoms reflect an inhalant-induced mood disorder. The symptoms improve with time for the great majority of people.

9.2.7. Medical Problems

9.2.7.1. Clinical Picture

The inhalants interfere with the normal functioning in many body systems.[1,3] However, because the use is generally intermittent and relatively short-lived, and the typical user is young and healthy, permanent sequelae are relatively rare. Nonetheless, the range of problems must be noted, as deaths do occur. The medical disorders associated with the inhalants include the following:

1. Cardiac irregularities, or arrhythmias, including fatal ventricular fibrillation, can be seen with inhalants, especially with aerosols. Most arrhythmias are successfully treated with abstinence and short-term use of antiarrhythmias drugs. Cardiomyopathy has also been reported in the context of chronic inhalation of glues.[3,4]
2. Hepatitis and liver failure have been noted following chronic exposure to inhalants, especially in the context of carbon tetrachloride, trichloroethylene, and chloroform.[1,26] Although liver changes are usually reversible, these substances might also increase the risk for liver cancer.
3. Many inhalants, especially toluene and benzene, are toxic to the kidney.[1,3,27] Problems include a distal-type tubular acidosis, glomerulonephritis, subsequent electrolyte abnormalities, and kidney damage secondary to muscle destruction with consequent rhabdomyolysis.[1,3]
4. Transient impairment of lung functioning, a result of lung irritation by inhalants, may be noted. However, while emphysema might develop, permanent lung damage has been difficult to document.[3]
5. Decreased production of all blood cells can occur, especially with the use of benzene and trichloroethylene.[1,3] In addition, methylene chloride and some of the nitrite compounds can impair the ability of hemoglobin to carry oxygen by converting this constituent of red blood cells to methemoglobin.[1] Some substances, especially benzene, might contribute to the development of acute myelocytic leukemia.[1,3]
6. Skeletal muscle weakness may develop as a result of muscle destruction, especially with toluene use.[3]
7. Transient, mild stomach or GI upsets can be seen with any of these substances.
8. Peripheral neuropathies have been reported, with *n*-hexane, methyl butyl ketone, naphtha, and lead.[4]
9. There is evidence that these substances might produce permanent CNS damage, a contention supported by reports of cerebral and cerebellar atrophy.[1,3,4]
10. These substances might be capable of inducing premature labor in pregnant women,[1] and there is a probability that the inhalants can cause adverse fetal effects, as they easily cross to the developing fetus[1,3,28,29]

9.2.7.2. Treatment

Most of these medical problems are transient and disappear with general supportive care. In the case of severe liver or kidney damage, the treatment is the same as that used for insults to these organs from other sources. Any patient with an encephalopathy should be carefully evaluated for other causes of the dementia.

REFERENCES

1. Crowley, T. J., & Sakai, J. T. Inhalant-related disorders. In B. J. Sadock & V. A. Sadock (Eds.), *Comprehensive Textbook of Psychiatry* (8th ed.). Baltimore, MD: Williams & Wilkins, 2004, pp. 1025–1032.
2. Klaassen, C. D. Nonmetallic environmental toxicants: Air pollutants, solvents and vapors, and pesticides. In J. G. Hardman, L. E. Limbird, & A. G. Goodman (Eds.), *The Pharmacological Basis of Therapeutics* (10th ed.). New York: McGraw-Hill, 2001, pp. 1877–1902.
3. Sharp, C. W., & Rosenberg, N. L. Inhalants. In J. H. Lowinson, P. Ruiz, R. B. Millman, & J. G. Langrod (Eds.), *Substance Abuse: A Comprehensive Textbook* (4th ed.). Baltimore, MD: Williams & Wilkins, 2004, pp. 336–366.
4. Brouette, T., & Anton, R. Clinical review of inhalants. *The American Journal on Addictions 10:*79–94, 2003.
5. Fleschler, M. A., Tortolero, S. R., Baumler, E. R., Vernon, S. W., & Weller, N. F. Lifetime inhalant use among alternative high school students in Texas: Prevalence and characteristics of users. *American Journal of Drug and Alcohol Abuse 28:*477–495, 2002.
6. American Psychiatric Association. *The Diagnostic and Statistical Manual of Mental Diseases* (4th ed., text revision). Washington, DC: American Psychiatric Press, 2000.
7. Gerasimov, M. R., Ferrieri, R. A., Schiffer, W. K., Logan, J., Gatley, S. J., Gifford, A. N., Alexoff, D. A., Marsteller, D. A., Chea, C., Garza, V., Carter, P., King, P., Ashby, C. R., Jr., Vitkun, S., & Dewey, S. L. Study of brain uptake and biodistribution of [^{11}C]toluene in non-human primates and mice. *Life Sciences 70:*2811–2828, 2002.
8. Gerasimov, M. R., Schiffer, W. K., Marstellar, D., Ferrieri, R., Alexoff, D., & Dewey, S. L. Toluene inhalation produces regionally specific changes in extracellular dopamine. *Drug and Alcohol Dependence 65:*243–251, 2002.
9. Riegel, A. C., Ali, S. F., & French, E. D. Toluene-induced locomotor activity is blocked by 6-hydroxydopamine lesions of the nucleus accumbens and the mGluR2/3 agonist LY379268. *Neuropsychopharmacology 28:*1440–1447, 2003.
10. Cairney, S., Maruff, P., Burns, C. B., Currie, J., & Currie, B. J. Neurological and cognitive recovery following abstinence from petrol sniffing. *Neuropsychopharmacology 30:* 1019–1027, 2005.
11. Kikuchi, A., & Wada, K. Factors associated with volatile solvent use among junior high school students in Kanto, Japan. *Addiction 98:*771–784, 2003.
12. Howard, M. O., Cottler, L. B., Compton, W. M., & Ben-Abdallah, A. Diagnostic concordance of DSM-III-R, DSM-IV, and ICD-10 inhalant use disorders. *Drug and Alcohol Dependence 61:*223–228, 2001.
13. Johnston, L. D., O'Malley, P. O., Bachman, J. G., & Schulenberg, J. E. *Monitoring the Future National Survey Results on Drug Use, 1975–2003: Vol. 1, Secondary School Students* (NIH Publication No. 04-5507). Bethesda, MD: National Institute on Drug Abuse, 2004.
14. Waraich, B. K., Chavan, B. S., & Raj, L. Inhalant abuse: A growing public health concern in India. *Addiction 98:*1169–1172, 2003.
15. Mackesy-Amiti, M. E., & Fendrich, M. Trends in inhalant use among high school students in Illinois: 1993–1995. *American Journal of Drug and Alcohol Abuse 26:*569–590, 2000.
16. Maxwell, J. C. Deaths related to the inhalation of volatile substances in Texas: 1988–1998. *American Journal of Drug and Alcohol Abuse 27:*689–697, 2001.
17. Substance Abuse and Mental Health Services Administration. *Results from the 2002 National Survey on Drug Use and Health. National Findings* (Office of Applied Studies, NHSDA Series H-22, DHHS Publication No. SMA 03-3836). Rockville, MD, 2003.
18. Beauvais, F., Wayman, J. C., Jumper-Thurman, P., Plested, B., & Helm, H. Inhalant abuse among American Indian, Mexican American, and Non-Latino white adolescents. *American Journal of Drug and Alcohol Abuse 28:*171–187, 2002.

19. Maclean, S. J., & D'Abbs, P. H. N. Petrol sniffing in Aboriginal communities: A review of interventions. *Drug and Alcohol Review 21:*65–72, 2002.
20. Fox, J. C. Hydrocarbons and volatile substances. In O. J. Ma & D. M. Cline (Eds.), *Emergency Medicine Manual* (6th ed.). New York, NY: McGraw-Hill, 2004, pp. 527–529.
21. Gable, R. S. Comparison of acute lethal toxicity of commonly abused psychoactive substances. *Addiction 99:*685–696, 2004.
22. Taylor, J. C., Norman, C. L., Bland, J. M., Ramsey, J. D., & Anderson, A. R. *Trends in Deaths Associated with Abuse of Volatile Substances 1971–1995* (10th annual report). London: St. George's Hospital, 1997.
23. Bowen, S. E., Daniel, J., & Balster, R. L. Deaths associated with inhalant abuse in Virginia from 1987 to 1996. *Drug and Alcohol Dependence 53:*239–245, 1999.
24. Hernandez-Avila, C. A., Ortega-Soto, H. A., Jasso, A., Hasfura-Buenaga, C. A., & Kranzler, H. R. Treatment of inhalant-induced psychotic disorder with carbamazepine versus haloperidol. *Psychiatric Services 49:*812–815, 1998.
25. Yamanouchi, N., Okada, S., Kodama, K., Sakamoto, T., Sekine, H., Hirai, S., Murakami, A., Komatsu, N., & Sato, T. Effects of MRI abnormalities on WAIS-R performance in solvent abusers. *Acta Neurologica Scandinavica 96:*34–39, 1997.
26. Meadows, R., & Verghese, A. Medical complications of glue sniffing. *Southern Medical Journal 89:*455–462, 1996.
27. Erramouspe, J., Galvez, R., & Fischel, D. R. Newborn renal tubular acidosis associated with prenatal maternal toluene sniffing. *Journal of Psychoactive Drugs 28:*201–204, 1996.
28. Gospe, S. M., Jr., & Zhou, S. S. Toluene abuse embryopathy: Longitudinal neurodevelopmental effects of prenatal exposure to toluene in rats. *Reproductive Toxicology 12:*119–126, 1998.
29. Jones, H. E., & Balster, R. L. Inhalant abuse in pregnancy. *Obstetrics and Gynecology Clinics of North America 25:*153–167, 1998.

CHAPTER 10

Over-the-Counter (OTC) Drugs and Some Prescription Drugs

10.1. INTRODUCTION

10.1.1. General Comments

Almost any substance has the potential for misuse (defined as voluntary intake to the point of causing physical or psychological harm). Previous chapters present information on the more classical drugs of abuse, while this chapter focuses on the misuse of over-the-counter (OTC) medications and some prescription drugs, including the anti-parkinsonian medications, diuretics, and antipsychotics.

The OTC drugs discussed in the following sections include nonprescription hypnotics (which contain antihistamines) and nonprescription antianxiety drugs (which usually contain substances similar to the OTC hypnotics; Section 10.2); nonprescription cold and allergy products (Section 10.3); OTC analgesics, also called nonsteroidal anti-inflammatory drugs (NSAID) (which contain aspirin, phenacetin, and aspirin-like products (Section 10.4); laxatives (Section 10.5); nonprescription stimulants, and diet pills (Section 10.6);[1] anabolic steroids (Section 10.7); and some thoughts on misuse of prescription medications. Because of the wide array of substances involved, each section essentially comprises a mini-chapter that includes subsections relevant to that class of drugs.

The history of OTC medications is long and complex.[2,3] Controls on drug availability are relatively recent, and at the turn of the twentieth century anyone could purchase opium, cocaine, and other potent substances without a prescription. Currently, although most nonprescription drugs have been incompletely evaluated and some are of questionable efficacy, these "dietary supplements" are not regulated by the Food and Drug Administration and are listed as "generally considered safe".[3] However, many are capable of producing physical and emotional pathology when taken either in excessive doses or in combination with other medications or with alcohol, and some impact on the metabolism of other drugs.[4,5]

The OTC market is large, lucrative, and continues to grow. These substances have been used by up to 50% of the population in the US, have generated over $12 billion in income,[3] and have represented one third of the National Health budget. These huge expenditures reflect a general movement from prescription to OTC agents, as well as the sale of more traditional vitamins, minerals, and OTC medications. Unfortunately, health-care practitioners and the general public have limited knowledge of the dangers of these substances, with most people receiving their information from advertisements. The result is heavy use and frequent misuse of these drugs, with subsequent pathology coming to light in both emergency and general practice settings.

10.1.2. Epidemiology and Patterns of Misuse

There are more than 500,000 different OTC preparations, and six out of every eight medications purchased in the United States fall into this category.[1] OTC substances are taken by all elements of society and must be considered a part of the differential diagnosis for patients seen in the clinician's office or the emergency room.

10.2. ANTIHISTAMINIC DRUGS (SEDATIVES/HYPNOTICS AS INGREDIENTS IN OTC COLD AND SINUS PREPARATIONS)

10.2.1. General Comments

All of the OTC sleep medications now contain 25–50 mg of an antihistamine such as diphenhydramine (Benadryl, Tylenol PM, Sominex, Nytol) or doxylamine (Unisom).[6,7] Some of these agents also contain aspirin or acetaminophen. In the past, many of these drugs (e.g., Sominex) included scopolamine (0.125–0.5 mg), but the atropine-type drugs have now been removed from these medications. Antihistamines are also found in many OTC cold, allergy, and sinus preparations.

Controlled studies indicate that OTC sleep aids and sedatives (such as Compoz) help decrease symptoms but are significantly less effective than the Bzs, such as temazepam (Restoril). However, when Compoz was compared with aspirin and with a placebo, patients taking Compoz had increased rates of side effects, including daytime sleepiness and dizziness.

10.2.2. Pharmacology

These drugs, first discovered in the late 1930s, have major effects on three types of histamine receptors (H_1, H_2, and H_3) in the brain and in the rest of the body.[7–9] One variety of histamine receptors (H_2), affects the amount of acid produced in the stomach and responds to drugs such as cimetidine (Tagamet), whereas the H_3 type has few known clinical implications.

It is the H_1 histamine receptor antagonists that have the broadest uses and are the most likely to be involved in abuse and dependence. These medications fit into five categories that are represented by drugs such as hydroxyzine (marketed as Vistaril or Atarax as calming or sedative agents) and meclizine (Bonine and Antivert) for motion sickness and dizziness; diphenhydramine (Benadryl) for the treatment of allergies and to help induce sleep, as well as dimenhydrinate (Dramamine) for motion sickness or for Meniere's disease; promethazine (Phenergan) for nausea or to help induce sleep; cyproheptadine (Periactin) for itching, skin rashes and similar disorders; and drugs such as chlorpheniramine (Chlor-Trimeton) or dexbrompheniramine (Drixoral) for colds and allergies. In the late 1980s, another type of H_1 blocker was developed that is effective in decreasing the symptoms of allergies, but that does not cross to the brain, and therefore, produces little or no sedation [e.g., loratidine (Claritin) or fexofenadine (Allegra)].

Antihistamines share an ability to counteract the effects of the body's release of the neurochemical histamine, as related to allergic reactions. Therefore, H_1 antihistaminic drugs diminish the response of blood vessels to histamine, with resulting decreases in inflammation and less marked alterations in blood vessel size. The antihistamines also affect cholinergic, serotonergic, and dopaminergic systems.[7,10]

A second major impact of drugs that cross to the brain is sedation, the most common side effect seen with the usual doses of the antihistamines. Antihistamines can have overall calming effects, but carry the unwanted reactions of decreased alertness, impaired vigilance, increased reaction time, and an inability to think clearly.[9,11] A small proportion of people, especially children, have an opposite (paradoxical) reaction, characterized by insomnia and agitation. Other properties of some antihistamines include anticholinergic effects, especially for diphenhydramine, hydroxyzine, and promethazine that can contribute to confusion, blurred vision, and urinary retention.

All of the antihistamines are well absorbed after oral administration. Almost all achieve peak blood levels within 2–3 h, and most have an effective time of 4–6 h (with up to 24 h for the prescription drugs hydroxyzine) (Vistaril or Atarax). Almost all antihistamines are metabolized in the liver, where they are likely to stimulate enzymes capable of metabolizing other drugs—with the result that the doses of additional medications sometimes have to be increased. The half-life of most antihistamines, including diphenhydramine, is approximately 4–8 h.

10.2.3. Epidemiology, Natural History, and Dependence

It has been estimated that almost 20 million Americans have used OTC hypnotics or sedatives, and about 5 million have taken one of the substances in the preceding 6 months. The rate of use is higher in women, and two thirds of users are over age 35, with 50% over 50. For the OTC tranquilizers, the average user tends to be younger, usually under 35. Recent reports have indicated a high rate of deliberate misuse of cough syrup mixtures containing antihistamines along with decongestants and codeine-like substances.

Several antihistamines (e.g., diphenhydramine) have been shown to have rewarding properties that promote repeated self-administration.[12] The feeling of stimulation, euphoria, and visual hallucinations reinforce repeated use among individuals who subsequently continue taking the drug despite consequences, spend a lot of time taking the substance, give up important events in order to use the drug, and so on, i.e., classical signs of DSM-IV dependence.[10,13,14] Despite case reports of a potential "cholinergic rebound syndrome" that might resemble withdrawal, such a syndrome has not been well documented with antihistamines, although modest levels of tolerance have been observed.[8]

10.2.4. Emergency Problems

Emergencies usually result from inadvertent overdose, deliberate misuse of the drugs in an attempt to achieve visual hallucinations, the combination of an antihistamine (e.g., pyrabenzamine) with an opioid [e.g., pentazocine (Talwin)—a mixture known as Ts and blues], or drug–drug interactions. Therefore, the most frequently noted syndromes in the emergency room are toxic reactions and states of confusion. In addition, there are a few, usually reversible, medical problems, as described below.

10.2.4.1. Toxic Reactions

See Sections 1.7.1, 2.2.1, 6.2.1, and 13.2.

The toxic reaction for the OTC antianxiety and hypnotic drugs is usually time-limited, disappearing in 2–48 h.[8,13,14] The clinical picture can be confusing to the clinician and life-threatening to the patient if multiple substances have been taken, as can occur with cough syrup mixtures or combination "cold" pills such as Coricidin. The onset of symptoms, which can consist of both antihistaminic and anticholinergic effects, varies from a few minutes, as seen in an overdose, to the more gradual evolution of signs of confusion and physical pathology in an elderly patient regularly consuming close to the "normal" doses of an OTC sedative. The patient, rarely a member of the "street culture," usually presents in a state of agitation or may exhibit varying degrees of a confusion.

The key characteristics of this overdose relate to the ability of higher doses of antihistamines to produce intense stimulation with associated confusion and convulsions. At the same time, many antihistamines have anticholinergic effects that cause dilated pupils, a flushed face, an increased heart rate, and the retention of urine in the bladder.[15] If death occurs, it is likely to be mediated through a failure in both cardiac and respiratory functioning along with convulsions.

Therapy for the toxic reaction involves general support.

10.2.4.2. Delirium, Dementia, and Other Cognitive Disorders (292.81, 292.82, or 292.83 in DSM-IV)

See Section 1.7.3.

A patient presenting with confusion and marked sedation could be labeled as having a toxic reaction. The clinical picture, course, and treatment are identical to those outlined in Section 10.2.4.1.

10.2.4.3. Psychosis

See Section 1.7.4.

Although this topic is discussed separately for ease of reference, the "psychosis" here is simply an intense toxic reaction. It consists of confusion that can be associated with hallucinations. The treatment and the prognosis are the same as outlined in Section 10.2.4.1.

10.2.4.4. Anxiety and Depression

See Section 1.7.6.

Severe anxiety or depression are unlikely to occur at normal doses, although a patient might present with anxiety regarding muddled thinking related to these drugs. Reassurance should be enough to allay the patient's fears and to decrease the level of discomfort.

10.2.4.5. Medical Problems

In animals, the chronic oral administration of antihistamines may be associated with a heightened risk for liver tumors. These drugs have also been reported to produce fetal abnormalities in animals, and should be avoided during pregnancy. Finally, antihistamines are listed among the drugs capable of producing a rapid and serious destruction of muscle cells, rhabdomyolysis.[16]

10.3. COLD, COUGH, AND ALLERGY PRODUCTS

These substances contain antihistamines (see Section 10.2), OTC analgesics, decongestants, expectorants, and cough suppressants. Additional relevant information is presented in more detail in Sections 10.2, 10.4, and 10.6, as the major clinical syndromes are similar to those seen with the stimulants, analgesics, or the antihistamines. For elixirs, some symptoms could also be related to the effects of alcohol, which can be present in concentrations of 25% (50 proof) or higher.

OTC products marketed for the treatment of colds and allergies are likely to contain substances that decrease nasal congestion (decongestants). All of these agents are amphetamine-like and produce most of their actions by stimulating a specific type of receptor, thus acting as alpha-adrenergic boosting (or agonist) drugs.[17] Here, whether administered orally as Actifed (pseudoephedrine plus triprolidine, an antihistamine) or pseudoephedrine alone (Sudafed), or taken as a nasal spray [e.g., oxymetazoline (Afrin), xylometazoline (Otrivin), or tetrahydrozoline (Tyzine, the same as Visine when given in drops for the eyes)], similar basic effects occur. Stimulation of the specific receptors results in an increase in air flow in nasal passages as a result of a decrease in the volume of the mucosal lining of the upper respiratory tract.[17] Unfortunately, repeated administration of these agents is associated with tolerance, and there might be a rebound increase in resistance to airflow, perhaps secondary to a decreased sensitivity of the receptors or to temporary damage the drug might do to the mucosal lining itself.[17]

These adrenaline-like substances can produce symptoms of anxiety, palpitations of the heart, and in some individuals, hallucinations or delusions at higher doses.[18,19] Similar hyperstimulation can be observed with a number of products prescribed for asthma. Additional problems associated with these stimulating drugs include an increase in blood pressure, abnormal heartbeats or arrhythmias, and potentially lethal interactions with other drugs such as the monoamine oxidase inhibitors (e.g., phenelzine or Nardil).

Another important OTC group worthy of brief discussion is the opioid-like substances that are used to decrease cough.[20] These agents are similar to codeine, as already described in Chapter 6. The cough suppressants include dextromethorphan, an ingredient in many OTC cough syrups, and, in other parts of the world, zipeprol.[13,14,18,19,21] Dextromethorphan is the d-isomer of the codeine-like substance, methorphan, and acts in the CNS through antagonism of NMDA receptors, producing a level of cough suppression close in efficacy to codeine, but without as many GI side effects.[21] When the OTC cough-suppressant-containing drugs are taken in high doses, the intoxication, tolerance, and subsequent withdrawal syndrome resemble those for codeine, and dextromethorphan has been used as a treatment for opioid withdrawal.[22] Patients can also develop intense confusion, anxiety, and hallucinations, especially when OTC products that contain mixtures of antihistamines, stimulant-like drugs, and opioid-like substances are consumed.

Treatment of toxic reactions and dependence on these substances is usually focused on symptom relief. In addition, CNS depression, especially respiratory impairment, may follow excessive doses of cough suppressants that contain codeine-like substances. In that instance, one can expect to see a mild form of some of the reactions noted for the opioids (see Section 6.2.1). Finally, many decongestants and antiasthma inhalers contain adrenaline-like substances (e.g., ephedrine, or Ma-Huang), the misuse of which can exacerbate psychiatric syndromes, including depressions and psychotic disorders, problems that need to be addressed in treatment. These are also discussed in Section 10.6

10.4. OTC ANALGESICS, INCLUDING NONSTEROIDAL ANTI-INFLAMMATORY DRUGS

10.4.1. General Comments

These OTC products contain aspirin, aspirin-like substances (such as phenacetin or acetaminophen), additional anti-inflammatory and fever-fighting drugs such as ibuprofen and naproxen, and, sometimes, caffeine. They are used for relief from minor pains, such as headache, and—in the case of aspirin, ibuprofen, and naproxen—for the treatment of some chronic inflammatory disorders such as arthritis.

10.4.2. Pharmacology

These agents are all referred to as nonselective cyclooxygenase (COX) inhibitors.[23] Aspirin is an analgesic, antipyretic, and an anti-inflammatory substance that is well absorbed orally. Actions occur, at least in part, through inhibition of prostaglandin synthesis. Phenacetin (rarely marketed on its own and usually given as part of a mixture with other substances) and its active metabolite acetaminophen (Tempra or Tylenol), are both members of a class of drugs, the *para*-aminophenols, first identified in the late 1800s. These medications are less likely to produce stomach upset compared to aspirin. They do have painkilling and fever-fighting properties, but are weak in their anti-inflammatory actions. All these substances are rapidly absorbed when taken orally, develop peak blood levels within 30–60 min, have a half-life of approximately 2 h, and are metabolized by the liver.

The third group of OTC analgesics that are classically considered as NSAID are mostly propionic acid derivatives. These agents, all effective as anti-inflammatory, analgesic, and fever-fighting drugs, include ibuprofen (Motrin), naproxen (Aleve), fenoprofen (Nalfon), and ketoprofen (Orudis). Similar to the other analgesics, these are rapidly absorbed when taken by mouth, they are efficiently metabolized by the liver, and the breakdown products are excreted in the urine. Some of the analgesics also contain - caffeine (see Chapter 11) or anti-acidic compounds such as sodium bicarbonate.

The side effect profiles for the NSAID compounds such as naproxen and ketoprofen are fairly similar. Most of them are capable of producing some level of gastric irritation (although less than that seen with aspirin), most diminish platelet functioning or number, and each carries some level of danger regarding potential impairment in either kidney and/or liver functioning. Some of these drugs (e.g., naproxen) can produce drowsiness, and none of the NSAIDs has been proven to be safe in pregnancy.

10.4.3. Epidemiology and Patterns of Misuse

In any given year, at least 33 million people in the United States use these medications, 20 million of whom taking the drugs in any given month. In one survey of athletes, 15% ingested these products daily, and the rate of administration exhibited no marked age or sex pattern.[24] In a survey of drug-related emergency room visits, 64% of those having a major problem with analgesics were taking aspirin, and 46% of those drug-involved emergencies were suicide attempts. In addition, misuse of phenacetin and acetaminophen has become a major health hazard, contributing to 13% of the cases of kidney dialysis and transplantation in Western countries. As a result, phenacetin has been removed from most OTC preparations in most parts of the world.

10.4.4. Emergency Problems

The major emergency problems for OTC analgesic misusers are toxic overdoses and medical disorders resulting from chronic use. Older individuals are especially liable to misuse analgesics and, by virtue of their age, are at high risk for adverse reactions.

10.4.4.1. Toxic Reactions

See Section 1.7.1.

10.4.4.1.1. Clinical Picture

Overdose of OTC analgesics containing aspirin usually results in a profound acid–base imbalance, ringing in the ears, dizziness, confusion, sweating, fever, thirst, and electrolyte problems.[23] This picture is most often seen in adolescents engaging in a deliberate overdose, usually in a spur-of-the-moment reaction to a life situation. Death can occur at blood levels of 30 mg/dl or doses of 300 mg/kg in the context of renal failure, pulmonary edema, convulsions, and coma at doses between 10 and 30 g or higher.[25,26] Overdoses of other OTC drugs such as acetaminophen can involve hepatic and renal tubular necrosis, bronchospasm, bleeding, as well as hypoglycemia.[13,23,27]

10.4.4.1.2. Treatment

Most clinical pictures tend to be relatively benign and respond to general supportive measures. Others, however, can be life-threatening. All the general steps for treating overdoses apply (e.g., Chapter 2, Section 2.2.1). These include maintaining the airway, controlling arrhythmias and seizures, combating shock, supporting vital signs, activated charcoal, and IV fluids. For aspirin, alkalinization of the serum and urine with sodium bicarbonate can be helpful, and for acetaminophen, *N*-acetylcysteine (140 mg/kg via a nasal-gastric tube, then 70 mg/kg every 4 h) can serve as an antidote.[26] Diuresis (see Section 2.2.1.2) is rarely needed.

10.4.4.2. Delirium, Dementia, and Other Cognitive Disorders

See Section 1.7.3.

An intense confusion occurring with OTC analgesics is usually the result of acid–base or electrolyte imbalance, as part of an overdose. It is temporary and clears with supportive care.

10.4.4.3. Psychosis

A psychosis is rarely, if ever, seen with these drugs unless they are a part of a combination of substances where additional ingredients (e.g., stimulants) produce psychotic symptoms.

10.4.4.4. Anxiety and Depression

These are rarely seen with these drugs, although some mild symptoms have been reported, especially with indomethacin (Indocin), perhaps because prostaglandin inhibition might produce dopamine supersensitivity.[28,29]

10.4.4.5. Medical Problems

10.4.4.5.1. Clinical Picture

The medical problems seen with analgesics vary from acute, usually benign, reactions such as a rash, to more permanent kidney and liver problems related to chronic drug misuse. Acutely, aspirin may cause GI upset, bleeding, minor changes in blood coagulability, asthmatic attacks, and skin reactions. There are data indicating that, even in therapeutic doses of 4 g/day, acetaminophen combined with moderate to high doses of ethanol can produce a toxic metabolite that can result in severe liver-cell damage and death.[27,30]

Chronic use of OTC analgesics can be associated with anemia, peptic ulcers, severe upper GI bleeding, renal disease, and possibly a neuropathy, although these may be less likely with acetaminophen. Phenacetin and other NSAIDs, in chronic high doses, can produce kidney failure and chronic anemia, although this picture usually develops in the context of misuse of OTC analgesics containing multiple substances.[23,31] The ibuprofen- and naproxen-type drugs can produce ulcers of the GI tract, are associated with potentially important alterations in blood levels of other drugs (including some anticoagulants) when given simultaneously, and, at least theoretically, might cause liver damage, especially at high doses.

10.4.4.5.2. Treatment

The treatment is usually symptomatic and supportive, based on the individual clinical picture.

10.5. LAXATIVES

10.5.1. General Comments

Laxatives (usually producing laxation, or the evacuation of formed stool) consist of a wide variety of substances that act to stimulate the bowel through diverse methods, including increasing bulk in the colon, enhancing intracolonic fluid and electrolytes, and directly stimulating bowel motility.[32] These drugs can be roughly divided into dietary fiber and bulk-forming laxatives, saline and osmotic laxatives, and colonic stimulants.

10.5.2. Pharmacology

The pharmacology differs with the type of laxative. Bulk-forming products, such as Metamucyl and Cologel, usually contain psyllium or methylcellulose, and often have a 1- to 2-day latency between their use and therapeutic effects. Saline and osmotic products such as Epsom salt, Fleet Phospho-Soda, castor oil (ricinoleic acid), and Milk of Magnesia increase the fluid in the colon and work more quickly, with a latency between use and result from less than 1 h to as long as 3 h. The stimulant laxatives contain bisacodyl (Ducolax), senna (Cascara or Senokot), or sennosides (Ex-Lax), and often work "overnight" with a latency of from 6 to 8 h. In recent years, another component of laxatives, phenolphthalein, has been withdrawn from the market due to the possibility that it causes cardiac and respiratory distress in susceptible individuals.[32] Finally, there is a series of substances containing docusate (e.g., Colace or some forms of Ex-Lax) that, although not technically laxatives, do help treat constipation by softening the stool.

There are a predictable series of side effects of these agents, many of which are discussed in Section 10.5.4 that follows.

10.5.3. Epidemiology and Patterns of Misuse

Laxative use, especially by older people and by younger individuals with bulimia, has become entrenched in Western societies.[32,33] More than 30% of people over age 60 take a dose of a cathartic at least once per week with the goal of achieving daily bowel movements, even though there is little convincing evidence that such regularity is necessary or desirable for everyone. There are presently almost 200 OTC laxative preparations in the United States that generate sales of over $34 million.

10.5.4. Emergency Medical Problems

Laxatives do not directly cause changes in the level of consciousness, and most have no direct effect on the CNS. Consequently, the major problems are medical.[32]

1. The effects of laxative misuse include diarrhea, nausea and vomiting, abdominal pain, thirst, muscular weakness, cramps secondary to hypokalemia, and the characteristic radiological appearance of a distended and flaccid colon.[34–36]
2. Mineral-oil laxatives, such as castor oil, may impede the absorption of some minerals and fat-soluble vitamins, thus producing a hypovitaminosis syndrome.
3. Saline cathartics can result in dehydration and in electrolyte imbalance, with major consequences for individuals with preexisting cardiac or kidney disorders. These saline and osmotic laxatives often contain magnesium salts (e.g., Milk of Magnesia and Epsom salts) that can add to electrolyte problems.
4. Other disorders that can be seen after a chronic overuse of laxatives include melanosis coli, fecal impaction from a flaccid colon, osteomalacia, and protein loss.[33]
5. The stimulant-type laxatives, such as bisacodyl, can produce gastric irritation and burning of the rectum, especially with prolonged use.
6. Stimulant laxatives containing anthraquinone can cross in mother's milk to the nursing infant, and can also possibly contribute to nephritis and GI pain.
7. Laxatives can also hinder the absorption of other medications.

10.6. STIMULANTS AND WEIGHT-REDUCING PRODUCTS

See Chapters 5 and 11, and Section 10.8.

10.6.1. General Comments

These substances, which usually contain caffeine, ephedrine, or phenylpropanolamine as their major active ingredients, are mostly used by people who work long hours, such as cross-country truck drivers, students preparing for exams, as well as people trying to lose weight. They are stimulant-like, and capable of producing all of the DSM-IV dependence criteria problems.[1,37] Similar emergency problems can be seen with the OTC asthma products, especially those that contain theophylline, epinephrine, or stramonium. The weight-reducing drugs are of limited, if any, value in long-term weight control, because, as is true of the prescription stimulants, any weight reduction tends to be temporary. Most OTC weight-control products contain either a relatively weak sympthomimetic-type drug (e.g., phenylpropanolamine), a local anesthetic (benzocaine), or a bulk producer (methylcellulose).

10.6.2. Pharmacology

The properties of one component of these drugs, caffeine (discussed in greater detail in Chapter 11), have been recognized for centuries.[38] Found naturally in teas, coffees, colas, and cocoa, caffeine has mild CNS stimulating effects. With doses in excess of 100 mg (one to two cups of coffee contain 150–280 mg), people begin to experience a slightly increased thought flow, enhancement of motor activity, and decreased drowsiness and fatigue. Accompanying these psychological changes are increases in heart rate and in blood pressure, along with GI irritability. Fatal overdosage from caffeine would require about 10 g (70–100 cups of coffee). The drugs that contain caffeine as their major ingredient include NoDoz (which has 100–200 mg/tablet), Tirend (100–200 mg), and Vivarin (200 mg/tablet). Other drugs include Summit, Pep-Back, Caffedrine, and Wakoz.[39]

Another drug, ephedrine, has become an increasingly popular OTC agent in recent years, sold on its own as Ma-Huang or as Herbal Ecstasy. Used in Chinese native medicine for over 5,000 years, this alpha- and beta-adrenergic receptor agonist was originally extracted from more than 12 species of Ephedra plants that also contain a variety of other stimulant-like substances such as the decongestant pseudoephrine (see Section 10.3).[17,37,40,41] Ephedrine, a drug with a half-life of 3–6 h, is excreted in the urine, has a structure similar to amphetamine, and produces feelings of stimulation along with relaxation of the breathing tubes, and decreased appetite. In addition to Ma-Huang, a variety of other OTC products contain ephedrine for asthma control, including Bronkaid and Primatene, and it is also sold as Ripped Fuel for appetite suppression and energy enhancement.

Regarding weight-reducing medications, phenylpropanolamine is a sympathomimetic, or adrenaline-like, agent similar to amphetamine that produces an adrenaline-type response along with weak CNS stimulation.[17,42] Most OTC diet preparations contain 25–75 mg of this or of norpseudoephedrine, including Acutrim, Appendrine, Control, Dexatrim, Diadal, Thinz, and Unitrol. In the suggested dosages, these products are of questionable efficacy in decreasing appetite over extended periods of time. The drug is associated with nervousness, restlessness, insomnia, headaches, palpitations, and increased blood pressure.

Also regarding weight loss, benzocaine is a local anesthetic that is included in some weight-control products in an attempt to decrease hunger. There is no evidence that this drug is effective. Methylcellulose produces bulk and thus a feeling of fullness in the stomach. However, this substance is no more effective than a low-calorie, high-residue diet, and it does have the danger of producing esophageal obstruction.

There are a number of other stimulant-like drugs discussed in Chapter 5. These include khat, which is consumed in an herbal form in many countries in Africa and in the Middle East.[43,44]

10.6.3. Epidemiology and Patterns of Misuse

Few data are available regarding the patterns of misuse of weight-control substances. However, these drugs are widely used, with yearly sales of

6 billion doses in the United States, at a cost of $400 million.[17,42,45,46] A general population survey indicated 11% of women and 3% of men have used these products, including 25% of overweight women.[47] Phenylpropanolamine and related substances are found in >50 OTC diet aids, plus a similar number of prescription drugs.

Sixteen million Americans have used OTC stimulants other than caffeinated beverages.[37] Two thirds of the users are male, but all ethnicities and socioeconomic groups are represented. There is an increased rate of use of caffeine-containing OTC pills among students.

10.6.4. Emergency Problems

The most frequent emergencies related to the caffeine-containing drugs include anxiety symptoms and medical problems. There is no evidence of flashbacks, although at very high doses drugs that contain ephedrine or phenylpropanolamine might cause stimulant-like psychoses. In high enough doses, these changes can produce a state of confusion, but such an occurrence is rare.

10.6.4.1. Anxiety Symptoms and Psychoses (e.g., 292.89 in DSM-IV)

10.6.4.1.1. Clinical Picture

Stimulants can bring about an increase in blood pressure, a rapid heart rate, palpitations, and panic symptoms that may be perceived by the individual as a heart attack. All stimulants can produce anxiety and mild manic-like symptoms during intoxication.[37,41]

In high enough doses, phenylpropanolamine can produce emergency situations similar to those outlined for the CNS stimulants (Section 5.2).[48] Case reports indicate that the OTC stimulant-like weight-reducing products can cause temporary psychoses almost identical to those described for amphetamines and cocaine in Section 5.2.4. In addition, depression and mania-like states have also been noted after chronic misuse. The clinical characteristics, diagnostic procedures, and treatments are identical to those described in Section 5.2.4.

10.6.4.1.2. Treatment

The treatment is the same as that for any drug-induced anxiety or psychotic syndrome as described in Chapters 5 and 7.

1. Carry out a physical examination, including an EKG, to rule out physical pathology.
2. Draw blood (10 cc) or collect urine (50 ml) for a toxicological screen.
3. Center treatment on gentle reassurance.
4. For psychoses, temporary use of antipsychotic medications might be required to control symptoms.

10.6.4.2. Medical Problems

In high doses, these stimulant-like drugs can produce many of the medical problems reported for amphetamine and cocaine in Chapter 5. These include

1. Intracranial (including subarachnoid and intracerebral) bleeding (also known as a hemorrhagic stroke). This might develop as a consequence of both vasoconstriction and high blood pressure, and has been reported both for ephedrine and phenylpropanolamine.[42,49]
2. Adverse cardiovascular events including arrhythmias, myocardial infarction, and sudden death.[37,46,49] There have also been case reports that ephedra might cause a myocarditis.[50,51]
3. Seizures can develop in the context of high doses of these drugs.[49]
4. An increase in blood pressure and palpitations (potentially mimicking a panic attack).[40,49]
5. Acute hepatitis, especially with ephedra.[37]
6. Esophageal obstruction with methylcellulose, especially in individuals who already have esophageal or gastric disease. The obstruction should be treated symptomatically.

10.7. ANABOLIC STEROIDS

10.7.1. General Comments

People have long searched for a fast and effective way to increase muscle mass and strength.[52–54] In this light, in the early 1900s, a famous neurologist injected himself with an extract of animal testosterone and reported subjective feelings of enhanced strength and work capacity. Even though these effects were probably more related to his expectations than true drug actions, the search for a muscle-building hormone continued, and a marked advancement occurred with the synthesis of the male sex hormone, testosterone, in 1935.

By the early 1950s, the muscle-building (nitrogen-saving or anabolic) properties of various substances were recognized as being of potential help to athletes. It was hoped that endurance and strength would result from the increased development of muscle in the absence of fat. Thus, variations of these synthetic testosterones were soon used by Soviet weight lifters, with the spreading of this approach to the United States and to other countries by 1960, and subsequent scandals at the 1976, 1988, and 2004 Olympics.[54] The substances involved were often male-hormone-like steroids that were produced to bring about a maximum of muscle development with a minimum of sex hormone side effects. Anabolic steroid use has spread widely among athletes as well as in teenagers (both male and female) hoping to be able to compete better in sports and to appear more sexually attractive.

Self-administration of these steroids usually begins in adolescence.[55,56] Most users deliberately alternate between periods of administration and abstinence in order to optimize perceived benefits while minimizing problems. One approach involves a pattern or cycle of "pyramiding" where the dose of the drug is slowly increased to a peak, and then slowly decreased in order to achieve abstinence. An alternate approach is called "stacking" where multiple types of drugs are combined during a cycle.[56]

10.7.2. Pharmacology and Laboratory Tests

There are at least eight anabolic steroids taken either by mouth or IM available in the United States, with even more on the black market outside the United States or sold in veterinary clinics.[52,54] Preparations include stanozolol (Winstrol), oxymetholone (Androl-50), methyltestosterone (Virilon and other names), fluoxymesterone (Halotestin), danazol (Danocrine), as well as several drugs that include nandrolone and testosterone itself. These drugs do, indeed, increase muscle mass, especially if used with concomitant exercise.[57,58]

In their injectable forms, these substances are often taken at between 100 mg/week and 200 mg/day. Oral forms are usually self-administered between 10 and 40 mg/day. The usual cycle occurs for periods of between 4 and 12 weeks, often involving the intake of multiple anabolic drugs.[54]

The user can be identified through the observation of a number of physical characteristics and laboratory tests. A prominent sign is a dramatic increase in muscle mass over a short period of time.[52,53] Other signs include severe acne, jaundice, unwanted changes in secondary sex characteristics such as the development of breasts in men, the lowering of the voice, more extensive hair distribution, and hypertrophy of the clitoris in women.[55,57,59,60] An additional physical sign can be swelling (edema) of the hands and feet or of other areas of the body secondary to water retention.

Repeated use of these substances can produce DSM-IV dependence symptoms.[56,61–64] People may spend a great deal of time using these drugs, continue to take them despite problems, give up important events in their lives, develop tolerance, and might demonstrate signs of a rebound syndrome (perhaps withdrawal) when the drugs are stopped.

Laboratory tests reflect the usual patterns of physical problems likely to be observed. The frequent user may demonstrate an increase in the usual liver function tests, total cholesterol (including both high- and low-density forms), abnormalities in blood sugar, and a decrease in sperm count for males.

The major medical disorders seen with stimulants include exacerbation of preexisting heart disease or hypertension, and precipitation of pain or bleeding in individuals with ulcers. Treatment is symptomatic.

10.7.3. Epidemiology

It has been estimated that 3–12% of boys, and as many as 2% of girls in high school have ever used anabolic steroids.[55,56] The 2003 Monitoring the Future Study reported that almost 4% of high school seniors had ever used these drugs, including 2% in the prior year, and almost 1.5% in the prior month.[65] The probability of taking anabolic steroids is, of course, even higher among athletes, including those playing football, track, or weight lifters.[53,55] Among gay men attending a gym in the UK, 15% reported having used these substances, and rates are also increased among individuals who have conduct disorder and those who report using other drugs.[55,59,60] In general, use appears to be a bit lower among males outside the US (estimated between 1 and 6% in Australia, Canada, South Africa, and Sweden), although rates for females (about 1–2%) are similar to the US[53]

10.7.4. Emergency Problems

In addition to dependence with psychological characteristics and perhaps a physiological component, most of the difficulties associated with anabolic steroids fall into the general categories of anxiety and depressions, the development of aggression or psychotic symptoms, and medical complications.

10.7.4.1. Psychoses and Aggression

Repeated intoxication with anabolic steroids has been reported to be associated with feelings of paranoia, at times occurring without insight. The paranoid feelings, coupled with irritability and hostility, have been reported to be associated with violent outbursts, causing physical harm to those around the users[59,66] Treatment of physical aggression involves protecting the individual from harming others, education, and reassurance of the probability that symptoms will disappear when the drugs are stopped.

10.7.4.2. Anxiety and Depression

Weight builders can develop severe depression, feelings of guilt, and loss of appetite, along with impaired sleeping patterns during continued heavy use. These conditions, resembling major depressive episodes, are likely to disappear with time alone after abstinence. In addition, one survey reported that perhaps one quarter to one third of people who use anabolic steroids also develop manic-like symptoms of hyperactivity and grandiosity.

10.7.4.3. Medical Problems

The repeated intake of anabolic steroids exposes the individual to a number of serious potential medical consequences, with the specifics depending on their gender and age.[55,60,64] Men can develop testicular atrophy as their own testosterone production is decreased in response to the high level of the synthetic hormone. Male users may also experience difficulty in urination because of changes in the prostate gland (with a possible increase in the risk for cancer). They may also show an accentuation of the male baldness pattern, develop impotence and/or a decreased libido, and experience other sex changes. If the drugs are begun at an early age, both boys and girls can develop premature sexual characteristics, perhaps an early growth spurt, but a premature shutdown of the areas of long bones responsible for growth with a resulting short adult stature.

In both genders, these drugs produce an oiliness to the skin that can be associated with acne. Women are likely to demonstrate features of masculinization and menstrual irregularities, as well as a shrinkage of the uterus and of the breast tissue.

Several of the anabolic substances are capable of causing changes in the liver. Clinicians might come across increases in some liver function tests, including lactate dehydrogenase (LDH) and alkaline phosphatase. A form of hepatitis and jaundice can develop, liver cysts can be observed, and there is an increased risk for liver cancer.

The increase in cholesterol is likely to be associated with narrowing of the arteries and subsequent heart attacks. Elevated synthetic testosterone levels can also interfere with the body's ability to regulate glucose, thus, exacerbating any preexisting diabetic problems and further complicating the increased risk for heart problems. A predisposition for stroke has also been reported to be associated with these drugs.

10.8. MISUSE OF SOME PRESCRIPTION DRUGS

In the previous sections of this chapter, I have referred to a number of prescription drugs that closely resemble some OTC agents. Thus, some of the antihistaminic agents are OTC, but others are prescribed. Similarly, some hypnotics are prescribed, but sedating antihistamines are OTC. In this section, I briefly present data regarding misuse (sometimes iatrogenic in nature), abuse, and dependence on some of these prescribed agents. These thoughts grew out of my feeling that as the practice of medicine becomes increasingly complex and access to specialists more restricted, more nonpsychiatric clinicians are prescribing psychotropic medications, and the opportunity for suboptimal use patterns is likely to grow.

Patients can misuse any drug, especially those that cross to the brain and produce changes in mood or in feeling states. Thus, there are reports of inappropriate use of the antimalarial agent chloroquine, repeated misuse of insulin, deliberate highs achieved from some muscle relaxants, and problems with inappropriate self-administration of drugs that affect brain neurochemical receptors but are rarely thought of as having an abuse potential, such as bromocriptine (Parlodel).[67–69]

This section, however, focuses mostly on drugs used for the treatment of psychiatric disorders as well as those with predominant anticholinergic effects, and a few other potential drugs of abuse. The information offered here supplements the data on prescription medications that fall into the more usual categories of drugs of abuse such as depressants (e.g., Bzs and barbiturates as described in Chapter 2), stimulants (e.g., amphetamine, methamphetamine, and methylphenidate as described in Chapter 5), and prescription pain pills (as described in Chapter 6), as well as caffeine and nicotine as described in Chapter 11.

10.8.1. Some General Thoughts about Medications Prescribed for Psychiatric Disorders

In medicine, drugs are best prescribed once there are data to indicate their ability to alter the prognosis and improve the level of functioning for specific conditions. Using the same approach in psychiatry, it is not possible to prescribe a drug that is best for sadness without knowing the appropriate diagnosis (e.g., major depressive disorder, side effects of medications, complications of medical conditions such as thyroid disease, and so on). Similarly, specific types of medications are prescribed for specific anxiety disorders, not for the general symptom of anxiety. Parallel comments can be offered regarding the appropriate use of medications to deal with psychotic symptoms such as hallucinations and delusions.

While the emphasis in this text is on problems associated with the self-administration of substances, it is important to share some of my concerns regarding some prescribing practices. Most practitioners have had limited training on how to best handle psychiatric symptoms or chronic pain syndromes. Feeling a bit out of our element, there is a natural tendency to try to treat a symptom with a medication without taking the time required to develop a differential diagnosis and to arrive at a plan based on the probable syndrome (not just symptom) involved. The results can be problematic for the patient, as the prescription of psychiatric medications requires carefully establishing the diagnosis, setting clear treatment goals, reviewing the Physician's Desk Reference and standard texts to be certain of the appropriate dose range, and selecting the optimal medication based not only on the category of drug, but the side effects most likely to be tolerated by the patient.

Serious consequences can develop if these steps are not followed. For example, this year I evaluated a 75-year-old woman who had been placed on an antipsychotic medication (chlorpromazine or Thorazine) to help her sleep—an inappropriate use of this medication, yet one that produced Parkinsonian side effects. I also saw a 60-year-old male who developed a major depressive episode in the context of being prescribed inappropriately high levels of opioids for back pain, and who became suicidal when he believed he was not responding to an antidepressant (he was actually given 10 mg of nortriptyline (Pamelor) when the effective dose would usually be 150–200 mg). A third recent case was an 80-year-old woman who was concerned about an upcoming hip surgery where (in the absence of a major depressive episode) her physician responded to her sadness by placing her on a new generation antipsychotic medication (olanzapine or Zyprexa). This produced serious side effects of severe sedation, instability of gait, and confusion in a woman who should have been given education and reassurance.

The practice of medicine is challenging, and the time pressures can be oppressive. However, many problems with prescription psychiatric medications could be avoided if the clinician placed an emphasis on full diagnostic syndromes (rather than symptoms), and prescribed the appropriate medication in the optimum dose.

The following are some guidelines regarding the use of psychiatric medications.

10.8.2. Psychiatric Medications Prescribed for Major Depressive Disorders

Severe depressions that last every day, all day, for weeks on end and that interfere with functioning are likely to be major depressive episodes.[70] Even here, a careful workup must establish that the depressive symptoms lasted throughout the day, occurred for a minimum of 2–4 weeks, and developed outside the context of the temporary sadness that can develop with repeated intoxication with depressants such as alcohol, or of withdrawal from stimulants such as cocaine or amphetamines.[71–73] When an individual has a major depressive disorder, he is likely to benefit from education, counseling, and from specific psychological treatments such as cognitive therapy, but might also require antidepressant medications for 6–9 months. Adequate doses of these agents must be used, a treatment trial of at least 3 weeks is required to observe the intensity of the response, and patients must be carefully monitored for side effects and for changes in their clinical condition. There are about 15 medications that could be appropriate for major depressive episodes, with the choice of the specific drugs resting with their side effect profiles and the patient's condition, without much evidence that one drug is more effective than any other. Examples of antidepressant medications include fluoxetine (Prozac), paroxetine (Paxil), citalopram (Celexa), nortriptyline (Pamelor), desipramine (Norpramin), and trazodone (Deseryl), to name only a few.

All patients meeting the criteria for an independent (i.e., not substance induced) major depression should be considered for an adequate trial of antidepressant medications.[74] However, it is important to remember that antidepressant drugs have significant dangers, including potential death from overdose. Therefore, these medications are not to be prescribed to treat individual symptoms; rather, their major indication is the full syndrome of major depressive disorders. There are too many side effects to justify their proscription to help people sleep (trying to take advantage of the sedative side effects of many of these drugs), or to help individuals to lose weight [taking advantage of the appetite suppressant properties of some drugs such as fluoxetine (Prozac)]. Nor have antidepressants been proven to be effective for the mood swings likely to be observed during and shortly after acute depressant or stimulant withdrawal.

Few patients develop abuse or dependence on the antidepressant drugs. There is no evidence that most of these agents cause high levels of tolerance or produce clinically significant withdrawal syndromes. However, some of these drugs, especially the monoamine oxidase inhibitors (MAOIs) such as tranylcypromine (Parnate) and phenelzine (Nardil), can produce feelings of excitement and increased energy. Thus, there are case reports of individuals who continued to use these substances after the disappearance of a depression, sought out the medication despite problems, and might have demonstrated a significant withdrawal syndrome when the drug was abruptly stopped.

10.8.3. Antipsychotic Medications Usually Used for Schizophrenia and for Mania

Antipsychotic drugs, such as haloperidol (Haldol) or risperidone (Risperdal), have potent effects on several brain chemicals, especially dopamine and serotonin. Thus, it is not surprising that they have many side effects including sedation, problems in temperature regulation, difficulty thinking clearly, and several acute (but reversible) problems with severe muscle stiffness (dystonia) and/or motor restlessness (akathisia). In addition, this group of medications has been found to produce a potentially permanent neurological disorder involving movements of the face, lips, hands, and trunk, especially after repeated doses (tardive dyskinesia).

Despite these dangers, the antipsychotic drugs can be life saving when used properly.[75] Men and women with long-term psychotic disorders such as schizophrenia often experience a marked decrease in hallucinations and/or delusions and an increase in their ability to interact with people when placed on appropriate doses of antipsychotics. Another disorder for which antipsychotic medications are appropriate for a short period of time is mania, a rapid onset of extreme excitement that includes rapid thoughts, inappropriate feelings of being special or having unusual powers, along with sleeplessness, spending sprees, and inappropriate social behaviors that can cause severe life impairment. Often alternating with extended periods of severe depression, this manic phase of manic–depressive disorder can create severe social problems and can even cause death through exhaustion. Temporary use of the antipsychotic drugs, frequently followed by lithium, is often an essential aspect of appropriate treatment.

There are a few additional conditions for which antipsychotic drugs can also be justified. Drugs such as quetiapine (Seroquel), olanzapine (Zyprexa), haloperidol, and other antipsychotic agents can also be used appropriately for short periods of several days to perhaps 2 weeks for controlling behaviors in a severe but temporary drug-induced psychotic syndrome. Even here, however, it is important to distinguish between the long-term pattern of psychotic symptoms that would be observed in schizophrenia and temporary hallucinations and/or delusions that are *only* observed during intoxication with stimulants. For the latter, only short-term use of antipsychotics is warranted.

At the same time, the antipsychotic medications are too toxic to be used for a number of other conditions. These drugs, including the more sedating agents, have *no* place in the treatment of anxiety or nervousness. Nor can these agents ever be appropriately used to help nonpsychotic patients sleep. Similarly, there are no data to indicate that antipsychotic drugs can help otherwise healthy people think more clearly or reason their way through difficult situations. These are antipsychotic agents, pure and simple, and have few other indications in psychiatry or in medicine.

The antipsychotic drugs are rarely perceived by people as causing pleasurable effects. However, the misuse of these substances can occur in the context of "pill testing" among young people trying to experiment with the effects of substances found in the medicine cabinet. In one series of such individuals, deliberate misuse of antipsychotic drugs (e.g., haloperidol) was associated with a subsequent altered state of consciousness and some severe physical side effects including tremor, muscle stiffness and spasms, and tooth grinding. The treatment of these physiological components usually consists of the IM administration of anti-parkinsonian drugs or of antihistamines, which are likely to cause a rapid clearing of the clinical picture.

10.8.4. Medications Used in the Treatment of Anxiety Disorders

Anxiety and nervousness are symptoms, not diagnoses. Feelings of tension can be warning signs that tasks need to be accomplished, and they can be a normal response to life stress. These anxiety conditions, however, are quite distinct from the major anxiety disorders outlined in diagnostic manuals, such as panic disorder, generalized anxiety disorder, agoraphobia, social phobia, and other conditions. For each of these major anxiety disorders, the syndromes are likely to develop prior to the age of 30 (often in the teens) and to increase to the point of repeatedly interfering with life functioning. Once established, these are likely to be lifelong conditions, although the intensity of symptoms is likely to wax and wane over time. Patients with these disorders can benefit from being taught new ways of thinking (cognitive therapy), as well as through behavioral approaches that incorporate relaxation training or self-hypnosis to help them become more relaxed in the presence of phobic situations. Many conditions associated with the major anxiety disorders improve markedly without pharmacological interventions.

When medications are used for anxiety, it is important to note that specific types of drugs are appropriate for specific disorders. Thus, panic disorder often responds to antidepressant medications, with these pharmacological agents acting on the brain areas involved in panic attacks rather than on depressive symptoms. Obsessive–compulsive disorder is likely to respond to a specific type of antidepressant that, like fluoxetine (Prozac), impacts on the brain chemical serotonin, whereas generalized anxiety disorders are likely to benefit from non-Bz antianxiety drugs such as buspirone (Buspar).

The diagnostic criteria and appropriate treatments for the major anxiety disorders are beyond the scope of this brief review. What is important here is to recognize that lifelong anxiety disorders are distinct from temporary symptoms of nervousness such as isolated panic attacks or some phobic behaviors observed during periods of life-stress. The long-term anxiety disorders are also different from anxiety problems noted in the context of intoxication with amphetamines or cocaine or during the course of withdrawal from alcohol or from other depressant drugs.

The major point is that there are no generic drugs for the treatment of nervousness. Similarly, no medications are necessarily indicated just because someone developed a panic attack. Each of the medications used for the treatment of anxiety disorders carries costs and side effects, and many, including the Bzs such as alprazolam (Xanax, described in Chapter 2), run the risk of producing psychological and physical dependence. When a man or a woman has a major anxiety disorder, medications might be warranted. However, when symptoms are only observed as part of life-stresses or of drug intoxication or withdrawal, careful evaluations are required to determine whether long-term medications similar to those used for major anxiety disorders are justified. Often, the anxiety symptoms will improve within weeks of abstinence without these drugs.

10.8.5. Anticholinergic Drugs, Including Those Used for Parkinson's Disease

10.8.5.1. General Comments

Probably the most common prescription drugs misused for a "high" but not yet described in this text are the anticholinergic-type anti-parkinsonian agents.[76–78] These drugs are used to treat abdominal spasms and pain, to dilate the eyes, and to reverse the tremor and muscle stiffness seen in Parkinson's disease and ones that develop as side effects of antipsychotic drugs. In prior years, anticholinergic agents were also used for their sedative side effects as the major ingredient in OTC sleep medications, but they were withdrawn from this use because of excessive dangers.

The prototypes of the anticholinergic drugs originally came as natural ingredients found in plants. These included *Atropina belladonna*, or deadly nightshade (for atropine) *Scopolia carniolica* (for scopolamine), and *Datura stramonium* or jimson weed. These agents, as well as the more frequently used synthetic substances, all affect the actions of the brain neurotransmitter acetylcholine. Used for a variety of prescription purposes, the anticholinergic drugs are misused for their ability to produce euphoria, clouded thinking, and an altered level of consciousness.

10.8.5.2. Pharmacology

There are two major types of cholinergic receptors in the body, nicotinic and muscarinic, each with multiple subtypes.[79,80] The anticholinergic drugs discussed in the following text all have their major effects on muscarinic receptors, and thus, might better be termed anti-muscarinic agents. Most of these substances are well absorbed through oral ingestion, and when applied locally some can have marked local effects on the size of the pupil of the eye and the functioning of the muscles that control the eyelids. For drugs taken orally, effects in both the brain and the periphery of the body result in an increase in breathing and in heart rate, a decrease in both bladder and intestinal constrictions, a decrease in hand tremor, and a variety of other effects. Thus, some of the drugs are used to dilate the eyes (including atropine), others are marketed to treat abdominal pain involving spasms of the intestines (e.g., propantheline or Probanthane, dicyclomine or Bentyl, and oxybutynin or Ditropan). Others can be administered as a patch for absorption through the skin for the treatment of motion sickness (scopolamine or Transderm Scop) and for the treatment of the tremor of Parkinson's disease or for antipsychotic drug-related parkinsonian symptoms. The latter indications are relevant for trihexyphenidyl (Artane) and the other drugs described in the following paragraphs.[79,81]

Most of the anticholinergic drugs are metabolized primarily in the liver, although some are excreted unchanged directly through the urine. The half-lives of these drugs vary, including the 4-h half-life observed for atropine itself.

Some widely prescribed agents are trihexyphenidyl (Artane) and benztropine (Cogentin) as well as biperiden (Akineton). The potential misuse of these substances reflects their wide level of prescription (they are among the 10 most prescribed drugs in the United States). A dose of 10–15 mg of trihexyphenidyl has been reported by patients to cause an increased sense of well-being (i.e., euphoria), as well as increased social interactions and a transient feeling of the relief of depression. It can also cause visual hallucinations.

Changes in the cholinergic nervous system may produce feelings of euphoria. Evidence of the potential misuse of these substances was first presented in 1960, when a patient deliberately increased the trihexyphenidyl dose from 8 mg/day to 30 mg/day, with subsequent interference in functioning. Four additional cases were presented in 1974 as part of a description of toxic reactions, and cases of misuse, particularly of trihexyphenidyl and benztropine, have consistently surfaced since the late 1980s. It is now estimated that as many as 7–10% of mental health outpatients taking these drugs misuse them for a "high."

10.8.5.3. Emergency Problems

Most of the difficulties encountered with anticholinergic agents are the complications of intoxication and toxic reactions.

10.8.5.3.1. Toxic Reactions

The onset of symptoms varies from a few minutes after ingestion to a more gradual evolution of signs of confusion. Agitation and anxiety are usually accompanied by a rapid heart rate, dry mouth, difficulty swallowing, abdominal distention, urinary retention, dilated pupils, blurred vision, sensitivity to light, flushed and dry skin, along with a rash covering the face and the neck.[15] Blood pressure can be elevated or can drop. The patient is often agitated, confused, and in the context of disorientation, can develop hallucinations, especially visual. In an overdose, if these symptoms are not appropriately treated, a collapse in blood pressure and circulation, respiratory failure, coma, and death can occur.

Therapy for the toxic reaction involves general supports, symptomatic treatment of physiological reactions such as the elevated body temperature, and a direct attack on the anticholinergic syndrome. Some factors to consider are listed in the following material, but their order of importance may change with specific clinical situations.

1. Attention must be paid to the maintenance of an adequate airway, adequate circulation, and the control of any traumatic lesions or bleeding. This treatment is described in greater depth in Sections 2.2.1.2 and 5.2.1.2.
2. A physical exam and careful monitoring of vital signs is essential.
3. Because these drugs are usually taken orally, saline gastric lavage using a nasogastric tube might be beneficial if a toxic overdose has occurred. The procedure should be continued until a clear return from the stomach is noted. However, if the patient is comatose or semi-comatose, lavage may be done safely only with an inflated cuff on a tracheal tube. Activated charcoal can be administered.
4. Relatively normal body temperature must be maintained by using a hypothermic blanket or ice soaks, if necessary.
5. Control of cardiac arrhythmias may be required.
6. Seizures may require treatment with a benzodiazepine (e.g., 2–4 mg lorazepam).[15]
7. The anticholinergic syndrome can be treated directly by the antidote physostigmine (Antilirium), given by slow IV injection (no more than

1 mg/min) of 0.5–2 mg (0.5–1.0 mg/kg for children).[79] This should be used only if conventional, supportive care is not enough. The dose can be repeated in 15 min if the patient does not respond, and once improvement is noted, can be given again every 1–3 h until the symptoms abate. Care must be taken as the treatment can precipitate a very slow heart rate. With this regimen, one can expect improvement in the mental status and the physiological symptoms, although there will be no reversal in pupillary dilation until the anticholinergic drugs wear off.

8. It is wise to avoid all other drugs to control behavior, if possible, especially those with anticholinergic side effects. However, if the patient is exceptionally excitable, one might use diazepam (Valium) in doses of 5–20 mg given orally, or chlordiazepoxide (Librium) in doses of 10–25 mg orally. The dose may be repeated in an hour or more, if necessary.

10.8.5.3.2. Delirium, Dementia, and Other Cognitive Disorders

Among individuals with higher sensitivity to anticholinergic agents, as well as those receiving higher doses, various levels of confusion can be observed. The key to identifying this condition is to observe the rapid heart rate, dry mouth, and dry, warm skin that are typical of an anticholinergic reaction. Treatment involves general supports and the usual approaches as given previously, for the treatment of the overdose.

10.8.5.3.3. Psychoses

Psychotic symptoms observed with anticholinergic drugs almost always develop as part of a confused state, or as one of the symptoms observed in the toxic reaction. Thus, the clinical picture, background, and treatment approaches are described previously.

10.8.5.3.4. Anxiety

Agitation and anxiety can develop as part of the usual confusion and increased heart rate that can be observed with anticholinergic drugs. The treatment approach is to offer education and reassurance and to stop prescription of these agents in such vulnerable individuals. Such reactions are said to occur more commonly among young children and older people.

REFERENCES

1. Berardi, R. R., DeSimone, II, E. M., Newton, E. D., Oszko, M. A., Popovich, N. G., Rollins, C. J., Shimp, L. A., & Tietze, K. J. *Handbook of Non-Prescription Drugs* (14th ed.). Washington, DC: American Pharmaceutical Association, 2004.
2. Pies, R. Adverse neuropsychiatric reactions to herbal and over-the-counter "antidepressants". *Journal of Clinical Psychiatry 61:*815–820, 2000.

3. Carlos Poston, II, L. W. S., Fan, L., Rakowski, R., Ericsson, M., Bunn, C. C., & Foreyt, J. P. Legal and regulatory perspectives on dietary supplements and foods. *Drugs and Society 15:* 65–85, 2000.
4. Beaubrun, G., & Gray, G. E. A review of herbal medicines for psychiatric disorders. *Psychiatric Services 51:*1130–1134, 2000.
5. Pyevich, D., & Bogenschutz, M. P. Herbal diuretics and lithium toxicity. *American Journal of Psychiatry 158:*1329, 2001.
6. Nemeroff, C. B., & Putnam, J. S. Antihistamines. In B. J. Sadock & V. A. Sadock (Eds.), *Comprehensive Textbook of Psychiatry* (8th ed.). Baltimore, MD: Lippincott, Williams & Wilkins, 2004, pp. 2772–2774.
7. Brown, N. J., & Roberts, L. J. Histamine, brodylsinin, and their antagonists. In J. G. Hardman, L. E. Limbird, & A. G. Gilman (Eds.), *The Pharmacological Basis of Therapeutics*, (10th ed.). New York: McGraw-Hill Medical Publishers, 2001, pp. 645–667.
8. Cox, D., Ahmed, Z., & McBride, A. J. Diphenhydramine dependence. *Addiction 96:*516–517, 2001.
9. Vuurman, E. F., Rikken, G. H., Muntjewerff, N. D., DeHalleux, F., & Ramaekers, J. G. Effects of desloratadine, diphenhydramine, and placebo on driving performance and psychomotor performance measurements. *European Journal of Clinical Pharmacology 60:*307–313, 2004.
10. Halpert, A. G., Olmstead, M. C., & Beninger, R. J. Mechanisms and abuse liability of the anti-histamine dimenhydrinate. *Neuroscience Biobehavioral Review 26:*61–67, 2002.
11. Wilken, J. A., Kane, R. L., Ellis, A. K., Rafeiro, E., Briscoe, M. P., Sullivan, C. L., & Day, J. H. A comparison of the effect of diphenhydramine and desloratadine on vigilance and cognitive function during treatment of ragweed-induced allergic rhinitis. *Annals of Allergy, Asthma & Immunology 91:*375–385, 2003.
12. Jun, J. H., Thorndike, E. B., & Schindler, C. W. Abuse liability and stimulant properties of dextromethorphan and diphenhydramine combinations in rats. *Psychopharmacology 172:*277–282, 2004.
13. Kirages, T. J., Sule, H. P., & Mycyk, M. B. Severe manifestations of coricidin intoxication. *American Journal of Emergency Medicine 21:*473–475, 2003.
14. Baker, S. D., & Borys, D. J. A possible trend suggesting increased abuse from Coricidin exposures reported to the Texas Poison Network: Comparing 1998 to 1999. *Veterinary and Human Toxicology 44:*169–171, 2002.
15. Ma, O. J. Anticholinergic toxicity. In O. J. Ma & D. M. Cline (Eds.), *Emergency Medicine Manual* (6th ed.). New York: McGraw-Hill Medical Publishers, 2004, pp. 476–478.
16. Coco, T. J., & Klasner, A. E. Drug-induced rhabdomyolysis. *Current Opinion in Pediatrics 16:*206–210, 2004.
17. Hoffman, B. B. Catecholamines, sympathomimetic drugs, and adrenergic receptor antagonists. In J. G. Hardman, L. E. Limbird, & A. G. Gilman (Eds.), *The Pharmacological Basis of Therapeutics* (10th ed.). New York: McGraw-Hill Medical Publishers, 2001, pp. 215–268.
18. Gauvin, D. V., Vanecek, S. A., Baird, T. J., Vallett, M., Briscoe, R. J., Carl, K. L., Holloway, F. A., & Sannerud, C. A. The stimulus properties of two common over-the-counter drug mixtures: Dextromethorphan + ephedrine and dextromethorphan + diphenhydramine. *Journal of Psychopharmacology 12:*84–92, 1998.
19. Roberge, R. J., Hirani, K. H., Rowland, P. L., III, Berkeley, R., & Krenzelok, E. P. Dextromethorphan- and pseudophedrine-induced agitated psychosis and ataxia: Case report. *Journal of Emergency Medicine 17:*285–288, 1999.
20. Mattoo, S. K., Basu, D., Sharma, A., Balaji, M., & Malhotra, A. Abuse of codeine-containing cough syrups: A report from India. *Addiction 92:* 1793–1787, 1997.
21. Gutstein, H. B., & Alsil, H. Opioid analgesics. In J. G. Hardman, L. E. Limbird, & A. G. Gilman (Eds.), *The Pharmacological Basis of Therapeutics*, (10th ed.). New York: McGraw-Hill Medical Publishers, 2001, pp. 569–619.

22. Bisaga, A., Gianelli, P., & Popik, P. Opiate withdrawal with dextromethorphan. *American Journal of Psychiatry 154:*584, 1997.
23. Roberts, L. J., & Morrow, J. D. Analgesic-antipyretic, and anti-inflammatory agents and drugs employed in treating gout. In J. G. Hardman, L. E. Limbird, & A. G. Gilman (Eds.), *The Pharmacological Basis of Therapeutics* (10th ed.). New York: McGraw-Hill Medical Publishers, 2001, pp. 687–731.
24. Warner, D. C., Schnepf, G., Barrett, M. S., Dian, D., & Swigonski, N. L. Prevalence, attitudes, and behaviors related to the use of nonsteroidal anti-inflammatory drugs (NSAIDs) in student athletes. *Journal of Adolescent Health 30:*150–153, 2002.
25. Lo, A., Shalansky, S., Leung, M., Hollander, Y., & Raboud, J. Patient characteristics associated with nonprescription drug use in intentional overdose. *Canadian Journal of Psychiatry 48:*232–236, 2003.
26. Mausner, K. L. Analgesics. In O. J. Ma & D. M. Cline (Eds.), *Emergency Medicine Manual* (6th ed.). New York: McGraw-Hill Medical Publishers, 2004, pp. 505–511.
27. Gyamlani, G. G., & Parikh, C. R. Acetaminophen toxicity: Suicidal vs. accidental. *Critical Care 6:*155–159, 2002.
28. Clunie, M., Crone, L. A., Klassen, L., & Yip, R. Psychiatric side effects of indomethacin in parturients. *Canadian Journal of Anaesthesia 50:*586–568, 2003.
29. Browning, C. H. Nonsteroidal anti-inflammatory drugs and severe psychiatric side effects. *International Journal of Psychiatry in Medicine 26:*25–34, 1996.
30. Zimmerman, J. J., & Maddrey, W. C. Acetaminophen (paracetamol) hepatotoxicity with regular intake of alcohol: Analysis of instances of therapeutic misadventure. *Hepatology 22:*767–773, 1995.
31. Chetty, R., Baoku, Y., Mildner, R., Banerjee, A., Vallance, D., Haddon, A., & Labib, M. Severe hypokalaemia and weakness due to Nurofen misuse. *Annals of Clinical Biochemistry 40:*422–423, 2003.
32. Jafri, S., & Pasricha, P. J. Agents used for diarrhea, constipation, and inflammatory bowel disease. In J. G. Hardman, L. E. Limbird, & A. G. Gilman (Eds.), *The Pharmacological Basis of Therapeutics* (10th ed.). New York: McGraw-Hill Medical Publishers, 2001, pp. 1037–1058.
33. Berardi, R. R. (Ed.). Gastrointestinal disorders. In R. R. Berardi, E. M. DeSimone II, G. D. Newton, *et al.* (Eds.), *Handbook of Nonprescription Drugs* (14th ed.). Washington, DC: American Pharmaceutical Association, 2004.
34. Korzets, Z., Hasdan, G., Podjarny, E., & Bernheim, J. Excessive fluid gain in a chronic laxative abuser: "Pseudo-idiopathic" oedema. *Nephrology, Dialysis, Transplantation 17:*161–162, 2002.
35. Duncan, A., & Forrest, J. A. Surreptitious abuse of magnesium laxatives as a cause of chronic diarrhea. *European Journal of Gastroenterology and Hepatology 13:*599–601, 2001.
36. Wald, A. Is chronic use of stimulant laxatives harmful to the colon? *Journal of Clinical Gastroenterology 36:*386–389, 2003.
37. Miller, S. C., & Waite, C. Ephedrine-type alkaloid-containing dietary supplements and substance dependence. *Psychosomatics 44:*508–511, 2003.
38. Strain, E. C., & Griffiths, R. R. Caffeine-related disorders. In B. J. Sadock & V. A. Sadock (Eds.), *Comprehensive Textbook of Psychiatry* (8th ed.). Baltimore, MD: Lippincott, Williams & Wilkins, 2004, pp. 1201–1210.
39. Popovich, N. G. (Ed.). Other medical disorders. In R. R. Berardi, E. M. DeSimone II, G. D. Newton, *et al.* (Eds.), *Handbook of Nonprescription Drugs* (14th ed.). Washington, DC: American Pharmaceutical Association, 2004.
40. Traboulsi, A. S., Viswanathan, R., & Coplan, J. Suicide attempt after use of herbal diet pill. *American Journal of Psychiatry 159:*318–319, 2002.
41. Jacobs, K. M., & Hirsch, K. A. Psychiatric complications of ma-huang. *Psychosomatics 41:*58–62, 2000.

42. Kernan, W. N., Viscoli, C. M., Brass, L. M., Broderick, J. P., Brott, T., Feldmann, E., Morgenstern, L. B., Wilterdink, J. L., & Horwitz, R. I. Phenylpropanolamine and the risk of hemorrhagic stroke. *The New England Journal of Medicine 343:*1826–1832, 2000.
43. Griffeths, P., & Gossap, M. A transcellular pattern of drug use: Khat. *British Journal of Psychiatry 170:*281–284, 1997.
44. Gurley, B. J., Gardner, S. F., & Hubbard, M. A. Content versus label claims in ephedra-containing dietary supplements. *American Journal of Health System Pharmacology 57:*963–969, 2000.
45. Couper, F. J., Pemberton, M., Jarvis, A., Hughes, M., & Logan, B. K. Prevalence of drug use in commercial tractor-trailer drivers. *Journal of Forensic Science 47:*562–567, 2002.
46. Samenuk, D., Link, M. S., Homoud, M. K., Contreras, R., Theohardes, T. C., Wang, P. J., & Estes, N. A., III. Adverse cardiovascular events temporally associated with ma huang, an herbal source of ephedrine. *May Clinical Proceedings 77:*12–16, 2002.
47. Blanck, H. M., Khan, L. K., & Serdula, M. K. Use of nonprescription weight loss products: Results from a multistate survey. *The Journal of the American Medical Association 286:* 930–935, 2001.
48. Goodhue, A., Bartel, R. L., & Smith, N. B. Exacerbation of psychosis by phenylpropanolamine. *American Journal of Psychiatry 157:*1021–1022, 2000.
49. Haller, C. A., & Benowitz, N. L. Adverse cardiovascular and central nervous system events associated with dietary supplements containing ephedra alkaloids. *The New England Journal of Medicine 343:*1833–1838, 2000.
50. Leikin, J. B., & Klein, L. Ephedra causes myocarditis. *Journal of Toxicology Clinical Toxicology 38:*353–354, 2000.
51. Kurt, T. L. Hypersensitivity myocarditis with ephedra use (letter). *Journal of Toxicology Clinical Toxicology 38:*351, 2000.
52. Snyder, P. J. Androgens. In J. G. Hardman, L. E. Limbird, & A. G. Gilman (Eds.), *The Pharmacological Basis of Therapeutics* (10th ed.). New York: McGraw-Hill Medical Publishers, 2001, pp. 1635–1648.
53. Kutscher, E. C., Lund, B. C., & Perry, P. J. Anabolic steroids: A review for the clinician. *Sports Medicine 32:*285–296, 2002.
54. Eisenberg, E. R., & Galloway, G. P. Anabolic-androgenic steroids. In J. H. Lowinson, P. Ruiz, R. B. Millman & J. G. Langrod (Eds.), *Substance Abuse: A Comprehensive Textbook* (4th ed.). Baltimore, MD: Williams & Wilkins, 2004, pp. 421–458.
55. Wichstrom, L., & Pedersen, W. Use of anabolic-androgenic steroids in adolescence: winning, looking good or being bad? *Journal of Studies on Alcohol 62:*5–13, 2001.
56. Keane, H. Anabolic steroids and dependence. *Contemporary Drug Problems 30:*541–562, 2003.
57. Bardin, D. W. The anabolic action of testosterone. *The New England Journal of Medicine 335:*52–53, 1996.
58. Bhasin, S., Storer, T. W., Berman, N., Callegari, C., Clevenger, B., Phillips, J., Bunnell, T. J., Tricker, R., Shirazi, A., & Casaburi, R. The effects of supraphysiologic dose of testosterone on muscle size and strength in normal men. *The New England Journal of Medicine 335:*1–7, 1996.
59. Kanayama, G., Pope, H. G., Jr., Cohane, G., & Hudson, J. I. Risk factors for anabolic-androgenic steroid use among weightlifters: A case–control study. *Drug and Alcohol Dependence 71:*77–86, 2003.
60. Bolding, G., Sherr, L., & Elford, J. Use of anabolic steroids and associated health risks among gay men attending London gyms. *Addiction 97:*195–203, 2002.
61. Brower, K. J. Anabolic steroids: Potential for physical and psychological dependence. In C. E. Yesalis (Ed.), *Anabolic Steroids in Sport and Exercise* (2nd ed.). Champaign, IL: Human Kinetics, 2000, pp. 279–304, 287–288.
62. Kleinman, C. C., & Petit, C. E. Legal aspects of anabolic steroid use and abuse. In C. E. Yesalis (Ed.), *Anabolic Steroids in Sport and Exercise* (2nd ed.). Champaign, IL: Human Kinetics, 2000, pp. 333–359, 344.

63. Brower, K. J. Anabolic steroid abuse and dependence. *Current Psychiatric Report 4:*377–383, 2002.
64. Kanayama, G., Cohane, G., Weiss, R. D., & Pope, H. G., Jr. Past anabolic-androgenic steroid use among men admitted for stance abuse treatment: An underrecognized problem? *Journal of Clinical Psychiatry 64:*156–160, 2003.
65. Johnston, L. D., O'Malley, P. M., Bachman, J. G., & Schulenberg, J. E. *Monitoring the Future National Survey Results on Drug Use, 1975–2003. Vol. 1: Secondary School Students* (NIH Publication No. 04-5507). Bethesda, MD: National Institute on Drug Abuse, 2003.
66. Pope, H. G., Jr., & Katz, D. L. Psychiatric effects of exogenous anabolic-androgenic steroids. In O. M. Wolkowitz & A. J. Rothschild (Eds.), *Psychoneuroendocrinology for the Clinician.* American Psychiatric Press, 2003, pp. 331–358.
67. Reeves, R. R., & Parker, J. D. Somatic dysfunction during carisoprodol cessation: Evidence for a carisoprodol withdrawal syndrome. *Journal of the American Osteopathic Association 103:*75–80, 2003.
68. Bailey, D. N., & Briggs, J. R. Carisoprodol: An unrecognized drug of abuse. *American Journal of Clinical Pathology 117:*396–400, 2002.
69. Boyd, A. Bromocriptine and psychosis: A literature review. *Psychiatric Quarterly 66:*87–95, 1995.
70. American Psychiatric Association. *The Diagnostic and Statistical Manual of Mental Disorders* (4th ed., test revision). Washington, DC: American Psychiatric Press, 2000.
71. Schuckit, M. A., Tipp, J. E., Bucholz, K. K., Nurnberger, J. I., Jr., Hesselbrock, V. M., Crowe, R. R., & Kramer, J. The life-time rates of three major mood disorders and four major anxiety disorders in alcoholic and controls. *Addiction 92:*1289–1304, 1997.
72. Raimo, E. B., & Schuckit, M. A. Alcohol dependence and mood disorders. *Addictive Behaviors 23:*933–946, 1998.
73. Preuss, U. S., Schuckit, M. A., Smith, T. L., Danko, G. P., Dasher, A. C., Hesselbrock, M. N., Hesselbrock, V. M., & Nurnberger, J. I., Jr. A comparison of alcohol-induced and independent depression in alcoholics with histories of suicide attempts. *Journal of Studies on Alcohol 63:*498–502, 2002.
74. Rush, A. J. Mood disorders: Treatment of depression. In B. J. Sadock & V. A. Sadock (Eds.), *Comprehensive Textbook of Psychiatry* (8th ed.). Philadelphia, PA: Lippincott, Williams & Wilkins, 2004, pp. 1652–1660.
75. Kane, J. M., & Marder, S. R. Schizophrenia: Somatic treatment. In B. J. Sadock & V. A. Sadock (Eds.), *Comprehensive Textbook of Psychiatry* (8th ed.). Philadelphia, PA: Lippincott, Williams & Wilkins, 2004, pp. 1467–1475.
76. Frauger, E., Thirion, X., Chanut, C., Natali, F., Debruyne, D., Saillard, C., Pradel, V., Reggio, P., & Micallef, J. Misuse of trihexyphenidyl (Artane, Parkinane): Recent trends (Article in French). *Therapie 58:*541–547, 2003.
77. Buhrich, N., Weller, A., & Kevans, P. Misuse of anticholinergic drugs by people with serious mental illness. *Psychiatric Services 51:*928–929, 2000.
78. Hirose, S. Insomnia related to biperiden withdrawal in two schizophrenic patients. *International Clinical Psychopharmacology 15:*357–359, 2000.
79. Brown, J. H., & Taylor, P. Muscarinic receptor agonists and antagonists. In J. G. Hardman, L. E. Limbird & A. G. Gilman (Eds.), *The Pharmacological Basis of Therapeutics* (10th ed.). New York: McGraw-Hill Medical Publishers, 2001, pp. 155–174.
80. Nemeroff, C. B., & Putnam, J. S. Anticholinergics and amantadine. In B. J. Sadock & V. A. Sadock (Eds.), *Comprehensive Textbook of Psychiatry* (8th ed.). Philadelphia, PA: Lippincott, Williams & Wilkins, pp. 2727–2731, 2004.
81. Halpern, J. H. Hallucinogens and dissociative agents naturally growing in the United States. *Pharmacology & Therapeutics 102:*131–138, 2004.

CHAPTER 11

Xanthines (Caffeine) and Nicotine

11.1. GENERAL COMMENTS

This chapter deals with two of the most widely used legal drugs of abuse. Despite the relatively benign acute effects at low doses, the high prevalence of repeated and intense use results in frequent morbidity and (for tobacco) high-level mortality. Both of these substances are stimulant-like in their effects but are discussed here, rather than in Chapter 5, because of their unique pharmacological mechanisms of action. The chapter deals first with the xanthines, including caffeine, and then goes on to a discussion of nicotine.

11.2. XANTHINES (CAFFEINE)

11.2.1. General Comments

Coffee, tea, and, to a lesser extent, colas and cocoa all contain caffeine-like psychoactive substances. For many years, people have recognized that caffeine can stimulate and elevate mood, while enhancing work capacity.[1–3]

The history of tea can be traced back to China in about 2800 BC, and the precursor of coffee began as an outgrowth of consumption of caffeine-containing berries almost 1,000 years ago in the Arab world.[1–4] The modern use of caffeine-containing beverages in Europe dates back to 1600 or earlier, and excessive intake has long been recognized as a potential problem, with resulting efforts to limit sales of coffee and tea through taxation.[3] In the late 1800s, caffeine was added to popular beverages such as Coca-Cola, Dr. Pepper, and Pepsi Cola, a practice that became mandated in 1914 in the United States, where caffeine was used to replace cocaine derivatives in these drinks.[2]

In more recent times, the United States Food and Drug Administration has debated whether caffeine should be viewed as a drug, or if it is appropriate to continue its notation as a substance Generally Recognized as Safe

(GRAS).[2] In this context, the energizing effects, enhanced mental concentration, and other effects have been reported to produce medicinal properties, including the treatment of some forms of headache, Parkinson's disease, breathing problems in neonates, some consequences of diabetes, and to help counter some effects of alcohol.[5–10]

11.2.2. Pharmacology and Physiology

There are at least 60 species of plants that have been found to produce caffeine and related substances.[3] These include *Thea sinensis* for tea, *Theobroma cacoa* (used for cocoa and chocolate), *Caffea arabica* for coffee, and *Cola acumenata*, which is a source of guru nuts in Sudan and which can also be used in cola preparations.[1,5] The three substances discussed in this section are caffeine (found in coffee, tea, maté, guarana, yoco, cocoa, colas, and chocolate), theobromine (found primarily in chocolate), and theophylline (found in most of these beverages and, because of its relatively high potency, also marketed as an antiasthmatic agent on its own and as a compound in aminophylline).[3] Most xanthine-containing beverages also have significant amounts of oils (perhaps contributing to some of the gastric irritation and enhanced stomach acid output caused by coffee), tannin (perhaps responsible for the constipating properties of tea), and a variety of other substances.[1]

The levels of xanthines in the most popular beverages and some OTC and prescription drugs have been established.[1,3] Among the beverages, the highest level of caffeine is in brewed (85–110 mg per cup) or drip (110–140 mg) coffee, with less caffeine in a cup of instant coffee or tea (about 70 mg), and still less in 12 oz of a cola (20–50 mg). Three cups of coffee (~300 mg) produces peak blood levels of ~30 μm.[5] There are about 5–10 mg of caffeine and 25 mg of theobromine (a less potent relative of caffeine) in a cup of cocoa, and similar amounts in chocolate.[1–3] Even decaffeinated coffee still contains 2–4 mg of the drug.[2] As discussed in greater detail in Chapter 10, many OTC pain pills contain between 30 and 60 mg of caffeine, cafergot (a combination of ingredients used to treat migraine headaches) has 100 mg, and pills used to help people stay awake such as Nodoz and Vivarin, as well as some OTC appetite suppressants such as Dexatrim, contain between 100 and 200 mg of caffeine.[2]

The xanthines (also known as *xanthine derivatives* and *methylxanthines*) are closely related alkaloids derived from plants.[1,2] They are readily and almost completely absorbed from the GI tract, are widely distributed in the body with a peak plasma level in 30–60 min, and are metabolized mostly in the liver, with less than 5% excreted unchanged in the urine, and a plasma half-life of 3–7 h.[1,2,11] However, the rate of metabolism of caffeine can be affected by other substances with, for example, a more rapid breakdown in the case of tobacco smoking and oral contraceptives, and the half-life is considerably longer in premature infants.[1,11] There is one longer lasting active metabolite, paraxanthine.[1]

The modes of action of caffeine are complex because multiple neurochemical systems are involved. Most prominent is the antagonist action at adenosine binding sites, thus, producing a decrease in the sedative actions of that neurotransmitter.[5,12–14] Although there are several adenosine receptors responsive to the blocking effects of caffeine, it is the A_1 variety that is probably the most relevant for the motor-stimulating effects of this drug, with A_2 more likely to be related to reinforcement.[15] A second prominent effect occurs with the release of norepinephrine, and subsequent stimulating actions.[7] In addition, caffeine inhibits the actions of GABA receptors, increases cortisol, inhibits actions of melatonin, and may enhance dopamine and, subsequently, feelings of reward or reinforcement.[11,15–17] It is likely that similar responses are seen to equivalent doses of caffeine in any form, including coffee, cola, or as part of medication.

11.2.2.1. Prominent Effects and Intoxication (305.90 in DSM-IV)

The effects of caffeine, also known as 1,3,7-trimethylxanthine, and other xanthines are dose-related, with more mild (and frequently beneficial) results coming from low doses and more troublesome and even aversive effects from higher doses.[11] Caffeine enhances the ability to concentrate, alertness, attention, and an improved feeling of well-being, while decreasing sleepiness.[11,17,18] At the same time, however, even at relatively lower doses, some individuals experience anxiety, problems of falling asleep and staying asleep, and an irritable mood.[2,3] These problems are especially likely at doses of caffeine of 500 mg or higher per day, a pattern of consumption reported by 10% or so of Americans.[2]

Caffeine also produces a variety of physiological changes during intoxication. This drug increases cardiac contractility and decreases vascular resistance at lower doses, but increases resistance at higher drug levels.[1–3] In a similar dose–response relationship, lower levels of caffeine appear to decrease the heart rate secondary to vagal stimulation, but higher doses result in an increased pulse and can cause arrhythmias.[3,7] Clinically relevant doses of caffeine might also contribute to the possibility of heart disease through both an increase in low-density lipoprotein cholesterol (especially for boiled rather than filtered coffee) and through an increase in blood pressure.[3,16,19,20] Doses as low as 250 mg of caffeine are likely to increase the systolic pressure by between 6 and 8 mmHg (millimeters of mercury), and the diastolic pressure of from 4 to 7 mmHg. The effects on the respiratory system include an increase in breathing rate, secondary to direct stimulatory effects in the medulla or an increased brainstem CO_2 sensitivity, and a beneficial change similar to that of theophylline and aminophylline on the relaxation of smooth muscles in the bronchi, which, in the case of theophylline, can be helpful in asthma.[1]

The caffeine-like substances also have important effects on the kidneys and the GI system.[1] Increased production of urine occurs through a direct effect on the renal tubules in a manner similar to that noted for the thiazide diuretics.[1] GI problems are related to the increase in gastric acid secretion, perhaps through a direct effect on the system both by the oils in coffee and by caffeine, as well as indirectly, through the release of peripheral catecholamines.[1] Diarrhea and GI pain may be related to the direct effect of caffeine-like substances that stimulate the phasic contraction of gut muscle, as well as to a direct irritation of the mucosa and the enhancement of gastric acid secretion.[1,3] Although the usual effect of caffeine is an *increase* in esophageal sphincter pressure, individuals with preexisting impaired sphincter strength can experience "heartburn" after caffeinated beverage ingestion, perhaps because of increased gastric secretions of pepsin and acid.[3]

Additional organ system effects include an increase in the capacity for skeletal muscle work, with a subsequent increase in muscle tension.[1,3] There can also be a reactive hypoglycemia (perhaps secondary to catecholamine release).[3] As is true of most psychoactive substances, caffeine interacts with the actions and the metabolism of other substances, antagonizing the actions of the Bzs, perhaps through a direct effect on relevant receptors, and increasing the metabolism of other substances through a possible induction of microsomal enzyme systems in the liver.[1–3] Of course, the reverse can also be true; smokers, for example, probably metabolize caffeine more rapidly secondary to nicotine-related induction of relevant liver enzymes.[1] The caffeine-like substances antagonize the effects of opioids, and have a slight antagonistic effect on alcohol intoxication.[18]

Actions in the CNS are important in the attractiveness of these drugs. There appears to be a direct stimulation of the cerebral cortex, with a decrease in drowsiness and an increased flow of thought with doses as low as 80 mg of caffeine.[1,5] Paradoxically, caffeine appears to cause vasoconstriction in the CNS, and some xanthine derivatives might be useful in treating vascular headaches.[1] Through a combination of both central and peripheral actions, increasing doses of caffeine result in insomnia, restlessness, tremor, and anxiety. The interference with sleep involves a decrease in the deeper sleep levels, a possible shift of the REM type of sleep to later in the evening, and a fragmentation of the usual sleep pattern.[1,3] The resulting effects on behavior are discussed in greater depth in the following sections. The symptoms listed previously form the basis of the DSM-IV diagnosis of Caffeine Intoxication (305.90).[21]

11.2.2.2. Tolerance and Dependence

As discussed in Chapter 2, tolerance is a complex phenomenon involving changes in metabolism, CNS responses, and through behavioral mechanisms. Physical dependence is directly related to adaptation of the brain to chronic exposure to the substance, but it has behavioral components as well.[22] The effects of caffeine are similar to (although weaker than) those produced by amphetamines, and are perceived as being at least moderately reinforcing.[3,22]

Caffeine-related disorders were not noted by the American Psychiatric Association until the publication of DSM-III in 1980, and DSM-IV does not list caffeine abuse, dependence, or withdrawal (only intoxication and caffeine-induced syndromes).[21] However, as described in Section 11.2.4, mild withdrawal symptoms of headache, fatigue, yawning, and nausea have been described in as many as 30–50% of regular users.[2,4,23] In addition, caffeine can produce tolerance.[22] It is likely that some people exceed limits they have set on the amount of caffeine they will use, and others report persistent desires and unsuccessful efforts to cut down on intake. Thus, at least a majority of the DSM-IV dependence criteria might apply to some individuals who repeatedly use high doses of caffeine.

It is more difficult to demonstrate DSM-IV abuse based on failure to fulfill major role obligations, use of caffeinated beverages in a physically hazardous situation, and legal difficulties. However, the irritability, anxiety, mood swings, and insomnia that can be associated with caffeine use might interfere with functioning and, thus, apply to one of the four potential abuse criteria. The clinician who believes that a specific patient has dependence or abuse related to caffeine could consider using the DSM-IV codes for "other or unspecified" substance withdrawal (292.0), dependence (304.90), or abuse (305.90).

11.2.3. Epidemiology and Natural History

It is estimated that two billion kilograms of coffee are consumed each year worldwide.[2,3,16,19,20] Between 85–96% of adults in the United States have ever ingested caffeinated beverages, most in the form of coffee, although 51% have ever used caffeinated soft drinks. The average American consumes 200–400 mg of caffeine per day.[1–3]

More detailed data on the pattern of use are available from the DSM-IV field trial in the early 1990s.[24] Using a random-digit dialing approach in the Northeast, the authors reported that 96% of the sample had ever consumed caffeinated beverages on at least a weekly basis, and 83% of respondents were currently consuming caffeine at that frequency. These include 78% of the population who had ever drunk coffee at least once per week (62% currently), 36% who had ever taken tea at that frequency (24% currently), and 71% who had ever taken caffeinated sodas weekly (47% currently). As might be predicted, the proportion of current users and the frequency and intensity of use of caffeine is likely to be higher among individuals who are dependent on other drugs such as alcohol and among individuals with psychiatric disorders such as schizophrenia.[25]

Although most caffeine consumers drink two or three cups of coffee a day or the equivalent, between one fourth and one third ingest 500–600 mg of caffeine daily.[2] The pattern of consumption appears to be higher in males, in Caucasians, people with lower education, as well as in those with lower levels of religious beliefs, and it tends to increase after age 18. There also appears to be a direct correlation between the level of caffeine used and the use of Bzs and other antianxiety medications. As is true of most of the substances described in this text, the desire to tolerate the side effects and to seek out the active effects of the drug is familial and may be genetically influenced.[2,26]

Typically, the use of caffeine in the form of colas begins in childhood, and consumption of brewed beverages, including coffee and tea, begins in the early to late teens.[2] The peak prevalence of use appears to be in the 20s and 30s, after which the proportion of the population consuming this drug stabilizes and then decreases.[2] Among caffeine users, about 40% had stopped some form of intake of this drug at some time in their lives, including 14% who had stopped permanently at the time of evaluation.[24] Most people who ceased intake named health concerns such as cardiac arrhythmias, other heart problems, and fibrocystic disease of the breast, along with psychological concerns such as insomnia and anxiety as the major reason.

11.2.4. Emergency Problems

11.2.4.1. Toxic Reactions

See Sections 1.7.1 and 5.2.1.

11.2.4.1.1. Clinical Picture

An overdose of caffeine can, but rarely does, result in death.[1,5,7,27] Very high doses of this drug, for example, 5–10 g or the equivalent of up to 100 cups of coffee, usually taken through the ingestion of OTC and prescription medications containing caffeine, result in potentially serious problems (see also Section 10.6). Most patients present with hyper-stimulation and anxiety, dizziness, tinnitus (a ringing in the ears), vomiting, abdominal pain, and feelings of derealization can progress to seizures, visual hallucinations and confusion.[1,3] The cardiovascular effects include elevated blood pressure, tachycardia, and extrasystoles (and possible lethal fibrillation), as well as an increased respiratory rate. Death has been reported after the ingestion of between 6 and 12 g of caffeine (along with other substances), with resulting pulmonary edema, enlarged liver, probable arrhythmias, and a dilated GI tract. Blood levels in lethal overdoses vary widely, but are probably in excess of 500 μm.[5]

11.2.4.1.2. Treatment

The treatment is symptomatic. Attention should be given to facilitate adequate respiration, and control of body temperature, convulsions, arrhythmias, and hypertension.

11.2.4.2. Withdrawal (DSM-IV Appendix for proposed criteria; DSM-IV code 292.0)

See Section 1.7.2.

11.2.4.2.1. Clinical Picture

The withdrawal symptoms seen after the chronic intake of a relatively mild substance such as caffeine are probably a mixture of the pharmacology of this drug and some learned behaviors. In fact, a recent report found no obvious cases of withdrawal among over 1700 subjects who consumed an average of five cups per day.[4] It has been reported, however, that some individuals might be especially sensitive to an abstinence syndrome.[26] No matter what the etiology, the rapid cessation of heavy caffeine intake may be associated with a variety of mild symptoms, including headache, increased levels of muscle tension, irritability, anxiety, a decreased ability to concentrate, and fatigue.[4,23] These begin within hours, peak on days 2–4, and improve greatly by 1 week after abstinence.[2,23]

11.2.4.2.2. Treatment

The key step is to rule out possible caffeine withdrawal whenever patients complain of muscle tension, anxiety, or related symptoms. As is true with most relatively mild rebound or withdrawal syndromes, treatment involves reassurance and the passage of time.

11.2.4.3. Delirium, Dementia, and Other Cognitive Disorders

See Section 1.7.3.

11.2.4.3.1. Clinical Picture

It is unlikely that caffeine is a frequent cause of clinically significant confusion. However, high doses (perhaps in excess of 500–600 mg a day) can cause agitation and possibly feelings of confusion, and that these substances should be considered a part of the differential diagnosis in all such clinical pictures.[2]

11.2.4.3.2. Treatment

Treatment involves stopping the substances in the expectation of relatively rapid improvement.

11.2.4.4. Psychosis

Psychotic pictures are rarely, if ever, observed as a direct effect of the caffeinated beverages. However, these substances may exacerbate preexisting psychotic disorders.[25] There is also the danger of caffeine-induced alterations in the metabolism and distribution of antipsychotic medications in schizophrenics, with subsequent lower blood levels of these drugs.

11.2.4.4.1. Clinical Picture

A possible clinical worsening of schizophrenia-type disorders after caffeine ingestion may be related to direct CNS effects of these substances or, perhaps, to an antagonism of the effects of antipsychotic medications, as precipitation of these substances in solution has been observed *in vitro*.[25,28] Despite these problems, between 15 and 20% of psychiatric patients consume 500–750 mg of caffeine per day.[2,3] These figures underscore the necessity of taking a careful history of caffeine intake from all psychiatric patients (in whom caffeine may exacerbate symptoms), as well from general medical and psychiatric patients (for whom caffeine should be considered part of the differential diagnosis of anxiety).

11.2.4.4.2. Treatment

Treatment involves the recognition of caffeinated beverages as possible exacerbating factors in psychiatric disorders. Decreasing and then stopping caffeine intake can be expected to result in improvement in a matter of hours to days.

11.2.4.5. Flashbacks

Probably because of the relatively mild effects of caffeine, flashbacks are not seen.

11.2.4.6. Anxiety, Depression, and Insomnia (e.g., 292.89, 292.84, 292.89 in DSM-IV)

See Sections 1.7.6 and 5.2.6.

11.2.4.6.1. Clinical Picture

Regarding anxiety, caffeinated beverages (as well as the prescribed xanthines, such as theophylline) can induce a classic panic and other anxious clinical pictures.[1,13,24,29] With caffeine doses in excess of 500–600 mg per day, the symptoms of "caffeinism" resemble those of panic attacks, and must be included in the differential diagnosis of all anxiety conditions.

Consistent with the general dictum that substances of abuse are likely to exacerbate preexisting psychiatric problems, caffeinated beverages may worsen preexisting anxiety syndromes. At least half of those with panic disorder or agoraphobia with panic, report that coffee exacerbates their symptoms, with 20% relating that caffeine can actually precipitate a panic attack.[30]

Administration of between 240 and 720 mg of caffeine can precipitate panic attacks in panic-disorder patients but not in controls, with one report relating that over two thirds of patients with panic experience symptoms similar to panic episodes with 10 mg/kg body weight of caffeine.

Of course, caffeine can also interfere with both falling and staying asleep, especially as people grow older.[2] High doses may produce a manic-like picture,[31] and this drug can intensify mood symptoms, and possibly exacerbate eating disorders. These observations underscore the necessity of taking a careful history of caffeine intake from all psychiatric patients.

11.2.4.6.2. Treatment

The half-life of many of the caffeinated substances is between 3 and 7 h.[1] Therefore the symptoms are usually relatively mild, treatment involves observation, education, and waiting until the symptoms dissipate. Antianxiety medications are rarely required.

11.2.4.7. Medical Problems

Consistent with many drugs of abuse (e.g., cannabinoids, opioids, and stimulants), there are potential healthful effects of caffeine. These include the ability to help focus attention, antagonize some of the more mild effects of alcohol, stimulate respirations in premature infants, and (combined with other medications) help in relieving the symptoms of migraine headaches.[7,9,32] Regular caffeine drinkers may have a decreased risk for Parkinson's disease, and this drug has been touted as potentially useful in alleviating some of the motor impairments associated with that disorder.[5,33] Similarly, high consumption of coffee may reduce the risk for type 2 diabetes,[34,35] and for gallstone disease.[36]

Yet, there are risks associated with the regular consumption of caffeine. These include:

1. As noted above, xanthines can result in increased blood pressure, tachycardia, and arrhythmias.[19]
2. Another relatively frequent problem involves GI upset, including pain (seen in perhaps 20% of heavy coffee drinkers), diarrhea (also seen in 20%), and peptic ulcers, as well as exacerbation of esophagitis with associated heartburn.[37]
3. Neuromuscular problems can include a feeling of restlessness in the legs and arms, as well as a hand tremor.[1–3]
4. Both direct and indirect effects on the CNS can result in insomnia (reported by 40% of regular heavy users), headache (reported by 20–25%), and anxiety and agitation as described earlier.[17,38]
5. More serious and life-threatening problems can also occur. There is a possible association between caffeine and cancer of the bladder,

lower urinary tract, colon, and pancreas, as well as increased problems with fibrocystic disease of the breast.[1,39]

6. The long-held belief that caffeine is relatively safe in pregnancy has recently been challenged.[1,40]
7. Caffeine not only readily crosses the placenta to the developing fetus but also is found in milk of lactating mothers.[1] Thus, the pediatrician must be aware of potential behavioral and physiological symptoms in nursing babies.

11.3. NICOTINE

11.3.1. General Comments

Nicotine ingestion is an ancient and widespread practice. References to this drug are found in Mayan stone carvings from AD 600, as the drug was used by North, Central, and South American natives, usually through tobacco smoking, chewing, or salves.[41] The goal was to achieve a transcendental experience, often as part of a ceremony of offerings to the gods and of warding off evil. It is possible that the older forms of tobacco were more potent and may have contained high concentrations of several psychoactive substances. Tobacco ingestion was taken back to the Old World following the explorations by Columbus in the 1490s, and it soon spread throughout Europe and thence to Africa and to Asia over the next 50–100 years. Problems were soon recognized, and control of use through taxation dates back to at least 1604 under King James of England.

As discussed in Section 11.3.2.2, nicotine causes a typical dependency process.[42,43] It resembles all the other substances of abuse in that people can be unable to stop or control use, ingest the substance despite knowledge of its serious dangers, deny problems even after they are obvious to those around them, are likely to relapse once use ceases, and genetic factors may influence the risk for dependence.[44–46] Regarding the latter, twin research suggests heritabilities of between 30 and 53% for initiation, persistence of use, and dependence, and genetically distinct rodent lines have been shown to have marked differences in reaction to nicotine and in self-administration of tobacco smoke.

11.3.2. Pharmacology

In Western cultures, nicotine is ingested primarily through smoking, nasal insufflation, or chewing of products of the tobacco plant. In the predominant mode of administration, smoking, almost 4,000 substances are inhaled, including nitrogen oxides, ammonia, and aldehydes (e.g., acetaldehyde), with the specifics depending on the temperature of burning.[41,47] A smaller number of substances are ingested by chewing or through intranasal administration of snuff.

The three major components of *Nicotinia tobacum* (named after Jean Nicot, who promoted nicotine for its medicinal value) are tars (also known as total particulate matter or TPM), carbon monoxide (CO), and nicotine. The tars contain possible cancer-causing aromatic amines, nitrosamines, and polycyclic aromatic hydrocarbons, the latter of which also induce liver enzymes with subsequent changes in the metabolism of other substances.[41,47] The CO causes a decreased ability of the blood to carry oxygen, and thus, an increase in red blood cell number (polycythemia), and it is probably a major contributor to heart disease, perhaps through the promotion of atherosclerosis. Additional potentially important constituents of tobacco smoke include ammonia, hydrogen cyanide, alcohols, acetaldehyde, formaldehyde, metallic ions, and some radioactive compounds. The prominent psychoactive component of tobacco ingestion, however, is nicotine, and unless otherwise specified, this chapter deals primarily with this substance.

Nicotine, a colorless drug that turns brown on exposure to air, was first isolated in 1828. It is probably the major (although not the only) reinforcer of tobacco ingestion and the probable rate-limiting substance in tobacco intake, as most smokers and chewers modify their use on the basis of the nicotine content.[41,47] This alkaloid is one of the few naturally occurring liquids of its class, and is rapidly absorbed through the lungs, the skin, or the digestive tract. A puff of smoke results in measurable nicotine levels in the brain within seconds, and there are about 10 puffs per cigarette. Thus, a pack per day administers 200 doses of this potent drug.[47]

The average cigarette contains between 8 and 10 mg of nicotine, with perhaps slightly lower levels for filter cigarettes, although these "low-tar" products may have heightened levels of CO.[47] The smoke is only 1–2% pure nicotine, and only about 1–3 mg of the drug actually reaches the smoker's blood stream.[41,47] Snuff contains 4.5–6.5 mg of nicotine per "dip," and nicotine gums contain between 2 and 4 mg per stick.[41] After ingestion, peak plasma concentrations are usually 25–60 ng/ml, with a half-life of disappearance from the plasma of 30–120 min.[41,47] Overnight abstinence results in plasma levels of 5–10 ng/ml.[47] African Americans appear to develop higher blood levels, perhaps reflecting slower clearance and/or higher intake of nicotine per cigarette.[48] It is hypothesized that these ethnic differences might contribute to greater problems quitting smoking and a higher risk for lung cancer among African American individuals.

At first glance, the actions of nicotine in the brain appear relatively straightforward. Widely distributed throughout the CNS are receptors sensitive to the neurochemical acetylcholine that also react to nicotine itself.[41,49–51] Similar (although not identical) receptors are located in the junction between nerves and skeletal muscles and in ganglia around the body that control ANS functioning.[41,47] Many of the changes in body functions as well as the pleasurable reinforcing effects of nicotine are the direct result of the actions of nicotine, and drugs that block nicotine receptors such as mecamylamine, can change the reaction to this drug in both animals and in humans.[50,52]

However, nicotine has different (even opposing) effects at different doses and under divergent conditions. These differences probably reflect the balance between the initial actions on the nicotinic–cholinergic receptor that is predominantly stimulatory, followed by a densensitization of receptor functioning, which is subsequently followed by an up-regulation of receptors and an increase in receptor density.[47]

Also contributing to the complexity of the reactions of the body to nicotine is the impact that this drug has on many different neurotransmitters, including serotonin and dopamine. Regarding the latter, it is hypothesized that the effects of nicotine on dopamine in the mesolimbic, dopamine-related reward system are closely involved with the rewarding (and thus dependence-producing) actions of these drugs.[53–56] The administration of nicotine also results in the release of epinephrine and of norepinephrine, and it produces a rise in a number of hormones including corticotropin releasing hormone (CRF), beta-endorphin, ACTH, and argenine vasopressin. Finally, there are some indications that nicotine affects glutamate (and thus NMDA receptors), GABA, and opioid receptors.[47,50,57]

Nicotine is oxidized primarily in the liver, to the less active longer lasting substance, cotinine, with a half-life of approximately 19 h.[58] However, a subgroup of people have a much slower rate of metabolism. Thus, smoking levels can be monitored through observation of plasma levels and of excretion of this metabolite.[41] The kidney then rapidly removes nicotine and cotinine from the body. Through the actions of nicotine on the liver, smokers are likely to induce enzymes with subsequent increased metabolic rates (and lower than expected blood levels) of a variety of drugs, including theophylline, warfarin (Coumadin) phenacetin, propranolol, some antidepressants, and caffeine. Nicotine is also reported to increase the needed doses of opioids and Bzs, and to decrease the antianginal and blood-pressure-lowering effects of drugs such as nifedipine (Procardia), atenolol (Tenormin), and propranolol (Inderal).

It is important to briefly discuss smokeless tobacco.[47,59] The most popular form, snuff, is cured, ground tobacco manufactured in three varieties: dry, moist, and fine cut. The second most popular form of smokeless tobacco is chewing tobacco, which is also prepared in three ways: loose-leaf, plug, and twist chewing tobacco. These substances are used by placing a pinch of snuff or a plug of chewing tobacco between the gum and the cheek, or chewing the leaves or the plug. The tobacco subsequently mixes with the saliva, and clinically significant levels of nicotine are absorbed through the oral mucous membrane linings. The mode of ingestion of snuff and chewing tobacco poses its own problems of irritation and increased cancer risks, as discussed in Section 11.3.4.7.

11.3.2.1. Predominant Effects and Intoxication (Nicotine Intoxication is not listed in DSM-IV)

As is true of all drugs discussed in this text, nicotine has prominent effects in the CNS. The nicotinic systems are important in learning, memory, and attention and general cognition.[49,50,60] Small doses might decrease anxiety and help alleviate feelings of stress,[50,61] while also decreasing appetite.[50] On a physiological level, the acute effects of nicotine include a stimulated-like EEG pattern with low voltage fast waves predominating, whereas in the periphery there can be changes in muscle tone and in deep tendon reflexes (DTRs), perhaps related to the direct effects on the spinal cord.

In the *digestive* tract, nicotine causes increased salivation and a decrease in the strength of stomach contractions (perhaps related to appetite suppression), but intake can result in nausea and vomiting through a direct effect on the vagus nerve and on the medulla. Acute effects on the *respiratory* system include local irritation, the deposit of potential cancer-causing substances, and a decrease in ciliary motion,[41] while in the *cardiovascular* system there is a 10–20 beat per minute increase in heart rate (perhaps related to a release of epinephrine and to effects on peripheral ganglia), a 5–10 mm increase in blood pressure, cutaneous vasoconstriction, an increase in the strength of heart contractions, and an elevation in platelet adherence.[41,47] Additional acute effects include an increase in growth hormone, cortisol, and antidiuretic hormone as described previously.[41]

11.3.2.2. Tolerance and Dependence (305.10 in DSM-IV; Nicotine Abuse is not listed)

Tolerance to nicotine does occur, but this process does not develop uniformly to all aspects of nicotine's actions.[47] For example, the most prominent changes occur for nausea, dizziness, vomiting, and perhaps behavioral arousal, with less for heart rate, tremors, and skin-temperature changes. Some aspects of tolerance begin to disappear within several days of abstinence, whereas others may be relatively long lasting.[41]

The repeated heavy use of nicotine-containing products is capable of producing all of the remaining items for DSM-IV dependence.[42,47] The risk for developing dependence increases with the intensity of smoking, with marked increases when use exceeds five cigarettes daily.[47] Reflecting lack of data on the subject, abuse criteria were not included in DSM-IV.

11.3.3. Epidemiology and Natural History

11.3.3.1. Epidemiology

The percentage of smokers in most Western cultures increased after World War I, reaching a peak in the mid-1960s, when it was estimated that 52% of American men and 32% of American women were regular smokers consuming 600 billion cigarettes per year.[41] In 1964, an Advisory Commission to the Surgeon General of the United States reported that tobacco intake was a major health hazard.[47] After this time, per capita consumption began to drop and, by 1975, the percentage of regular, current smokers among men had decreased to 39%, although women showed only a slight drop, to 29%. The decrease in consumption continued through the 1980s and beyond.[62]

More recent US data come from the 2001 National Survey on Drug Use and Health.[63] Overall about 70% of the population in the United States had ever used a cigarette (75% of men and 66% of women), but only 26% (29 and 23% of the two sexes) in the past month. Thus, there is a movement toward equilibration of smoking rates across men and women, although higher rates remain for men. These figures for current smokers are a bit higher than those reported for 1987, but lower than 1997. Regarding age, the highest rate of use in the prior month was 45% for those aged 18–25. It was estimated that about 61 million people in the United States were current or recent past smokers.

The proportion of smokers in the last month varies a bit across racial groups, including 37% of American Indians, 27% of Caucasians, 25% of Blacks, 23% for Hispanics, and 18% for Asians.[63] Rates are higher for high school dropouts (35%) compared to college graduates (14%), and those who smoke are more likely to consume four or five alcohol drinks per evening (43%) and to use illicit substances (20%) compared to nonsmokers (16 and 4%, respectively).[63]

The risk for nicotine dependence during a person's lifetime is about 24% in the United States[64] although some authors cite a figure as high as 30% for those aged 20 and over.[65,66] Approximately 10% of the population were nicotine dependent in the prior year.[63]

Recognizing the higher prevalence of smoking in relatively young populations, additional useful data come from the 2003 Monitoring the Future Study.[67] That group reported that in 2003, 54% of high school seniors reported ever having used cigarettes, compared to 43% in 10th grade and 28% in 8th grade. For smokeless tobacco, the figures were 17, 15, and 11%, respectively. During the prior 30 days, 24% of 12th graders had used a cigarette, versus 17% of 10th graders and 10% of 8th graders. The figures for smokeless tobacco were 7, 5, and 4%, respectively.

General population data regarding smokeless tobacco are also available from the recent National Survey on Drug Use and Health.[63] Here, 6.5% of males and <1% of females had used products like chewing tobacco or snuff in the previous year, and 6% of men and 0.5% of women in the last month.

Children of regular smokers have an elevated risk for smoking.[44,68–70] Family studies revealed a twofold to fourfold increased risk for smoking among individuals whose parents or siblings are smokers, and as briefly alluded to earlier, twin investigations have demonstrated a significantly higher level of similarity in smoking histories for identical compared to fraternal twins. In addition, an adoption study has demonstrated a significantly higher level of correlation in the number of cigarettes smoked per day between adopted children and their biological parents than is observed between such children and their adoptive parents.

Rates of smoking in most western countries are generally similar to the US, or a bit higher. For example, in Germany, 36% smoked in the last year, and about 10% were estimated to be nicotine dependent.[71] These include 14% versus 8% who smoked 2+ days of the week in the last month, and 25% versus 15% in the previous year.

11.3.3.2. Natural History

The usual clinical course of smoking does not appear to have changed much in recent decades. Smoking usually begins in early adolescence, and most young people experiment by age 12 or 13.[72,73] Initiation often occurs in response to social pressures, continues in the context of the positive or reinforcing effects of the drug, and then progresses as people try to avoid withdrawal. It has been estimated that once an individual has consumed five or more cigarettes, he or she has markedly increased the risk for long-term continued consumption, with dependence developing in a few months to a few years.[74] The chance of smoking in youth increases with signs of adjustment problems (e.g., academic failure), evidence of risk taking, and characteristics of extraversion.[47] The chances of developing dependence increases if parents or siblings smoke, if there is a history of a mood disorder, or if the initial effect of nicotine was especially pleasurable.

When asked, the majority of smokers and most smokeless tobacco users (up to 80%) say they want to stop.[47,75,76] These findings may reflect the recognition by most smokers that tobacco is socially undesirable and dangerous to health. Thus, it is not surprising that the natural history of smoking includes frequent attempts to abstain, along with as high a rate of relapse as there is with illicit drugs. About one third of smokers try to quit each year, 90% of these without treatment, but only 2.5–5% are successful.[47] Eventually, 50% of smokers do succeed in gaining long-term abstention, with lower rates in women, in younger individuals, and in African Americans.

Regular smoking is associated with a poorer quality of life than that of nonsmokers.[71] This includes life problems for 14% versus 8% who smoked 2+ days of the week in the last month, and 25% versus 15% in the previous year.

Finally, regarding the usual clinical course of the use of nicotine, it is worthwhile to comment briefly on the relationship between smoking and drinking.[45,77–80] Almost 80% of men and women who are alcohol dependent currently smoke, a rate that is significantly higher than that for the general population. In fact, even nonalcoholic drinkers are at least twice as likely to be smokers than are abstainers. Furthermore, people who are alcohol dependent and who smoke, report a significantly higher number of cigarettes per day. Unfortunately, concomitant use of nicotine and repeated heavy drinking increases the risk for many disorders, including cirrhosis and various forms of cancers.

People with alcoholism who are nicotine dependent are less likely than the average person who is alcohol dependent to develop abstinence from either drug.[78,81] It has been hypothesized that the intense use of both substances might "sensitize" an individual to more psychological and environmental clues regarding substance use, thus jeopardizing continued abstinence. Several studies have suggested that it might be appropriate to encourage people with alcoholism in treatment to also stop using nicotine. Clinicians have sometimes been reluctant to take on these joint tasks for fear that addressing both dependencies simultaneously might decrease the chances that an individual will be successful in either. Fortunately, there does not seem to be an increased risk for relapse or lower overall success rates when nicotine dependence treatment is added to alcoholism rehabilitation.

11.3.4. Emergency Problems

Although years ago nicotine was likely to be seen as a benign substance, this drug and its associated chemicals taken in through tobacco are responsible for a great amount of morbidity and mortality.

11.3.4.1. Toxic Reactions

See Section 1.7.1.

11.3.4.1.1. Clinical Picture

A fatal overdose of nicotine in adults can occur with 60 mg (as might be seen with an ingestion of some insecticides). Lower amounts (even from tobacco) are dangerous for children. In a less severe reaction (as might be seen in tobacco pickers), the symptoms can include nausea, salivation, abdominal pain, diarrhea, vomiting, headache, dizziness, decreased heart rate, and weakness.[41] In higher doses, these problems are followed by feelings of faintness, confusion, a precipitous drop in blood pressure, a decrease in respirations, onset of convulsions, and even death from respiratory failure.

11.3.4.1.2. Treatment

The treatment of a nicotine overdose is to control symptoms.[41] In addition to general support of respiration and blood pressure as well as the administration of oxygen, a number of maneuvers can be used to try to rid the body of the substance. Gastric lavage can be useful, as emptying is often delayed, and a slurry of activated charcoal can also help.[41] The excretion of nicotine is probably enhanced by acidifying the urine with ammonium chloride (500 mg orally every 3–4 h). Some authors recommend the use of short-acting barbituates to help control clonic muscle movements or seizures.

11.3.4.2. Withdrawal (292.0 in DSM-IV)

See Section 1.7.2.

11.3.4.2.1. Clinical Picture

There is little doubt in the mind of any heavy smoker that sudden cessation or an attempt to "cut down" can cause a withdrawal syndrome. The symptoms include nagging discomfort that can persist for many days, but the intensity is usually modest, although it varies greatly among people.[47,82] It has been hypothesized that most heavy smokers get to a point where they continue to administer nicotine to avoid withdrawal symptoms, more than to enjoy the substance itself.[2,41]

The withdrawal symptoms tend to begin within hours of stopping intake, increasing over the first day, peaking on days 2–4, and lasting up to a month.[47] Most patients complain of increased tobacco and food craving, irritability, anxiety, difficulty concentrating, and restlessness.[83,84] Some people note feeling depressed during withdrawal, symptoms that can be especially prominent in individuals who have had prior episodes of a major depressive disorder. Anxiety symptoms have also been reported, but at least one recent study questions whether these are more likely during nicotine withdrawal than at other times in a person's life.

More than three fourths of regular smokers report four or more withdrawal symptoms in the first week of abstinence, and there appears to be a relationship between prior tolerance to nicotine and the subsequent intensity of withdrawal symptoms. Additional difficulties reported in other investigations include evidence of EEG slowing with a decreased arousal pattern, a feeling of dullness or drowsiness, as well as feelings of hostility, headache, and sleep problems accompanied by an increase in REM latency and in total REM time.[72] Similar symptoms can be seen after abrupt cessation of nicotine gum—indicating that the syndrome observed by smokers is related to the development of physical dependence on nicotine itself. Constipation and/or diarrhea may also occur early in withdrawal, and there may be a significant weight gain, with one study indicating that, although the average weight gain is 2–3 kg, almost 10% of men and almost 15% of women gain 13 kg or more after smoking cessation. Craving for nicotine, an increased appetite, and weight gain can continue for 3–6 months in some people.[72]

11.3.4.2.2. Treatment

Treatment of the withdrawal symptoms is an important step toward "rehabilitation." Optimally, detoxification requires general supports, counseling (so the smoker knows he is not going through this alone and that the symptoms will improve), and usually the administration of nicotine as a gum, a patch, or a nasal spray in decreasing quantities over 3 weeks or so.[72,85] Some data support the usefulness of clonidine (Catapres) taken orally (0.1 mg TID) or as a 0.1–0.2 mg patch, and others indicate the effectiveness of bupropion (Zyban) 150–300 mg/day and possibly some other antidepressants.[86–88] Additional pharmacological and physiological approaches have been proposed for help in treating the symptoms of nicotine withdrawal, but these have not been intensively studied and have little clinical applicability at present.[72,89] Most of the usual approaches for rehabilitation relating to smoking cessation are described in greater depth in Chapter 14.

11.3.4.3. Delirium, Dementia, and Other Cognitive Disorders

With the exception of the toxic reaction described previously, nicotine is not expected to precipitate clinically relevant levels of confusion. However, decreased cognition can develop as a result of a number of medical consequences of smoking. These include a low level of brain oxygen as seen in chronic obstructive lung disease, or emphysema.

11.3.4.4. Psychosis

No known clinically significant psychotic state has been reported with nicotine in modern times. This topic is of historical value, however, in light of the possibility that more potent tobacco forms may have been used by North American natives to achieve transcendental states along with visual hallucinations.

There is, however, an intriguing relationship between smoking and at least one psychotic disorder, schizophrenia.[90–95] A number of theories for this phenomenon have been set forth, including possible effects of nicotine on dopamine, a neurochemical important in schizophrenia. In addition, the high rate of smoking in people with this disorder might impact on changes in psychotic symptoms, or smoking might be attractive as a way to decrease movement-related side effects of antipsychotic drugs for people who smoke.

11.3.4.5. Flashbacks

Flashbacks are not a problem known to exist with nicotine.

11.3.4.6. Anxiety and Depression (292.9 and possibly 298.89 and 292.84 in DSM-IV)

See Sections 1.7.6 and 7.2.6.

With the exception of the toxic reactions or overdose conditions described previously, it is unlikely that nicotine intake results in persistent panic attacks or other anxiety state in individuals not so predisposed. However, for a person under stress, the increased blood pressure and heart rate, as well as respiratory changes caused by nicotine could precipitate temporary anxiety symptoms, including panic attacks.[96–98] Treatment is symptomatic, and includes reassurance and informing the patient that his tobacco intake is exacerbating the problems.

In recent years, more data have accrued regarding the potential relationship between smoking and symptoms of depression.[83,99–101] Several articles have noted an increased prevalence of smoking among individuals with severe depression, as well as a correlation between a history of major depressive disorder and a greater difficulty in stopping smoking. These findings are of clinical interest, and they relate to theories that brain cells rich in acetylcholine interact with those primarily containing monoamines such as norepinephrine, thus having an important impact on the onset and course of major depressive disorders. In addition, nicotine inhibits the monoamine oxidase B enzyme, which could result in higher brain levels of all monoamines, and thus tobacco might be used as a "self-medication" for some people with mood disorders. However, a study of smoking and major depression among twins indicates the likelihood that the relationship between nicotine consumption and severe depression might reflect familial, and perhaps genetic, factors that predispose the same individual to both smoking and to major depressive episodes.[102]

For each of these conditions involving anxiety or depression, treatment for the nicotine portion of the symptoms is generic. Individuals should be reassured that their symptoms or intensification of prior conditions is temporary and will improve. In addition, clinicians should consider the cognitive and behavioral approaches for smoking cessation described in Chapter 14.

11.3.4.7. Medical Problems

With the possible exception of alcohol, tobacco has the highest cost to society of any substance of abuse. It has been estimated that tobacco use contributes to 3 million deaths per year in the world, including 400,000–450,000 premature deaths in the United States annually.[103] This yearly loss of American lives is greater than the total number of Americans killed in World War I, in Korea, and in Vietnam combined, and is approximately equal to the number who perished in World War II. This substance is in part responsible for at least 20% of all deaths in the United States and has been estimated to cut an average of 8 years off the lifespan of the average smoker, 45% of whom die of tobacco-related disorders.[72] A recent 15-year follow-up of almost 8,000 middle-aged men in Britain revealed that 7.8% of those who never smoked died during the decade and a half, compared to 23.3% of those who had begun smoking prior to the age of 30 and continued to use tobacco products during the follow-up period.[62] That study estimated that whereas 78% of the lifelong nonsmokers were likely to live to the age of 73, the same was true for only 42% of the smokers. An estimated 60% of direct healthcare costs are the consequence of smoking, with an overall price tag of $1 billion per year. Thus, tobacco consumption is one of the most important causes of preventable morbidity and mortality in the United States.

There are some potential healthful benefits of nicotine. They include a possible decreased risk for schizophrenia and possibly an inhibition of the deposition of 3 amyloid with a decreased risk for Alzheimer's disease.[95,104,105] However, the list of health problems associated with tobacco products is prodigious. These include:

1. Tobacco, especially through smoking, is associated with a significantly elevated rate of cancer, especially of the lung, the oral cavity, the pharynx, the larynx, and the esophagus.[47,71] At least 30% of cancer deaths in the United States are related to smoking, including 90% of bronchogenic cancers. It is also estimated that 84% of cancers of the larynx are related to smoking (a relative risk of between 2.0 and 27.5 in heavy smokers versus nonsmokers) and that there is a 13-fold increased risk for oral cancer, a twofold to threefold increased risk for bladder cancer, a twofold increased risk for pancreatic cancer, and the possibility of a fivefold increased risk for cancers of the kidney or the uterine cervix.[47] Heightened cancer risks are also obvious for snuff and for chewing tobacco users, up to 64% of whom have some precancerous cellular changes of the mouth (leukoplakia), with overall cancer risks similar to those noted for smokers.[59]
2. Smoking contributes to both cerebrovascular and cardiovascular problems, including strokes, heart attacks, and angina.[106,107] A third or more of coronary deaths in the United States are related to smoking, with evidence that the chances for a myocardial infarction increase approximately threefold in smokers.[107] This may relate to an increased arterial-wall stiffness that could contribute to atherosclerosis, as well as increases in blood pressure and other difficulties with vascular disease. Consistent with these factors is the twofold to threefold increased risk for abdominal aortic aneurysms among heavy smokers, as well as the twofold to threefold increased risk for both thromboembolic and hemorrhagic stroke. A lowering of these levels of risk is expected with cessation of smoking.[107] Although low-tar cigarettes might lower the level of cancer risk, they have little beneficial effect on the increased risk for heart disease.
3. Nicotine and other tobacco substances also affect the developing fetus and the neonate.[69,108,109] Many of these substances (especially nicotine) easily cross the placenta to the baby and are also found in breast milk. An increase in the fetal heart rate can be seen for 90 min after a pregnant woman smokes. Mothers who smoke heavily have almost a twofold increased risk of spontaneous abortion, are likely to deliver babies who are small for their gestational age, and have offspring with over a twofold increased risk of congenital abnormalities,

including patent ductus arteriosis, tetralogy of Fallot, and cleft palate and lips.[47] Although fewer data are available, the children of mothers who smoke heavily may demonstrate a higher risk of symptoms of hyperactivity and conduct disorder in childhood and in adolescence and may demonstrate higher risks for cancer later in life.[110–112] For men, smoking is also associated with abnormal sperm forms and evidence of chromosomal damage in lymphocytes.

4. Respiratory problems do not stop with cancer. Tobacco smoke decreases ciliary action, which may help explain the increased risk of bronchitis and of other infections in smokers.[47,113] If these problems persist, chronic obstructive lung disease (COLD), or emphysema, can be expected. Perhaps 80–90% of cases of COLD are related to smoking, with a relative risk of between 2.2 and 24.7 compared to the general population, depending on the number of packs smoked per day and the number of years the user has smoked. Problems with slower growth of lung function and mild airway obstruction have also been reported in teenage smokers.[113]
5. Other difficulties include an enhanced risk for the development and recurrence of GI ulcers,[47] with a relative risk of at least twofold for peptic ulcer disease. People who use nicotine products also have an increased risk for periodontal disease.
6. An additional difficulty comes from the effects of nicotine on sex hormones. The overall antiestrogen properties of this drug in women, a problem relating to increased rates of metabolism of this hormone, contribute to early menopause and high risks for osteoporosis.[114]
7. Smoke in the ambient air affects nonsmokers. This phenomenon of passive smoking involves nicotine, tars, and carbon monoxide both from exhaled smoke (mainstream) and from smoke emanating from the tip of the cigarette (sidestream smoke).[115] Problems in adults from passive smoking include eye irritation, headaches, cough and nasal symptoms, as well as more serious allergic and asthma attacks, an increase in angina symptoms, and even an increase in lung cancer for spouses of smokers who smoke one pack per day or more. Problems extend to children of smokers, as these young people carry a higher risk for bronchitis, pneumonia, middle-ear infections, and worsening of an asthma condition.
8. Additional observations have included an almost twofold increased risk for hearing loss in smokers.[116]

REFERENCES

1. Undem, B. J., & Lichtenstein, L. M. Drugs used in the treatment of asthma. In J. G. Hardman, L. E. Limbird, & A. G. Gilman (Eds.), *The Pharmacological Basis of Therapeutics* (10th ed.). New York: McGraw-Hill, 2001, pp. 733–754.

2. Strain, E. C., & Griffiths, R. M. Caffeine-related disorders. In B. J. Sadock & V. A. Sadock (Eds.), *Comprehensive Textbook of Psychiatry* (8th ed.). Baltimore, MD: Lippincott, Williams & Wilkins, 2004, pp. 1201–1210.
3. Juliano, L. M., & Griffiths, R. M. Caffeine. In J. H. Lowinson, P. Ruiz, R. B. Millman, & J. G. Langrod (Eds.), *Substance Abuse: A Comprehensive Textbook* (4th ed.). Baltimore, MD: Lippincott, Williams & Wilkins, 2004, pp. 403–420.
4. Sjaastad, O., & Bakketeig, L. S. Caffeine-withdrawal headache. The Vågå study of headache epidemiology. *Cephalalgia 24:*241–249, 2004.
5. Fisone, G., Borgkvist, A., & Usiello, A. Caffeine as a psychomotor stimulant: Mechanism of action. *Cellular and Molecular Life Sciences 61:*857–872, 2004.
6. Ascherio, A., & Chen, H. Caffeinated clues from epidemiology of Parkinson's disease. *Neurology 61:*S51–S54, 2003.
7. Holmgren, P., Nordén-Pettersson, & Ahlner, J. Caffeine fatalities – four case reports. *Forensic Science International 139:*71–73, 2004.
8. Richardson, T., Rozkovec, A., Thomas, P., Ryder, J., Meckes, C., & Kerr, D. Influence of caffeine on heart rate variability in patients with longstanding type 1 diabetes. *Diabetes Care 27:*1127–1131, 2004.
9. El Yacoubi, M., Ledent, C., Parmentier, M., Costentin, J., & Vaugeois, J. M. Caffeine reduces hypnotic effects of alcohol through adenosine A2A receptor blockade. *Neuropharmacology 45:*977–985, 2003.
10. Rosengren, A., Dotevall, A., Wilhelmsen, L., Thelle, D., & Johansson, S. Coffee and incidence of diabetes in Swedish women: A prospective 18-year follow-up study. *Journal of Internal Medicine 255:*89–95, 2004.
11. Lorist, M. M., & Tops, M. Caffeine, fatigue, and cognition. *Brain and Cognition 53:*82–94, 2003.
12. Halldner, L., Aden, U., Dahlberg, V., Johansson, B., Ledent, C., & Fredholm, B. B. The adenosine A(1) receptor contributes to the stimulatory, but not the inhibitory effect of caffeine on locomotion: a study in mice lacking adenosine A(1) and/or A(2A) receptors. *Neuropharmacology 46:*1008–1017, 2004.
13. Alsene, K., Deckert, J., Sand, P., & de Wit, H. Association between A_{2a} receptor gene polymorphisms and caffeine-induced anxiety. *Neuropsychopharmacology 28:*1694–1702, 2003.
14. Karcz-Kubicha, M., Antoniou, K., Terasmaa, A., Quarta, D., Solinas, M., Justinova, Z., Pezzola, A., Reggio, R., Müller, C. E., Fuxe, K., Goldberg, S. R., Popoli, P., & Ferré, S. Involvement of adenosine A_1 and A_{2A} receptors in the motor effects of caffeine after its acute and chronic administration. *Neuropsychopharmacology 28:*1281–1291, 2003.
15. Kaasinen, V., Aalto, S., Nagren, K., & Rinne, J. O. Dopaminergic effects of caffeine in the human striatum and thalamus. *Neuroreport 15:*281–285, 2004.
16. Lane, J. D., Pieper, C. F., Phillips-Bute, B. G., Bryant, J. E., & Kuhn, C. M. Caffeine affects cardiovascular and neuroendocrine activation at work and home. *Psychosomatic Medicine 64:*595–603, 2002.
17. Shilo, L., Sabbah, H., Hadari, R., Kovatz, S., Weinberg, U., Dolev, S., Dagan, Y., & Shenkman, L. The effects of coffee consumption on sleep and melatonin secretion. *Sleep Medicine 3:*271–273, 2002.
18. Liguori, A., & Robinson, J. H. Caffeine antagonism of alcohol-induced driving impairment. *Drug and Alcohol Dependence 63:*123–129, 2001.
19. Hartley, T. R., Lovallo, W. R., & Whitsett, T. L. Cardiovascular effects of caffeine in men and women. *The American Journal of Cardiology 93:*1022–1026, 2004.
20. Savoca, M. R., Evans, C. D., Wilson, M. E., Harshfield, G. A., & Ludwig, D. A. The association of caffeinated beverages with blood pressure in adolescents. *Archives of Pediatric and Adolescent Medicine 158:*473–477, 2004.
21. American Psychiatric Association. *The Diagnostic and Statistical Manual of Mental Disorders* (4th ed., text revision). Washington, DC: American Psychiatric Press, 2000.

22. Dager, S. R., Layton, M. E., Strauss, W., Richards, T. L., Heide, A., Friedman, S. D., Artru, A. A., Hayes, C. E., & Posse, S. Human brain metabolic response to caffeine and the effects of tolerance. *American Journal of Psychiatry 156:*229–237, 1999.
23. Evans, S. M., & Griffiths, R. R. Caffeine withdrawal: a parametric analysis of caffeine dosing conditions. *Journal of Pharmacology and Experimental Therapeutics 289:*285–294, 1999.
24. Hughes, J. R., & Oliveto, A. H. A systematic survey of caffeine intake in Vermont. *Experimental and Clinical Psychopharmacology 5:*393–398, 1997.
25. Hughes, J. R. McHugh, P., & Holtzman, S. Caffeine and schizophrenia. *Psychiatric Services 49:*1415–1417, 1998.
26. Kendler, K. S., & Prescott, C. A. Caffeine intake, tolerance, and withdrawal in women: A population-based twin study. *American Journal of Psychiatry 156:*223–228, 1999.
27. Holstege, C. P., Hunter, Y., Baer, A. B., Savory, J., Bruns, D. E., & Boyd, J. C. Massive caffeine overdose requiring vasopressin infusion and hemodialysis. *Journal Toxicol Clinical Toxicology 41:*1003–1007, 2003.
28. Carrillo, J. A., Herraiz, A. G., Ramos, S. I., & Benítez, J. Effects of caffeine withdrawal from the diet on the metabolism of clozapine in schizophrenic patients. *Journal of Clinical Psychopharmacology 18:*311–316, 1998.
29. Bruce, M., Scott, N., Shine, P., & Lader, M. Anxiogenic effects of caffeine in patients with anxiety disorders. *Archives of General Psychiatry 49:*867–869, 1992.
30. Breier, A., Charney, D. S., & Heinger, G. R. Agoraphobia with panic attacks. Development, diagnostic stability, and course of illness. *Archives of General Psychiatry 43:*1029–1036, 1986.
31. Ogawa, N., & Ueki, H. Secondary mania caused by caffeine (Letters to the Editor). *General Hospital Psychiatry 25:*136–144, 2003.
32. DiMonda, V., Nicolodi, M., Aloisio, A., Del Bianco, P., Fonzari, M., Grazioli, I., Uslenghi, C., Vecchiet, L., & Sicuteri, F. Efficacy of a fixed combination of indomethacin, prochlorperazine, and caffeine versus sumatriptan in acute treatment of multiple migraine attacks: A multicenter, randomized, crossover trial. *Headache 43:*835–844, 2003.
33. Ascherio, A., Zhang, S. J., Hernán, M. A., Kawachi, I., Colditz, G. A., Speizer, F. E., & Willett, W. C. Prospective study of caffeine consumption and risk of Parkinson's Disease in men and women. *Annals of Neurology 50:*56–63, 2001.
34. Agardh, E. E., Carlsson, S., Ahlbom, A., Efendic, S., Grill, V., Hammar, N., Hilding, A., & Östenson, C.-G. Coffee consumption, type 2 diabetes and impaired glucose tolerance in Swedish men and women. *Journal of Internal Medicine 255:*645–652, 2004.
35. Van Dam, R. J., & Feskens, E. J. M. Coffee consumption and risk of type 2 diabetes mellitus. *The Lancet 360:*1477–1478, 2002.
36. Leitzmann, M. F., Stampfer, M. J., Willett, W. C., Spiegelman, D., Colditz, G. A., & Giovannucci, E. L. Coffee intake is associated with lower risk of symptomatic gallstone disease in women. *Gastroenterology 123:*1823–1830, 2002.
37. Pehl, C., Pfeiffer, A., Wendl, B., & Kaess, H. The effect of decaffeination of coffee on gastro-oesophageal reflux in patients with reflux disease. *Alimentary Pharmacology and Therapeutics 11:*483–486, 1997.
38. Kelly, T. L., Mitler, M. M., & Bonnet, M. H. Sleep latency measures of caffeine effects during sleep deprivation. *Electroencephalography and Clinical Neurophysiology 102:*397–400, 1997.
39. Slattery, M. L., Caan, B. J., Anderson, K. E., & Potter, J. D. Intake of fluids and methylxanthine-containing beverages: Association with colon cancer. *International Journal of Cancer 81:*199–204, 1999.
40. Signorello, L. B., & McLaughlin, J. K. Maternal caffeine consumption and spontaneous abortion: A review of the epidemiologic evidence. *Epidemiology 15:*229–239, 2004.
41. Taylor, P. Agents acting at the neuromuscular junction and autonomic ganglia. In J. G. Hardman, L. E. Limbird, & A. G. Gilman (Eds.), *The Pharmacological Basis of Therapeutics* (10th ed.). New York: McGraw-Hill, 2001, pp. 193–214.

42. Strong, D. R., Kahler, C. W., Ramsey, S. E., & Brown, R. A. Finding order in the DSM-IV nicotine dependence syndrome: A rasch analysis. *Drug and Alcohol Dependence 72:*151–162, 2003.
43. Hughes, J. R. Distinguishing nicotine dependence from smoking. *Archives of General Psychiatry 58:*817–818, 2001.
44. Li, M. D., Cheng, R., Ma, J. Z., & Swan, G. E. A meta-analysis of estimated genetic and environmental effects on smoking behavior in male and female adult twins. *Addiction 93;*23–31, 2003.
45. Hopfer, C. J., Stallings, M. C., & Hewitt, J. K. Common genetic and environmental vulnerability for alcohol and tobacco use in a volunteer sample of older female twins. *Journal of Studies on Alcohol 62:*717–723, 2001.
46. Bowers, B. J., McClure-Begley, T. D., Keller, J. J., Paylor, R., Collins, A. C., & Wehner, J. M. Deletion of the ∝7 nicotinic receptor subunit gene results in increased sensitivity to several behavioral effects produced by alcohol. *Alcoholism: Clinical and Experimental Research 29:*295–302, 2005.
47. Schmitz, J. M., & DeLaune, K. A. Nicotine. In J. H. Lowinson, P. Ruiz, R. B. Millman, & J. G. Langrod (Eds.), *Substance Abuse: A Comprehensive Textbook* (4th ed.). Baltimore, MD: Lippincott, Williams & Wilkins, 2004, pp. 387–402.
48. Perez-Stable, E., Herrera, B., Jacob, P., III, & Benowitz, N. L. Nicotine metabolism and intake in black and white smokers. *Journal of the American Medical Association 280:*152–156, 1998.
49. Rassoulpour, A., Wu, H.-Q., Albuquerque, E. X., & Schwarcz, R. Prolonged nicotine administration results in biphasic, brain-specific changes in kynurenate levels in the rat. *Neuropsychopharmacology 30:*697-704, 2005.
50. Rose, J. E., Behm, F. M., Westman, E. C., Mathew, R. J., London, E. D., Hawk, T. C., Turkington, T. G., & Coleman, R. E. PET studies of the influences of nicotine on neural systems in cigarette smokers. *American Journal of Psychiatry 160:*323–333, 2003.
51. Tapper, A. R., McKinney, S. L., Nashmi, R., Schwarz, J., Deshpande, P., Labarca, C., Whiteaker, P., Marks, M. J., Collins, A. C., & Lester, H. A. Nicotine activation of (4 receptors: Sufficient for reward, tolerance and sensitization. *Science 306:*1029–1032, 2004.
52. Blomqvist, O., Hernandez-Avila, C. A., Van Kirk, J., Rose, J. E., & Kranzler, H. R. Mecamylamine modifies the pharmacokinetics and reinforcing effects of alcohol. *Alcoholism: Clinical and Experimental Research 26:*326–331, 2002.
53. Picciotto, M. R., & Corrigall, W. A. Neuronal systems underlying behaviors related to nicotine addiction: neural circuits and molecular genetics. *The Journal of Neuroscience 22:*3338–3341, 2002.
54. Brody, A. L., Olmstead, R. E., London, E. D., Farahi, J., Meyer, J. H., Grossman, P., Lee, G. S., Huang, J., Hahn, E. L., & Mandelkern, M. A. Smoking-induced ventral striatum dopamine release. *American Journal of Psychiatry 161:*1211–1218, 2004.
55. Klimek, V., Zhu, Y., Dilley, G., Konick, L., Overholser, J. C., Meltzer, H. Y., May, W. L., Stockmeier, C. A., & Ordway, G. A. Effects of long-term cigarette smoking on the human locus coeruleus. *Archives of General Psychiatry 58:*821–827, 2001.
56. Chen, H., Vlahos, R., Bozinovski, S., Jones, J., Anderson, G. P., & Morris, M. J. Effect of short-term cigarette smoke exposure on body weight, appetite and brain neuropeptide Y in mice. *Neuropsychopharmacology 30:*713-719, 2005.
57. Berggren, U., Fahlke, C., Eriksson, M., & Balldin, J. Tobacco use is associated with reduced central serotonergic neurotransmission in Type 1 alcohol-dependent individuals. *Alcoholism: Clinical and Experimental Research 27:*1257–1261, 2003.
58. Benowitz, N. L., Peez-Stable, E. J., Herrera, B., & Jacob, P., III. Slower metabolism and reduced intake of nicotine from cigarette smoking in Chinese-Americans. *Journal of the National Cancer Institute 94:*108–115, 2002.
59. Ebbert, J. O., Rowland, L. C., Montori, V. M., Vickers, K. S., Erwin, P. J., & Dale, L. C. Treatments for spit tobacco use: a quantitative systematic review. *Addiction 98:*569–583, 2003.
60. Sacco, K. A., Termine, A., Seyal, A., Dudas, M. M., Vessicchio, J. C., Krishnan-Sarin, S., Jatlow, P. I., Wexler, B. E., & George, T. P. Effects of cigarette smoking on spatial working

memory and attentional deficits in schizophrenia: Involvement of nicotinic receptor mechanisms. *Archives of General Psychiatry 62:*649–659, 2005.

61. Cheeta, S., Irvine, E. E., Tucci, S., Sandhu, J., & File, S. E. In adolescence, female rats are more sensitive to the anxiolytic effect of nicotine than are male rats. *Neuropsychopharmacology 25:*601–607, 2001.
62. Phillips, A. N., Wannamethee, S. G., Walker, M., Thomson, A., & Smith, G. D. Life expectancy in men who have never smoked and those who have smoked continuously: 15-year follow-up of large cohort of middle aged British men. *British Medical Journal 313:*907–908, 1996.
63. Substance Abuse and Mental Health Services Administration. *Results From the 2002 National Survey on Drug Use and Health: National Findings* (Office of Applied Studies, NHSDA Series H-22, DHHS Publication No. SMA 03-3836). Rockville, MD, 2003.
64. Breslau, N., Johnson, E.O., Hiripi, E., & Kessler, R. Nicotine dependence in the United States. *Archives of General Psychiatry 58:*810–816, 2001.
65. Anthony, J. C., & Echeagaray-Wagner, F. Epidemiologic analysis of alcohol and tobacco use: Patterns of co-occurring consumption and dependence in the United States. *Alcohol Research & Health 24:*201–208, 2000.
66. Anthony, J. C. Epidemiology of drug dependence. In K. L. Davis, D. Charney, J. T. Coyle, & C. Nemeroff (Eds.), *Neuropsychopharmacology: The Fifth Generation of Progress.* Philadelphia, PA: Lippincott Williams & Wilkins, 2002.
67. Johnston, L. D., O'Malley, P. M., & Bachman, J. R. *Monitoring the Future National Survey Results on Drug Use, 1975–2002,* Volume I: Secondary school Students (NIH Publication No. 03-5375). Bethesda, MD: National Institute on Drug Abuse, 2003.
68. Collins, A. C. Genetic influences on tobacco use: A review of human and animal studies. *International Journal of Addictions 25:*35–55, 1991.
69. Bricker, J. B., Leroux, B. G., Peterson, A. V., Jr., Kealey, K. A., Sarason, I. G., Andersen, M. R., & Marek, P. M. Nine-year prospective relationship between parental smoking cessation and children's daily smoking. *Addiction 98:*585–593, 2003.
70. Audrain-McGovern, J., Lerman, C., Wileyto, E. P., Rodriguez, D., & Shields, P. G. Interacting effects of genetic predisposition and depression on adolescent smoking progression. *American Journal of Psychiatry 161:*1224–1230, 2004.
71. Schmitz, N., Kruse, J., & Kugler, J. Disabilities, quality of life, and mental disorders associated with smoking and nicotine dependence. *American Journal of Psychiatry 160:*1670–1676, 2003.
72. Hughes, J. R., Fiester, S., Goldstein, M., *et al.* Practice guidelines for the treatment of patients with nicotine. *American Journal of Psychiatry 153(suppl):*1–29, 1996.
73. Abroms, L., Simons-Morton, B., Haynie, D. L., & Chen, R. Psychosocial predictors of smoking trajectories during middle and high school. *Addiction 100:*852–861, 2005.
74. Russell, M. A. H. The nicotine addiction trap: A 40-year sentence for four cigarettes. *British Journal of Addiction 85:*293–300, 1990.
75. West, R., McEwen, A., Bolling, K., & Owen, L. Smoking cessation and smoking patterns in the general population: A 1-year follow-up. *Addiction 96:*891–902, 2001.
76. Meyer, C., Rumpf, H.-J., Schumann, A., Hapke, U., John, U. Intentionally reduced smoking among untreated general population smokers: prevalence, stability, prediction of smoking behaviour change and differences between subjects choosing either reduction or abstinence. *Addiction 98:*1101–1110, 2003.
77. Cooney, J. L., Cooney, N. L., Pilkey, D. T., Kranzler, H. R., & Oncken, C. A. Effects of nicotine deprivation on urges to drink and smoke in alcoholic smokers. *Addiction 98:*913–921, 2003.
78. Jackson, K. M., Sher, K. J., Cooper, M. L., & Wood, P. K. Adolescent alcohol and tobacco use: Onset, persistence and trajectories of use across two samples. *Addiction 97:*517–531, 2002.
79. Bierut, L. J., Rice, J. P., Goate, A., Hinrichs, A. L., Saccone, N. L., Foroud, T., Edenberg, H. J., Cloninger, R., Begleiter, H., Conneally, P. M., Crowe, R. R., Hesselbrock, V., Li, T.-K., Nurnberger, J. I., Jr., Porjesz, B., Schuckit, M. A., & Reich, T. A genomic scan for habitual

smoking in families of alcoholics: Common and specific genetic factors in substance dependence. *American Journal of Medical Genetics, 124:*19–27, 2005.

80. Richter, K. P., Ahluwalia, H. K., Mosier, M. C., Nazir, N., & Ahluwalia, J. S. A population-based study of cigarette smoking among illicit drug users in the United States. *Addiction 97:*861–869, 2002.
81. Ferguson, J., Bauld, L., Chesterman, J., & Judge, K. The English smoking treatment services: One-year outcomes. *Addiction 100:*59–69, 2005.
82. Jacobsen, L. K., Krystal, J. H., Mencl, W. E., Westervald, M., Frost, S. J., & Pugh, K. R. Effects of smoking and smoking abstinence on cognition in adolescent tobacco smokers. *Biological Psychiatry 57:*56-66, 2005.
83. Dierker, L. C., Avenevoli, S., Stolar, M., & Merikangas, K. R. Smoking and depression: An examination of mechanisms of comorbidity. *American Journal of Psychiatry 159:*947–953, 2002.
84. Zubieta, J.-K., Heitzig, M. M., Xu, Y., Koeppe, R. A., Ni, L., Guthrie, S., & Domino, E. F. Regional cerebral blood flow responses to smoking in tobacco smokers after overnight abstinence. *American Journal of Psychiatry 162:*567–577, 2005.
85. Schneider, N. G., Olmstead, R., Vaghaiwalla Mody, F., Doan, K., Franzon, M., Jarvik, M. E., & Steinberg, C. Efficacy of a nicotine nasal spray in smoking cessation: A placebo-controlled, double-blind trial. *Addiction 90:*1671–1682, 1995.
86. George, T. P., Vessicchio, J. C., Termine, A., Bregartner, T. A., Feingold, A., Rounsaville, B. J., & Kosten, T. R. A placebo controlled trial of bupropion for smoking cessation in schizophrenia. *Biological Psychiatry 52:*53–61, 2002.
87. Hall, S. M., Humfleet, G. L., Reus, V. I., Munoz, R. F. & Cullen, J. Extended nortriptyline and psychological treatment for cigarette smoking. *American Journal of Psychiatry 161:*2100–2107, 2004.
88. Goldstein, M. G. Bupropion sustained release and smoking cessation. *Journal of Clinical Psychiatry 4:*66–72, 1998.
89. Ashenden, R., Silagy, C. A., Lodge, M., & Fowler, G. A meta-analysis of the effectiveness of acupuncture in smoking cessation. *Drug and Alcohol Review 16:*33–40, 1997.
90. Breslau, N., Schultz, L. R., Johnson, E. O., Peterson, E. L., & Davis, G. C. Smoking and the risk of suicidal behavior: A prospective study of a community sample. *Archives of General Psychiatry 62:*328–334, 2005.
91. Grant, B. F., Hasin, D. S., Chou, P., Stinson, F. S., & Dawson, D. A. Nicotine dependence and psychiatric disorders in the United States: Results from the National Epidemiologic Survey on Alcohol and Related Conditions. *Archives of General Psychiatry 61:*1107–1115, 2004.
92. Tregellas, J. R., Tanabe, J. L., Martin, L. F., & Freedman, R. fMRI response to nicotine during a smooth pursuit eye movement task in schizophrenia. *American Journal of Psychiatry 162:*391–393, 2005.
93. Smith, R. C., Singh, A., Infante, M., Khandat, A., & Kloos, A. Effects of cigarette smoking and nicotine nasal spray on psychiatric symptoms and cognition in schizophrenia. *Neuropsychopharmacology 27:*479–497, 2002.
94. Weiser, M., Reichenberg, A., Grotto, I., Yasvitzsky, R., Rabinowitz, J., Lubin, G., Nahon, D., Knobler, H. Y., & Davidson, M. Higher rates of cigarette smoking in male adolescents before the onset of schizophrenia: A historical-prospective cohort study. *American Journal of Psychiatry 161:*1219–1223,2004.
95. Zammit, S., Allebeck, P., Dalman, C., Lundberg, I., Hemmingsson, T., & Lewis, G. Investigating the association between cigarette smoking and schizophrenia in a cohort study. *American Journal of Psychiatry 160:*2216–2220, 2003.
96. Goodwin, R., & Hamilton, S. P. Cigarette smoking and panic: The role of neuroticism. *American Journal of Psychiatry 159:*1208–1213, 2002.
97. Isensee, B., Wittchen, H.-U., Stein, M. R., Hofler, M., & Lieb, R. Smoking increases the risk of panic: Findings from a prospective community study. *Archives of General Psychiatry 60:*692–700, 2003.

98. Johnson, J. G., Cohen, P., Pine, D. S., Klein, D. F., Kasen, S., & Brook, J. S. Association between cigarette smoking and anxiety disorders during adolescence and early adulthood. *Journal of the American Medical Association 284:*2348–2351, 2000.
99. McGee, R., Williams, S., & Nada-Raja, S. Is cigarette smoking associated with suicidal ideation among young people? *American Journal of Psychiatry 162:*619-620, 2005.
100. Malone, K. M., Waternaux, C., Haas, G. L., Cooper, T. B., Li, S., & Mann, J. J. Cigarette smoking, suicidal behavior, and serotonin function in major psychiatric disorders. *American Journal of Psychiatry 160:*773–779, 2003.
101. Breslau, N., Novak, S. P., & Kessler, R. C. Psychiatric disorders and stages of smoking. *Biological Psychiatry 55:*69–76, 2004.
102. Kendler, K. S., Neale, M. C., MacLean, C. J., Heath, A. C., Eaves, L. J. & Kessler, R.C. Smoking and major depression: A causal analysis. *Archives of General Psychiatry 50:*36–43, 1993.
103. Doll, R., Peto, R., Boreham, J., & Sutherland, I. Mortality in relation to smoking: 50 years' observation on male British doctors. *British Medical Journal 328:*1519–1528, 2004.
104. Zamani, M. R., & Allen, Y. S. Nicotine and its interaction with β-amyloid protein: a short review. *Biological Psychiatry 49:*221–232, 2001.
105. Newhouse, P. A., Potter, A., Kelton, M., & Corwin, J. Nicotinic treatment of Alzheimer's disease. *Biological Psychiatry 49:*268–278, 2001.
106. Howard, G., Wagenknecht, L. E., Burke, G. L., Diez-Roux, A., Evans, G. W., McGovern, P., Nieto, F. J., & Tell, G. S. Cigarette smoking and progression of atherosclerosis: The atherosclerosis risk in communities (ARIC) study. *Journal of the American Medical Association 279:*119–124, 1998.
107. Rosenberg, L., Palmer, J. R., & Shapiro, S. Decline in the risk of myocardial infarction among women who stop smoking. *New England Journal of Medicine 322:*213–217, 1990.
108. Parath, A. J. & Fried, P. A. Effects of prenatal cigarette and marijuana exposure on drug use among offspring. *Neurotoxicology and Teratology 27:*267–277, 2005.
109. Abreu-Villaca, Y., Seidler, F. J., & Slotkin, T. A. Does prenatal nicotine exposure sensitize the brain to nicotine-induced neurotoxicity in adolescence? *Neuropsychopharmacology 29:*1440–1450, 2004.
110. Brennan, P. A., Grekin, E. R., Mortensen, E. L., & Mednick, S. A. Relationship of maternal smoking during pregnancy with criminal arrest and hospitalization for substance abuse in male and female adult offspring. *American Journal of Psychiatry 159:*48–54, 2002.
111. Linnet, K. M., Dalsgaard, S., Obel, C., Wisborg, K. Henriksen, T. B., Rodriguez, A L., Kotimaa, A., Moilanen, I., Thomsen, P. H., Olsen, J., & Jarvelin, R. Maternal lifestyle factors in pregnancy risk of attention deficit hyperactivity disorder and associated behaviors: Review of the current evidence. *American Journal of Psychiatry 160:*1028–1040, 2003.
112. Thapar, A., Fowler, T., Rice, F., Scourfield, J., van den Bree, M., Thomas, H., Harold, G., & Hay, D. Maternal smoking during pregnancy and attention deficit hyperactivity disorder symptoms in offspring. *American Journal of Psychiatry 160:*1985–1989, 2003.
113. Gold, D. R., Wang, X., Wypij, D., Speizer, F. E., Ware, J. H., & Dockery, D. W. Effects of cigarette smoking on lung function in adolescent boys and girls. *New England Journal of Medicine 335:*931–937, 1996.
114. Jensen, J., Christiansen, C., & Rodbro, P. Cigarette smoking, serum estrogens, and bone loss during hormone-replacement therapy early after menopause. *New England Journal of Medicine 313:*973–975, 1985.
115. Steenland, K. Passive smoking and the risk of heart disease. *Journal of the American Medical Association 267:*94–99, 1992.
116. Cruickshanks, K. J., Klein, R., Klein, B. E. K., Wiley, T. L., Nondahl, D. M., & Tweed, T. S. Cigarette smoking and hearing loss. *Journal of the American Medical Association 279:* 1715–1719, 1998.

CHAPTER 12

Multidrug Abuse and Dependence

12.1. INTRODUCTION

12.1.1. General Comments

A review of the epidemiology sections of the previous chapters reveals that most people have had experience with alcohol, nicotine, or at least one illicit substance at some time in their lives.[1,2] The consumption of these substances has many implications, especially for drug interactions when two or more pharmacological agents are taken at the same time. The situation becomes even more complex in individuals who also consume over-the-counter (OTC) medications and prescription drugs. Each substance has a potential for impacting how other drugs are absorbed into the body, distributed throughout the tissues, metabolized, and how they affect organs such as the brain. Therefore, health-care providers need to take a careful history from all patients and clients regarding the recent and long-term intake patterns of alcohol, nicotine, illegal drugs, OTC medications, and prescription drugs. Such use patterns must be considered in initiating the appropriate treatment, and in minimizing the potential for side effects.

These problems are even more challenging in people with substance abuse or dependence. Whenever a difficulty related to one substance is noted, it is important to search for use, abuse, and dependence on other drugs. Even if criteria for a substance-use disorder are not apparent regarding the second or third drug, consumption of other substances can impact on the clinical course of the abuse or dependence on the first agent, and can alter the symptoms observed during intoxication or withdrawal. For example, an individual who is alcohol dependent but who also has a history of taking marijuana several times a week needs to abstain from all substances, because a return to marijuana following treatment for alcoholism is, at least theoretically, likely to increase the chances for relapse. This might occur because intoxication with the cannabinol decreases a person's focus and judgment, and because past consumption of both substances (alcohol and marijuana) together means that the sight, smell, and feelings associated with the cannabinol are likely to increase the craving for alcohol.

As described in previous chapters, although any combination of substances is possible, there are a number of drug mixtures that are especially likely to occur. First, more than 70% of people who are alcohol dependent are also current nicotine users, and most of these are dependent on cigarettes.[3] Second, people who are cocaine dependent are more likely than those in the general population to also demonstrate dependence on alcohol, in part because the combination produces a new substance in the body (cocaethylene) when the two substances are combined.[4] Third, many people who are opioid dependent inject a mixture of heroin and cocaine as a "speedball," perhaps using each drug to enhance the effects and decrease the side effects experienced with the other.[5] Additional combinations of drugs of abuse that are observed more often than would be predicted by chance include the high rate of intake of Bzs among individuals who are heroin or methadone dependent; the concomitant use of heavy doses of alcohol and methadone; and combinations of an antihistamine and pentazocine (Talwin), known as Ts and Blues.[6,7]

There are several situations in which dependence on multiple drugs may be especially likely to occur. The first involves the early onset and continuation into adulthood of severe and pervasive antisocial behaviors, a condition known as conduct disorder during childhood and the antisocial personality disorder (ASPD) in adulthood.[8] This disorder is characterized by a high level of impulsivity, difficulty learning from mistakes or punishment, and a lack of empathy for animals and for people. It is not surprising that the combination of these characteristics is associated with a rate of dependence on at least one drug of 70–80% or more in individuals with ASPD, along with a heightened likelihood for dependence on multiple substances.

A second situation in which dependence on multiple drugs is especially likely to occur as a result of the usual progression of experiences with substances that are increasingly scarce and/or more frowned upon by society.[9] Most people begin their substance-use careers with nicotine, caffeine, or alcohol, and, if they progress to other drugs, are next likely to use cannabinols, followed by exposure to one or more drugs from the categories of stimulants, hallucinogens, or other brain depressants such as Bzs. Thus, by the time a person uses drugs such as heroin or have exposed themselves to IV substances, they are likely to already have been acquainted with the actions of more available and less highly controlled drugs such as alcohol and the cannabinols. Therefore, it is likely that when their preferred drug is not available, or when they are experiencing unwanted symptoms associated with intoxication or withdrawal, they might be especially likely to increase their use of these prior drugs. For example, men and women who are opioid dependent are more likely to have histories of dependence on other drugs than is true for the usual individual who is alcohol dependent.

Reflecting these considerations, the clinician is often faced with the question of the appropriate diagnosis for an individual who fulfills criteria for dependence on more than one drug. DSM-IV offers very clear advice, telling us to list *every* substance-use disorder separately.[10] Thus, for example, the appropriate labeling of an individual who is dependent on alcohol, cocaine, and heroin is to list all three dependencies. It is important to note that the term "poly-substance dependence" is only to be used when an individual does not meet criteria for dependence on any one specific drug and only fulfills three of seven dependence criteria items when the substances are considered as a group.[11]

Finally, by way of introduction, it is possible to offer some general advice regarding the optimal approaches to treatment for individuals who are dependent on more than one drug. If the clinician has sufficient knowledge about the treatment of intoxication, withdrawal, and rehabilitation approaches appropriate for each drug individually, it is only a matter of common sense to use this information in real-life situations where more than one substance-use disorder is observed. In general, the focus is placed on the drug with the most severe sequelae (e.g., for withdrawal, depressants pose more dangers than the other relevant classes of drugs), adding additional treatments for the second drug as needed. An emphasis is also placed on the substance with the longest half-life (e.g., diazepam or methadone versus alcohol or heroin), where treating the withdrawal, for example, associated with diazepam for several weeks takes care of the problems for alcohol withdrawal as well. Common-sense modifications can then be added for the second or third drug. In these analyses it is important to remember that only two classes of drugs of abuse routinely justify the use of medications during withdrawal (depressants and opioids); the treatment of any type of intoxication or most substance-induced psychiatric syndromes whether related to one drug or several requires careful observation and general supports; with the exception of using opioid antagonists, overdose conditions are usually treated by supporting the vital signs regardless of the drug or combination involved (again keeping the emphasis on the drug with the most severe symptoms and longer half-life); and that the approaches for rehabilitation are more similar than different across drug categories. With these generalizations in mind, it is possible to offer information related to abuse and dependence on multiple substances, remembering that this represents a restatement of the issues already presented in the preceding chapters.

12.1.2. Natural History of Multidrug Abuse and Dependence

The patterns of substance use sometimes differ with the immediate environment, as exemplified by the greater access to drugs like crack cocaine in urban ghettos compared to middle-class suburbs where cocaine powder may be more available. Similarly, physicians and other health-care providers have more access to, and potential misuse of, some prescription drugs of abuse than people in most other professions.[12]

With these caveats in mind, it is still possible to offer some generalizations about likely patterns of concomitant drug misuse. As described previously, in Western societies, youth begin drug experiences with caffeine, nicotine, and alcohol.[13] If they go on to use other substances, the next drug is likely to be marijuana, followed in frequency by one of the hallucinogens, the depressants, or the stimulants, usually taken on an experimental basis, ingested orally, and with few immediately serious consequences. Individuals who go on to heavier intake may graduate to IV drug use, with a progression to opioids.[14]

This pattern of exposure has been viewed by some investigators as an age-related clustering of drugs, reflecting the use of whatever substance is most available and culturally acceptable at a given stage of life. Here, the drug pattern is not seen as a series of "stepping-stones," where the use of one drug neurochemically primes the person to seek out the next. Other researchers, however, have raised the possibility that use of drugs changes the person's biological makeup in a way that might enhance additional drug-seeking behavior.[15] The available data do not definitively rule out either theory.

12.1.3. Pharmacology

12.1.3.1. General Comments

All of the drugs of abuse affect the brain. In general, if a person takes two drugs, each of which have sedation as a side effect, the intoxication will demonstrate at least an additive effect of the sleepiness associated with Drug One plus the sleepiness from Drug Two. Sometimes, the drugs actually multiply (potentiate) the effects of each other, so that the overall sedation (or, for substances with adrenalineline actions, stimulation) is greater than one might have expected from either drug alone. Potentiation may be most likely to occur when two drugs of the same class (e.g., a Bz and alcohol or amphetamines and cocaine) are taken together.

While all positively reinforcing events are likely to impact on the brain neurotransmitter dopamine (and thus, all drugs of abuse have an effect on this neurochemical), different categories of drugs generally have their major effects on overlapping, but distinct, neurochemical systems. As a result, if the clinician studies the pharmacology section of each of the chapters, it is possible to estimate some of the interactions of neurotransmitters likely to be observed when drugs from multiple classes are taken together. For example, any two drugs that diminish the effect of acetylcholine (i.e., are anticholinergic) are likely to enhance the side effect profile (e.g., for anticholinergic drugs, feelings of confusion, blurred vision, dry mouth, urinary retention, and so on). This is commented upon at various points in the preceding chapters, especially regarding the need to take special care in prescribing medications to treat drug-induced symptoms when the prescribed drugs might increase some of the side effects observed from the drug of abuse.

All drugs of abuse are to a greater (e.g., alcohol) or lesser (e.g., inhalants) degree metabolized in the liver. When a first drug stimulates the liver to produce more enzymes to metabolize substances, it is probable that the rate of breakdown of the second drug will occur more rapidly. However, when the two drugs of abuse use the same enzyme system for metabolism and are taken at the same time, it is likely that both drugs will be broken down more slowly than expected.

These generalizations may be helpful when you are evaluating a patient who is taking multiple substances. The general approach is to use the information you have regarding Drug A, consider the information regarding Drug B, and make your best estimate of what is likely to occur regarding the intensity and duration of intoxication, toxic reactions or overdoses, withdrawal, and so on.

Another way of looking at these comments is to remember that the effects of a drug may be either increased or decreased through interactions with other drugs.

1. The effect of a drug is *decreased* when it is administered to an individual who, although *not* taking any other drug at the same time, has recently developed cross-tolerance to a similar drug. This can occur through metabolic tolerance (usually reflecting the increased production of the relevant metabolic enzymes in the liver), or through pharmacodynamic mechanisms (by which the effect of the substance on cells has been decreased). Thus, higher levels of the substance are needed to generate the expected clinical effects. A relevant example is the need for higher levels of anesthetics, hypnotics, antianxiety drugs, or analgesics in recently sober alcoholics.
2. The results are the opposite, however, when two drugs with similar effects are administered *concomitantly*. In this instance, both drugs must sometimes compete for the same enzyme and other protein systems, both in the liver and at the target cell, such as in the brain. One likely result is an increased half-life in the body for the drugs when both are administered at the same time, although this adaptation may be lost as tolerance develops after continued exposure to both agents. The overall effect with concomitant acute administration of such agents can be *potentiation*, through which, for example, the amount of depression of brain activity that results from the conjoint administration of two depressant drugs is more than would be expected from the actions seen with either drug alone. This can produce an unexpected lethal overdose for the individual who has had too much to drink and decides that a few extra sleeping pills will help him rest through the night.

12.1.3.2. Some Specific Examples

The pharmacological mechanisms for specific drug–drug interactions are somewhat unpredictable, underlining the dangers in multidrug misuse. However, it is possible to make some generalizations about combinations of particular types of drugs.

12.1.3.2.1. Depressants–Depressants

The mechanisms of action of most depressants are complex, but all affect the neurotransmitter GABA. There is ample evidence of cross-tolerance among the brain depressants, including documentation of this phenomenon regarding alcohol and Bzs.[16] At least part of the effect of alcohol occurs either directly or indirectly via GABA, and the number of Bz receptors in the frontal cortex may be altered in people with chronic alcoholism. Also, a Bz antagonist has been reported to block part of the anxiolytic and intoxicating actions of ethanol, at least in animals, although the interactions may not be as specific and selective as was first hoped. If, however, the two depressants (e.g., alcohol and barbiturates) are given at the same time, potentiation of respiratory depression develops, with resulting morbidity and even mortality.

12.1.3.2.2. Depressants–Opioids

Clinicians have long been interested in the relationship between alcohol-related problems and opioid-related difficulties.[17–19] In the early 1900s, the possible benefits of substituting alcohol for opioids among people who are dependent was considered, as well as the possibility of using opioids as a substitute for alcohol among people with alcoholism. These speculations were based in part on the partial cross-tolerance between the two classes of drugs, at least for the mild analgesic effects of ethanol. Also, opioid antagonists might ameliorate severe alcohol overdose (although this appears to be unrelated to the direct effects of the alcohol and may be more closely tied to aspects of "shock"), ethanol exerts at least some of its effects through endogenous opiate peptides or opiate receptors, and opioid antagonists such as naltrexone (Re-Via) are useful in treating alcoholism.[20] There might be some overlap of genes that predispose a person to opioid dependence and to alcoholism,[21,22] but the evidence is not yet convincing once one excludes the impact of the antisocial personality disorder (with which misuse of many substances can be expected).

Even though the depressants and the opioids do not have true cross-tolerance, one frequently sees a decreased efficacy of one drug when administered to an individual who has developed tolerance to a drug in the second class. Of greater clinical importance, however, is the fact that both opioids and depressants have depressing effects on the brain, so that each potentiates the actions of the other in overdose, increasing the likelihood of death.

Another link relates to the clinical correlates of comorbid alcohol and opioid disorders. Dependence on ethanol significantly decreases the survival among men and women in methadone maintenance, perhaps because concomitant administration of ethanol with methadone could result in increased brain concentrations of the latter (at least in animals). Misuse of alcohol also appears to predict the termination of treatment among people who are opioid dependent.[23]

12.1.3.2.3. Depressants or Opioids along with Stimulants

The brief discussion of epidemiology in Section 12.1.4 highlights the likelihood that some people with alcoholism also misuse stimulants. Similar generalizations can be made about people who are opioid dependent, where most men and women who were heroin dependent have had experience with cocaine as a speedball.

The concomitant use of depressant or opioid and stimulant drugs might decrease the side effects encountered with either drug alone. For example, the person who is depressant-drug dependent or the person with alcoholism may seek out stimulants to help him feel less sleepy after using his favorite drug, or the stimulant misuser may use alcohol or other depressants to help him feel less anxious and demonstrate less tremor while taking his preferred drug. The dangers rest with the unpredictability of the drug–drug interactions, as the CNS and metabolic systems attempt to maintain equilibrium (homeostasis) in the presence of multiple drugs with opposite effects.

12.1.3.2.4. Cannabinoids–Other Drugs

Cannabinoids and alcohol share some mechanisms of action, and marijuana has been reported to potentiate the CNS-depressing effect of alcohol.[24–28] Although these relationships require more research, it is unwise to take marijuana concomitantly with other substances, especially alcohol, because the combination is likely to enhance motor incoordination and CNS depression, a problem with serious implications for driving abilities.

12.1.4. Epidemiology and Patterns of Abuse and Dependence

The two national surveys discussed in each chapter highlight the high rate of exposure to alcohol, nicotine, caffeine, cannabinols, and other illicit substances in most Western societies.[1,2] These data imply that the use of multiple substances is quite common.

There is anecdotal evidence that the rates of multiple substance abuse and dependence are high, and over one half of the people presenting to drug clinics reported the use (not necessarily abuse or dependence) of three or more substances. Certain individuals appear to be at especially high risk for multidrug problems, including those with a history of psychiatric disorders such as schizophrenia or manic-depressive disorders, those "denied" access to their favorite drug (e.g., people in methadone maintenance programs), and those who deliberately use the more "exotic" substances, such as PCP.

In general, multidrug users tend to be young, can be from any socioeconomic background, and often show evidence of preexisting life maladjustment, sometimes severe enough to be labeled as a personality disorder.

12.1.5. Establishing a Diagnosis

It is important to remember that substance abuse and dependence are relatively common phenomena in our society, and they must be considered in the differential diagnosis of a wide variety of medical and psychological problems. To briefly review, in evaluating an individual who fits the criteria for the antisocial personality, one must note the likelihood that he or she is misusing multiple drugs. This is also probable for people in methadone maintenance programs, who also might increase their intake of alcohol and Bzs. On another level, anyone presenting to the emergency room with a drug overdose must be evaluated for the *possibility* of problems with multiple drugs, particularly someone who does not show the usual response to emergency room interventions. The key to making a diagnosis is to consider the possibility that multiple substances might be involved and to systematically gather the appropriate history.

12.2. EMERGENCY ROOM SITUATIONS

The most important clinical pictures seen with multiple drugs include toxic reactions (overdoses), drug withdrawal states, psychoses, and states of confusion. The discussion here is brief because once multidrug problems are identified, treatment involves combining the procedures outlined in other chapters for each substance alone.

12.2.1. Toxic Reactions

See Sections 1.7.1.

The approach to overdoses involving multiple drugs is fairly straightforward. First, the core of treatment is to support vital signs so that the body can metabolize and excrete the drugs and return to normal. The ABCs of such treatment (dealing with airway, breathing, and circulation) focus on control of symptoms, regardless of the specific drug involved.[29] Therefore, if two depressants or depressants and opioids are involved in the overdose, the patient will appear with depressed vital signs and require control of respirations and bolstering of blood pressure. If stimulants and opioids are ingested, the emergency treatment depends upon the vital sign changes that are most apparent—controlling high blood pressure and elevated body temperature and/or seizures if the stimulant picture predominates, and supporting blood pressure and respirations if the opioid predominates.

Whenever an opioid drug is likely to have contributed to the overdose, the clinician should administer an opioid antagonist (e.g., naloxone [Narcan], about 2 mg IV which can be repeated, as described in Chapter 6 on opioids). When Bzs are involved in an overdose, the clinician can consider an antagonist (e.g., flumazenil or Romazicon 0.2 mg IV over 3 min, with repeat doses over the next 10 min as needed up to a total of 3 mg), although, as described in Chapter 2, this drug must be used with care for patients who might have increased intracranial pressure or other contraindications.[30,31] Another general rule is to consider gastric lavage (using an endotrachial tube if needed for comatose patients), followed by the possible use of activated charcoal (1 g/kg) if there is evidence of recent oral administration of the drugs.

As you can see, a thorough knowledge of the characteristics likely to be associated with the overdose of any category of drugs is essential for determining the optimal combination of approaches to be used when multiple drugs are taken together in overdose. It is important to use the clinical symptoms observed as a guideline for which toxic reaction picture to address first.

The following sections give some brief examples of the types of overdoses the clinician might see.

12.2.1.1. Clinical Pictures and Treatments

Clinically relevant multidrug overdoses most often result from the concomitant administration of two depressants, opioids along with depressants, or mixtures of opioids with depressants or stimulants.

12.2.1.1.1. Multiple Depressants

See Sections 2.2.1 and 4.2.1.

The clinical manifestations and time course of overdoses with multiple depressants are likely to be best predicted by the drug with the longer half-life. For example, if a person overdoses on alcohol and the longer half-life drug, diazepam, the clinical course is likely to reflect diazepam.

The treatment regimen for mixed depressant overdoses is similar to the approach outlined in Section 2.2.1.2, including acute life-preserving steps and the use of general life supports, relying on the body to detoxify the substances. When a Bz is involved, the patient may improve with the Bz-antagonist flumazenil as described above. Dialysis or diuresis should be reserved for extremely severe cases that don't respond to other treatments. While the appropriate approach is likely to be best predicted by the depressant with the longer half-life, the length of drug effects when multiple depressants are involved is less predictable, as the metabolism of one may interfere with the break down of the other.

12.2.1.1.2. Depressants–Opioids

See Sections 2.2.1 and 6.2.1

The concomitant administration of opioids and depressants results in a depression of vital signs, levels of consciousness, and reflexes, the magnitude of which it is difficult to predict. The specific symptoms are combinations of those reported for the depressants and the opioids in Chapters 2 and 6.

Regarding treatment, acute emergency procedures (e.g., controlling airway and cardiac status) are followed, and naloxone (Narcan) is administered at doses of 0.4 mg IM or IV, with repeats given every 5 min for the first 15 min, and repeated every several hours thereafter, as needed, for control of the respiratory depression and the degree of stupor. Treatment with the Bz-antagonist/agonist flumazenil (Romazicon) should be considered as noted above.[32] Repeat doses might be required in 20–30 min. General supports are then continued until the body is able to destroy the drugs. These procedures are outlined in Sections 2.2.1.2 and 6.2.1.2.

12.2.1.2.3. Other Combinations

The treatment of other drug combinations is symptomatic in nature and follows the procedures outlined in the relevant chapters. It is worthwhile to note the importance of controlling hypertension, arrhythmias, and hypothermia when stimulants are involved, and considering physostigmine (Antilirium) when atropinic drugs [e.g., the anti-parkinsonian drugs, such as benztropine (Cogentin)] are part of the overdose.

12.2.2. Withdrawal from Multiple Drugs

See Section 1.7.2.

There are only three clinically relevant withdrawal syndromes, with each representing the opposite of the acute effects of the drugs of that class. Depressant withdrawal (relevant to alcohol, Bzs, barbiturates, and similar drugs prescribed for sleep) consists of an elevation of vital signs (blood pressure, heart rate, respiratory rate, and mild increases in body temperature), an increased risk for convulsions (less likely to be seen with alcohol), anxiety, insomnia, a hand tremor, and in a minority of patients, withdrawal delirium. This is the most clinically intense of the withdrawal syndromes, and should be the major focus of treatment even when concomitant withdrawal states are seen with the two other classes of drugs. When a patient is withdrawing from two depressants (e.g., alcohol and diazepam or Valium), withdrawal treatment should focus on the longer acting drug.

The next most physically intense withdrawal is seen with opioids, and is similar for almost all prescription pain pills on through heroin or methadone. When multiple opioids are involved, the withdrawal treatment should focus on the drug with the longer half-life, as the shorter half-life drug will be adequately taken care of in this approach. When opioid withdrawal occurs in conjunction with either a depressant or a stimulant, one is likely to observe a combination of withdrawal pictures, with the opioid component consisting of diarrhea, abdominal pain, a flu-like feeling, along with nausea and vomiting, as well as a runny nose, and the stimulant component characterized by somnolence and moodiness, and so on. As described in more detail in Chapter 6, in the usual instance the opioid-related symptoms are treated with drugs that address the specific complaints, including nonsteroidal anti-inflammatory drugs (e.g., naproxyn or Aleve) for pain, loperamide (Imodium) for diarrhea, and decongestants for upper respiratory symptoms.

The stimulant-withdrawal syndrome consists of sleeping too much, eating too much, and depression, along with an inability to concentrate or focus attention. Whether seen alone, or in combination of withdrawal from other groups of drugs (e.g., alcohol and cocaine or heroin and cocaine), the stimulant portion of the withdrawal is treated with education and reassurance, while the depressant and opioid withdrawal is likely to require short-term medications.

The other categories of drugs of abuse (e.g., cannabinoids or hallucinogens) are not likely to be associated with clinically relevant withdrawal phenomena, at least not any that require active pharmacological intervention.

Therefore, the approach to the treatment of withdrawal states involving multiple categories of drugs uses the common-sense combination of information offered within the chapters on depressants, opioids, and stimulants. The following sections discuss several of these concomitant withdrawal states in a bit more detail.

12.2.2.1. Clinical Pictures and Treatments

12.2.2.1.1. Multiple Depressants

The depressant withdrawal syndrome described in Section 2.2.2 is similar for all depressant drugs. However, a higher incidence of convulsions is seen with abstinence symptoms regarding Bzs or with barbiturates than with alcohol.[33–35] The latency of onset and the length of the acute withdrawal syndrome roughly parallel the half-life of the drugs, ranging from relatively short periods of time for alcohol to much longer withdrawals for drugs such as chlordiazepoxide (Librium) and phenobarbital. It is probably safest to treat withdrawal from the longer acting drug most aggressively, assuming that the second depressant will be adequately "taken care of" through this approach, but keeping an open eye for any unusual symptoms.

Adequate therapy for withdrawal from multiple depressants follows the guidelines outlined in Section 2.2.2.2, with the added caveat that the time course of withdrawal is less predictable.

1. Thus, it is unwise to decrease the levels of depressants at a rate faster than 10% a day, taking special care to reinstitute the last day's dose if there are increasingly serious signs of withdrawal.

2. It is usually possible to carry out a smooth withdrawal from multiple depressants by administering only one of the depressant drugs (the one with the longer half-life) to the point where the symptoms are markedly decreased on day 1. The patient is then weaned off the drug.

12.2.2.1.2. Depressants–Stimulants

See Sections 2.2.2, 4.2.2, and 5.2.2.

The withdrawal from depressants and stimulants more closely follows the depressant withdrawal paradigm, but probably includes greater levels of sadness, enhanced appetite, and lethargy than would be expected with depressants alone.

Regarding treatment, in the case of multiple dependencies on depressants and stimulants, it is the depressant withdrawal syndrome that produces the greatest amount of discomfort and is the most life threatening (Sections 2.2.2 and 4.2.2). Thus, although there may be higher levels of sleepiness and depression than usually seen with depressant withdrawal, most problems can be diminished by focusing on the treatment for depressant withdrawal.

12.2.2.1.3. Depressants–Opioids

See Sections 2.2.2, 4.2.2, and 6.2.2

The individual withdrawing from depressants and opioids usually demonstrates an opioid-type withdrawal syndrome (Section 6.2.2), along with heightened levels of insomnia and anxiety and a small depressant-related risk for convulsions and confusion (see Sections 2.2.2 and 4.2.2).

The optimal approach to treatment is again predicted from an understanding of the treatment of each withdrawal alone.

1. In the case of physical dependence on both depressants and opioids, it is advisable to administer both symptomatically based treatment for the opioid (e.g., Imodium, decongestants, etc.) and to more directly treat the depressant symptoms, as outlined in Sections 2.2.2.2 and 6.2.2.1.2, until the withdrawal symptoms have been abolished or greatly decreased.
2. If the patient is on methadone maintenance, most authors recommend stabilization with the opioid (Section 6.2.2.1.2), while the depressant is withdrawn at 10–20% a day (Section 2.2.2.2).
3. After the depressant withdrawal is completed, opioid withdrawal can then proceed (Section 6.2.2.1.2).

12.2.2.1.4. Opioids–Stimulants

Here the usual opioid abstinence syndrome dominates the picture, accompanied by lethargy, depressive symptoms, and problems concentrating.

The focus of treatment should be on opioid withdrawal (Section 6.2.2.1.2), along with reassurance that the mood impairment and difficulty focusing attention will improve with time.

12.2.3. Delirium, Dementia, and Other Cognitive Disorders

See Section 1.7.3.

Any drug in high enough doses can cause confusion and disorientation. In drug combinations, one can expect this clinical picture to be evanescent, and the general treatment plans outlined in the individual chapters should be followed. However, it is wise to remember that the course is less predictable with multiple drugs, and it is probable that the patient will be impaired for a longer time than would be expected with either drug alone.

12.2.4. Psychoses

See Section 1.7.4.

The drug-induced psychoses seen with stimulants (Section 5.2.4) or with depressants (Sections 2.2.4 and 4.2.4) are disturbing but temporary pictures, disappearing within a few days or weeks following abstinence. The treatments and likely time course are the same regardless of the class of drugs, and include short-term use of antipsychotic medications if needed. Few specific data are available on the psychoses produced by the administration of multiple groups of these substances. Treatment follows the guidelines in Section 5.2.4.

12.2.5. Flashbacks

Flashbacks are mostly seen with the hallucinogens and the cannabinoids, and the clinical course and treatments for recurrences after the use of these drugs in combination with others are the same as outlined in Sections 7.2.5 and 8.2.5 for the individual drugs.

12.2.6. Anxiety and Depression

See Section 1.7.6.

The clinical picture, course, and treatment for temporary anxiety and for depression resemble those seen for any one of the substances, including intoxication with alcohol or other depressants, and withdrawal from stimulants. The treatment is education, reassurance, and cognitive therapy, as outlined in the specific drug chapters.

12.2.7. Medical Problems

The concomitant administration of two substances over an extended period of time is likely to increase the risk for the development of medical consequences. However, the specific problems depend on the drugs involved as well as the individual's age, preexisting medical disorders, and concomitant nutritional status and levels of stress. When treating a patient who is dependent on multiple drugs, the clinician should review the sections on medical problems in each of the relevant chapters.

One special problem is seen in those people whose dependence has occurred in the context of attempts at controlling pain, usually by misusing depressants or analgesics from a doctor's prescription. Pain syndromes that are unresponsive to the usual measures (e.g., frequently back pain and chronic headache) are difficult to treat and are not well understood. It is important to gather a history of any dependence and of concomitant medical complaints in evaluating all people who are drug dependent. Following withdrawal, these identified individuals can be included as part of a drug treatment program, but they will also require additional care, such as that offered in specialized pain clinics.[36]

REFERENCES

1. Substance Abuse and Mental Health Services Administration. *Overview of Findings from the 2002 National Survey on Drug Use and Health* (NHSDA Series H-21, DHHS Publication No. SMA 03-3774). Rockville, MD: Office of Applied Studies, 2003.
2. Johnston, L. D., O'Malley, P. M., Bachman, J. G., & Schulenberg, J. E. *Monitoring the Future National Survey Results on Drug Use 1975–2003* (NIH Publication No. 04-5506). Bethesda, MD: National Institute on Drug Abuse, 2004.
3. Wetzels, J. J. L., Kremers, S. P. J., Vitória, P. D., & deVries, H. The alcohol–tobacco relationship: A prospective study among adolescents in six European countries. *Addiction 98:*1755–1763, 2003.
4. Harris, D. S., Everhart, E. T., Mendelson, J., & Jones, R. T. The pharmacology of cocaethylene in humans following cocaine and ethanol administration. *Drug and Alcohol Dependence 72:*169–182, 2003.
5. Coffin, P. O., Galea, S., Ahern, J., Leon, A. C., Vlahov, D., & Tardiff, K. Opiates, cocaine and alcohol combinations in accidental drug overdose deaths in New York City, 1990–98. *Addiction 98:*739–747, 2003.
6. Edwards, G. *Matters of Substance: Drugs—and Why Everyone's a User*. London: Penguin Books, 2004.
7. Brown, N. J., & Roberts, L. J., II. Histamine, bradykinin, and their antagonists. In J.G. Hardman, L.E. Limbird, & A. G. Gilman (Eds.), *The Pharmacological Basis of Therapeutics* (10th ed.). New York: McGraw-Hill, 2001, pp. 645–668.
8. Fu, Q., Heath, A. C., Bucholz, K. K., Nelson, E., Goldberg, J., Lyons, M. J., True, W. R., Jacob, T., Tsuang, M. T., & Eisen, S. A. Shared genetic risk of major depression, alcohol dependence, and marijuana dependence. Contribution of antisocial personality disorder in men. *Archives of General Psychiatry 59:*1125–1132, 2002.
9. Lynskey, M. T., Heath, A. C., Bucholz, K. K., Slutske, W. S., Madden, P. A., Nelson, E. C., Statham, D. J., & Martin, N. G. Escalation of drug use in early-onset cannabis users vs. co-twin controls. *Journal of the American Medical Association 289:*427–433, 2003.
10. American Psychiatric Association. *The Diagnostic and Statistical Manual of Mental Disorders* (4th ed., text revision). Washington, DC: American Psychiatric Press, 2000.
11. Schuckit, M. A., Danko, G. P., Raimo, E. B., Smith, T. L., Eng, M. Y., Carpenter, K. K. T., & Hesselbrock, V. M. A preliminary evaluation of the potential usefulness of the diagnoses of polysubstance dependence. *Journal of Studies on Alcohol 62:*54–61, 2001.

12. Morrison, J., & Wickersham, P. Physicians disciplined by a state medical board. *Journal of the American Medical Association 279*:1889–1893, 1998.
13. Kandel, D., & Yamaguchi, K. From beer to crack: Developmental patterns of drug involvement. *American Journal of Public Health 83:*851–855, 1993.
14. Labouvie, E., & White, H. R. Drug sequences, age of onset, and use trajectories as predictors of drug abuse/dependence in young adulthood. In C. B. Kandel (Ed.), *Stages and Pathways of Drug Involvement: Examining the Gateway Hypothesis*. Cambridge, MA: Cambridge University Press, 2002, pp. 19–41.
15. Pistis, M., Perra, S., Pillolla, G., Melis, M., Muntoni, A. L., & Gessa, G. L. Adolescent exposure to cannabinoids induces long-lasting changes in the response to drugs of abuse of rat midbrain dopamine neurons. *Biological Psychiatry 56:*86–94, 2004.
16. Koski, A., Ojanpera, I., & Vuori, E. Alcohol and benzodiazepines in fatal poisonings. *Alcoholism: Clinical and Experimental Research 26:*956–959, 2002.
17. Rittmannsberger, H., Silberbauer, C., Lehner, R., & Ruschak, M. Alcohol consumption during methadone maintenance treatment. *European Addiction Research 6:*2–7, 2000.
18. Lenne, M. G., Dietze, P., Rumbold, G. R., Redman, J. R., & Triggs, T. J. The effects of the opioid pharmacotherapies methadone, LAAM and buprenorphine, alone and in combination with alcohol, on stimulated driving. *Drug and Alcohol Dependence 72:*271–278, 2003.
19. Foster, K. L., McKay, P. F., Seyoum, R., Milbourne, D., Yin, W., Sarma, P. V. V. S., Cook, J. M., & June, H. L. GABA and opioid receptors of the central neucleus of the amygdala selectively regulate ethanol-maintained behaviors. *Neuropsychopharmacology 29:*269–284, 2004.
20. Kiefer, F., Jahn, H., Tarnaske, T., Helwig, H., Briken, P., Holzbach, R., Kampf, P., Stracke, R., Baehr, M., Naber, D., & Wiedemann, K. Comparing and combining naltrexone and acamprosate in relapse prevention of alcoholism. *Archives of General Psychiatry 60:*92–99, 2003.
21. Kendler, K. S., Karkowski, L. M., Neale, M. C., & Prescott, C. A. Illicit psychoactive substance use, heavy use, abuse, and dependence in a U.S. population-based sample of male twins. *Archives of General Psychiatry 57:*261–269, 2000.
22. Schuckit, M. A., Smith, T. L., & Kalmijn, J. The search for genes contributing to the low level of response to alcohol: Patterns of findings across studies. *Alcoholism: Clinical and Experimental Research 28:*1449–1458, 2004.
23. Magura, S., Nwakeze, P. C., & Demsky, S. Pre- and in-treatment predictors of retention in methadone treatment using survival analysis. *Addiction 93:*51–60, 1998.
24. Grinspoon, L., Bakalar, J. B., & Russo, E. Marihuana: Clinical aspects. In J. H. Lowinson, P. Ruiz, R. B. Millman, & J. G. Langrod (Eds.), *Substance Abuse: A Comprehensive Textbook* (4th ed.). Baltimore, MD: Lippincott, Williams & Wilkins, 2004, pp. 263–276.
25. Hungund, B.L., Szakall, I., Adam, A., Basavarajappa, B. S., & Vadasz, C. Cannabinoid CB1 receptor knockout mice exhibit markedly reduced voluntary alcohol consumption and lack alcohol-induced dopamine release in the nucleus accumbens. *Journal of Neurochemistry 84:*698–704, 2003.
26. Lallemand, F., Soubrie, P. H., & DeWitte, P. H. Effects of CB1 cannabinoid receptor blockade on ethanol preference after chronic ethanol administration. *Alcoholism: Clinical and Experimental Research 25:*1317–1323, 2001.
27. Ortiz, S., Oliva, J. M., Perez-Rial, S., Palomo, T., & Manzanares, J. Chronic ethanol consumption regulates cannabinoid CB1 receptor gene expression in selected regions of rat brain. *Alcohol and Alcoholism 39:*88–92, 2004.
28. Shillington, A. M., & Clapp, J. D. Beer and bongs: Differential problems experienced by older adolescents using alcohol only compared to combined alcohol and marijuana use. *American Journal of Drug and Alcohol Abuse 28:*379–397, 2002.
29. Najarian, S. L. General management of the poisoned patient. In O. J. Ma & D. M. Cline (Eds.), *Emergency Medicine Manual* (6th ed.). New York: McGraw-Hill, 2004, pp. 467–475.

30. Glaspy, J. N. Drugs of abuse. In O. J. Ma & D. M. Cline (Eds.), *Emergency Medicine Manual* (6th ed.). New York: McGraw-Hill, 2004, pp. 499–504.
31. Mausner, K. L. Sedatives and hypnotics. In O. J. Ma & D. M. Cline (Eds.), *Emergency Medicine Manual* (6th ed.). New York: McGraw-Hill, 2004, pp. 489–493.
32. Weinbroum, A. A., Flaishon, R., Sorkine, P., Szold, O., & Rudick, V. A risk-benefit assessment of flumazenil in the management of benzodiazepine overdose. *Drug Safety 17*:181–196, 1997.
33. Chand, P. K., & Murthy, P. Megadose lorazepam dependence. *Addiction 98:*1633–1636, 2003.
34. Gatzonis, S. D., Angelopoulos, E. K., Daskalopoulou, E. G., Mantouvalos, V., Chioni, A., Zournas, C., & Siafakas, A. Convulsive status epilepticus following abrupt high-dose benzodiazepine discontinuation. *Drug and Alcohol Dependence 59:*95–97, 2000.
35. McGregor, C., Machin, A., & White, J. M. In-patient benzodiazepine withdrawal: Comparison of fixed and symptom-triggered taper methods. *Drug and Alcohol Review 22:*175–180, 2003.
36. Stack, K., Cortina, J., Samples, C., Zapata, M., & Arcand, L. F. Race, age, and back pain as factors in completion of residential substance abuse treatment by veterans. *Psychiatric Services 51:*1157–1161, 2000.

CHAPTER 13

Emergency Problems: A Quick Overview

13.1. INTRODUCTION

13.1.1. Comments

If you have come to this chapter of the book after having read (or at least skimmed) Chapters 1–12, this chapter and the companion text (*Educating Yourself About Alcohol and Drugs*) can serve as a review.[1] If you are reading this chapter because an overview of emergency problems is the most important goal, I bid you welcome and hope that you will have a chance to go back and review the other topics in greater depth. No single chapter can summarize each topic in detail, nor can it offer the same span of references used in other sections of the book.

This chapter reviews general guidelines for drug emergencies. I approach the problem from the standpoint of *patient symptoms*, assuming a situation in which you do not know the specific drug involved.

13.1.2. Some General Rules for Dealing with Drug Issues

1. In any drug-related emergency you must, of course, first address life-threatening problems, gather a more substantial history, take other patient-care steps, and, finally, plan disposition and future treatment. The first priority is to support respiration, maintain adequate blood pressure, aggressively treat convulsions, and establish an IV line.
2. Do not prescribe medications unless you are fairly sure they are needed. Adding additional meds to an individual with a drug-related problem can result in unpredictable drug–drug interactions, which can be made worse by an intense level of arousal. However, when there is good reason for administering medications, it is important that they be given in doses adequate to produce clinical effects.

3. It is important to gather a complete history from the patient and an *additional resource person* whenever possible.
4. Your general *attitude* and demeanor can be important, especially if you are dealing with a panicked, confused, or psychotic patient. While carrying out your evaluations, it is important that you first clearly identify yourself and consistently behave in a self-assured and calm manner.
5. Finally, it is important to briefly review how to determine the relevant drug problem category (see Section 1.7):

   First: Any patient who has taken enough of a drug to show a serious compromise in vital signs should be regarded as having a toxic reaction or overdose. In the midst of this, he may have hallucinations (especially visual), delusions, or confusion, but all symptoms can be expected to return to normal once the toxic reaction has been adequately treated.

   Second: Patients who have stable vital signs, but are showing symptoms of any of the three classic abstinence syndromes are labeled as undergoing drug withdrawal. This is true even if they are confused and/or psychotic, as these can occur as part of depressant- or stimulant-related conditions.

   Third: Any patient with a drug-related condition, that includes stable vital signs and no obvious withdrawal but with clinically significant levels of confusion, is regarded as having a substance-induced delirium or dementia. In the midst of this, he may demonstrate hallucinations or delusions, but these will be expected to return to normal once the state of confusion is adequately treated.

   Fourth: An individual with stable vital signs and no clinically significant confusion or withdrawal, but showing hallucinations and/or delusions without insight, is regarded as having a psychosis. A similar approach is used for evaluating potential substance-induced mood and anxiety disorders.

   Thus, as is true in medicine in general, it is not only the specific signs or symptoms that are used to arrive at a diagnosis but also the constellation or grouping of symptoms along with their time course.[2]

13.1.3. An Overview of Relevant Laboratory Tests

There is no perfect laboratory panel appropriate for every drug-emergency patient. The best approach is to use your medical knowledge and common sense to dictate which tests must be ordered, so as to avoid unnecessary costs.

Table 1.6 lists some relevant blood chemistry and blood count values. In addition, you should consider a urinalysis (you might collect urine for a toxicological screen anyway) to look for evidence of kidney damage or of

Table 13.1
A Brief List of Relevant Blood Toxicologies

Drug	Toxic blood level
Chlordiazepoxide (Librium)	0.6–2.0 mg/dl
Diazepam (Valium)	0.5 mg/dl
Meperidine (Demerol)	100–500 g/dl
Meprobamate (Miltown, Equanil)	5.0–10.0 mg/dl
Morphine	0.1–0.5 mg/dl
Oxazepam (Serax)	0.5–1.5 mg/dl
Phenobarbital	3–10 mg/dl

infections; blood to screen for the hepatitis-related antigens for patients who have used drugs IV (in similar patients there is a need to rule out AIDS); a chest x-ray to screen for tuberculosis for all patients who have not received a film in the last 6 months; a baseline EKG for patients over the age of 35 and/or those who have any evidence of heart disease; and a serology evaluation for syphilis or a possible culture for gonorrhea for patients who have a history of sexual promiscuity or prostitution.[3–5]

A toxicological screen on blood and/or urine should be considered in all relevant patients. Some representative toxic levels are shown in Table 13.1. Take care in interpreting negative results, however, as signs of confusion, psychosis, and withdrawal (the latter from long-acting drugs such as diazepam or methadone) may persist for 4 weeks or longer, after blood and urine levels return to zero by most techniques.

13.1.4. An Introduction to Specific Emergency Problems

Table 13.2 lists some symptoms and signs that can be used in making an educated guess as to which drug was taken, and the likely future course of problems. However, these thoughts have not been tested in controlled investigations and, therefore, can only be used as a guideline.

For example, if a patient has decreased respiration and pinpoint pupils, one might consider it an opioid overdose. A second example is an individual with an elevated temperature, warm, dry skin, and fixed, dilated pupils; this is probably a toxic reaction involving an atropine-like anticholinergic drug.

These comments now proceed with a discussion of major emergency situations, first giving a definition, then making some generalizations about the drug state, and reviewing some of the substances that might be involved. The reader is encouraged to return to the chapters that deal with specific drugs for more detailed discussions.

13.2. TOXIC REACTIONS

See Section 1.7.1.

13.2.1. Clinical Picture

Here, the individual has ingested enough of a substance to produce life-threatening decrements in vital signs. In this discussion, I distinguish between these overdose conditions, where unstable or dangerous vital signs predominate, a *psychosis*, with hallucinations and delusions in an oriented individual, and a *delirium*, in which the major symptoms include confusion and disorientation.

Table 13.2
A Rough Guide to Symptoms and Signs in Drug Reactions

Symptom or sign	Reaction type	Possible drugs
Vital signs		
Blood pressure		
Increase	Toxic	Stimulants or lysergic acid diethylamide (LSD)
	Withdrawal	Depressants
Pulse		
Increase	Toxic	Stimulants
	Withdrawal	Depressants
Body temperature		
Irregular	Toxic	Inhalants
Increase	Toxic	Atropine-type, stimulants, or LSD
Decrease	Withdrawal	Opioids or depressants
Respiration		
Decrease	Toxic	Opioids or depressants
Eyes		
Pupils		
Pinpoint	Toxic	Opioids
Dilated	Toxic	Hallucinogens, withdrawal, opiates
Sluggish	Toxic	Glutethimide or stimulants
Unreactive	Toxic	Atropine-type
Sclera		
Injected (bloodshot)	Toxic	Marijuana or inhalants
Nystagmus	Toxic	Depressants
Tearing	Withdrawal	Opioids
Nose		
Runny (rhinorrhea)	Withdrawal	Opioids
Dry	Toxic	Atropine-type
Ulcers	Chronic use	Cocaine

(*Continued*)

Table 13.2
A Rough Guide to Symptoms and Signs in Drug Reactions—Cont'd

Symptom or sign	Reaction type	Possible drugs
Skin		
Warm/Dry	Toxic	Atropine-type
Moist	Toxic	Stimulants
Needle marks	Chronic use	Opioids, stimulants, or depressants
Gooseflesh	Toxic	LSD
	Withdrawal	Opioids
Rash over mouth or nose	Toxic	Inhalants
Speech		
Slow/Not slurred	Toxic	Opioids
Slurred	Toxic	Depressants
Rapid	Toxic	Stimulants
Hands		
Fine tremor	Toxic	Stimulants or hallucinogens
	Withdrawal	Opioids
Coarse tremor	Withdrawal	Depressants
Reflexes		
Increased	Toxic	Stimulants
Decreased	Toxic	Depressants
Convulsions	Toxic	Stimulants, codeine, propoxyphene, methaqualone
Lungs		
Pulmonary edema	Toxic	Opioids or depressants

13.2.2. Differential Diagnosis

Life-threatening overdoses are most likely to be seen with drugs that depress the CNS, such as *opioids* and *depressants*, or those that grossly overstimulate the brain, such as the *stimulants*. Because the treatments for the toxic reactions of these classes of drugs differ, it is important to identify the class of drug involved.

There are no major psychiatric syndromes that mimic the overdose, but medical disorders that can cause coma (e.g., hypoglycemia or severe electrolyte abnormalities) must be considered.

13.2.3. Treatment

The definitive treatment of shock-like states is complex and requires precise knowledge that is beyond the scope of this text. Briefly, it is necessary to address acute life supports and then to provide general patient care, allowing time for the body to metabolize the drug ingested.

13.2.3.1. Acute Life-Saving Measures[6,7]

1. Measure the vital signs.
2. Assure adequate ventilation:
   a. Straighten the head (if not contraindicated).
   b. Remove any obstructions from the mouth and throat.
   c. Do tracheal intubation if necessary (use an inflatable cuff tube, if at all possible, to allow for safer gastric lavage).
   d. Use a respirator, if necessary; 10–12 respirations per minute, avoiding oxygen if possible, as this may decrease spontaneous respirations.
   e. Maintain an adequate circulatory state.
3. Rule out serious bleeding, life-threatening trauma, and so on.
4. Start an IV:
   a. Use a large-gauge needle.
   b. Use a slow IV drip until the need for IV fluids has been established.
5. Control convulsions. In most instances, a single seizure will occur, but repeated convulsions (i.e., status epilepticus) requires aggressive treatment (e.g., IV diazepam slow infusion of 10 mg, which can be repeated in 20 min, if necessary).
6. Draw blood for chemical analysis:
   a. A minimum of 10 cc is needed for a toxicological screen.
   b. 30–40 cc is necessary for the usual blood count, electrolytes, blood sugar, and blood urea nitrogen (BUN).
7. Test for hypoglycemia and, if needed, administer 50 cc of 50% glucose IV.
8. Rule out cardiac arrhythmias.
9. For recent drug ingestion, consider inducing vomiting (only for a fully alert patient) or carry out gastric lavage.
   a. Do this only when the heart rate is stable, to avoid inducing a clinically significant vagal response.
   b. For the awake and cooperative patient, emesis can be induced with syrup of ipecac, which is given as 10–30 mg orally and repeated once in 15–30 min, if vomiting does not occur.
   c. If the patient is not awake and cooperative, or if emesis does not work, consider gastric lavage. For sleepy or comatose patients, lavage only after tracheal intubation. Use an inflatable cuff to prevent aspiration.
   d. Gastric lavage is best carried out only on individuals who have taken drugs orally within the last 4–6 or, at most, 12 h. The longer period is especially appropriate with phencyclidine (PCP), as this drug may be recycled and excreted in the stomach for

more than 6 h after the actual ingestion. Lavage should *not* be carried out if individuals have ingested corrosives, kerosene, strychnine, or mineral oil.

e. For adults, a nasogastric tube is usually used, and the patient is placed on his left side with the head slightly over the edge of the table.
f. After evacuating the stomach, administer an isotonic saline lavage until the returned fluid looks clear. It is preferable to use small amounts of fluid so as to not distend the stomach and increase the passage of the drug into the upper intestine. Lavage may be repeated 10–12 times, and it is best to save a sample of the washings for drug analyses.
g. Consider administering activated charcoal (1g/kg) or castor oil (60 ml) to decrease absorption.

10. Collect urine, which may require catheterizing the bladder. Send 50 ml of the urine for a toxicological screen.
11. If the patient's blood pressure remains dangerously low, you may consider plasma expanders or pressors as for any shock-like state, taking care to titrate the needed dose and being aware of any potentially life-threatening drug interactions.
12. If an opioid is involved, administer naloxone (Narcan) in doses of 0.2–0.4 mg (1 ml) IM or IV, as discussed in Section 6.2.1.2.[8] However, it is important to recognize the possibility of precipitating a severe opioid withdrawal syndrome in opioid-dependent individuals.
13. If a Bz is involved in the toxic reaction, consider using flumazenil (Romazicon) in doses of 1 mg IV over 3 min, or up to 5 mg over 10 min.[9,10] Special care must be taken to avoid precipitating seizures, and this drug should not be used if there is increased intracranial pressure.
14. If the overdose involves an atropine-like (anticholinergic) drug with a subsequent rapid heart rate, dry skin and mouth, and/or a rash, consider giving physostigmine, 1–4 mg, by slow IV injection.

13.2.3.2. Subacute Treatment

1. Measure vital signs regularly; every 15 min for the first 4 h; then monitor carefully (perhaps every 2–4 h) over the next 24–48 h, even if the patient's condition improves. Some of the substances clear from the plasma only temporarily and are then rereleased from fat stores, causing severe re-intoxication after the patient has improved. Also, for opioid overdoses, naltrexone is only active for a relatively short period.
2. Carry out a thorough physical examination.

3. Gather a detailed history of substance use, medical problems, and medications from the patient and from a resource person (e.g., the spouse).
4. Establish a flow sheet to monitor vital signs, medications, fluid intake, fluid output, and so on.
5. Measure baseline weight to serve as guide to fluid balance.
6. Dialysis or diuresis is rarely needed, and details are beyond the scope of this discussion.
7. If the patient is comatose, take the steps necessary for adequate care, including careful management of electrolytes and fluids, eye care, frequent turning of the patient, and careful tracheal toilet.

13.3. DRUG WITHDRAWAL STATES

See Section 1.7.2.

13.3.1. Clinical Picture

A sudden cessation or a rapid decrease in the intake of members of the three classes of drugs capable of producing physical dependence, can result in the withdrawal state. This, simplistically, is manifested by a heightened drive to obtain the drug and physiological symptoms that are usually in the direction opposite to those expected with intoxication.[1,9]

Withdrawal from drugs is rarely life threatening (except with the occasional case regarding depressants) unless the patient experiences the syndrome while in a seriously impaired physical state.

13.3.2. Differential Diagnosis

It is important to determine whether the withdrawal state is related to *stimulants*, to *depressants*, or to *opioids*, as aspects of the specific treatments differ. It is also necessary to identify any physiological disorders and to implement proper medical treatment.

13.3.3. Treatment

In addition to recognizing and treating all concomitant medical disorders, offer reassurance, rest, and good nutrition

1. Carry out a good physical examination, taking special care to rule out infections, hepatitis, AIDS, subdural hematomas, heart failure, and electrolyte abnormalities. A patient undergoing depressant withdrawal with impaired physical functioning has an increased chance of confusion or delirium during the withdrawal. Also, if any

physiological abnormality is overlooked at the inception of withdrawal, it may be difficult to tell whether abnormal vital signs are a response to the withdrawal or represent other physical pathology as the abstinence syndrome progresses.

2. Treatment of withdrawal depends on recognizing that the symptoms have developed because the drug of dependence has been stopped *too quickly*. Therefore, theoretically, the basic paradigm of treatment (at least for depressants and opioids) is to give enough of the drug (or one to which the individual has cross-tolerance) to greatly diminish the withdrawal symptoms on day 1. For dependence on relatively short half-life drugs (e.g., alcohol or heroin), the medication is then decreased by about 20% of the initial day's dose each day, over the subsequent 5 or so days. This is the optimal approach for depressant withdrawal (including alcohol), although laws in most states preclude the use of opioids for opioid withdrawal, which is usually treated with clonidine (Catapres) and symptom relief with Bzs, immodium, OTC analgesics, and decongestants. No medications are appropriate for stimulant withdrawal. Alternate approaches are discussed in the sections on withdrawal in relevant chapters.

13.4. DELIRIUM, DEMENTIA, AND OTHER COGNITIVE DISORDERS

See Section 1.7.3.

13.4.1. Clinical Picture

A state consisting of confusion and disorientation along with decreased general mental functioning can be caused by high, near toxic, doses of any drug. However, if the vital signs are unstable, this is best labeled and treated as a toxic reaction. As is true with any state of confusion, these reactions may be accompanied by illusions (which are misinterpretations of real stimuli such as inaccurate interpretations of shadows or machinery sounds), hallucinations (usually visual or tactile), or delusions. A similar picture is possible (but rare) during withdrawal from depressants, but in this situation typical withdrawal symptoms such as a rapid heart rate, tremor, and an increased blood pressure are apparent. This section assumes that the confusion is not a part of a toxic reaction or withdrawal in a patient presenting with evidence of a diminished cognitive functioning.

13.4.2. Differential Diagnosis

Any drug can cause confusion, but in clinical practice this problem is most likely to be seen in cases of intoxication with *depressants*, *anticholinergic* or *atropine-type drugs*, *inhalants*, and *PCP*.

When confusion is observed, it is important to consider the possibility of head trauma, vitamin deficiency, blood loss, or serious medical problems that might disrupt electrolyte balance. If these medical disorders are overlooked, life-threatening problems can develop.

13.4.3. Treatment

The treatment for these intoxication-related deliria or dementias consists of general life supports. If the problem is part of a toxic reaction, the treatment is identical to that outlined in Section 13.2.3. Although most intoxication-related states of confusion disappear within hours to days, some caused by vitamin deficiencies with alcohol dependence or by physical trauma can take many months to clear, and can be permanent.

The treatment of a delirium in the context of depressant withdrawal is presented in Chapter 4.

13.5. PSYCHOSIS

See Section 1.7.4.

13.5.1. Clinical Picture

As shown in this text, psychosis is a loss of contact with reality that occurs in a clear sensorium (i.e., the person is oriented to time, place, and person). The patient usually presents with hallucinations (classically auditory) and/or delusions (usually paranoid). Although clinically dramatic, such a drug-induced state is usually a self-limited problem, running its course within a matter of days to a month of abstinence for most drugs.

13.5.2. Differential Diagnosis

Any psychiatric disorder capable of producing a psychotic picture, especially schizophrenia, mania, a delirium or dementia if confusion is present, or a major depression, must be considered a part of the differential diagnosis. The drugs most frequently involved in temporary drug-induced psychoses are *stimulants*, as well as *alcohol*, and the other *depressants*.[11,12] When patients on PCP develop hallucinations and/or delusions, it is usually part of a temporary delirium.[13] Unless they are part of a toxic reaction, hallucinogen-induced visual hallucinations usually occur with insight, and are technically not psychoses as discussed here or in the DSM-IV.[2]

13.5.3. Treatment

The major goal is to protect the patient from harming himself or others, or from carrying out acts that would be embarrassing and cause difficulties later. At the same time, it is important to rule out other serious medical and psychiatric disorders. The patient who presents with hallucinations/delusions, therefore, usually requires hospitalization until the delusions clear. Temporary (several days to several weeks) treatment with antipsychotic medications (e.g., risperidone or Risperdal) can help control the psychotic symptoms.

13.6. FLASHBACKS

See Section 1.7.5.

13.6.1. Clinical Picture

This drug-induced state involves a recurrence of feelings of intoxication some time after the initial drug effects have worn off. This is usually a benign, self-limited condition.

13.6.2. Differential Diagnosis

Flashbacks are seen primarily with *marijuana* and the *hallucinogens*. However, it is also important to rule out the possibility of underlying psychiatric disorders, especially schizophrenia, a mood disorder, or a delirium or dementia.

13.6.3. Treatment

The approach to this condition is reassurance and education. If the person does not respond to reassurance, he may be administered a Bz such as diazepam (Valium) in doses of 10–20 mg orally, repeated as needed.

13.7. ANXIETY AND DEPRESSION

See Section 1.7.6.

13.7.1. Clinical Picture

All drugs of abuse cross to the brain and produce altered feelings and perceptions. Because the range of psychological feelings and emotions that can be expressed by a person is relatively limited, it is not surprising that intoxication and/or withdrawal from most of the drugs can produce psychotic symptoms and confusion (both of which are described in other sections of this chapter), as well as feelings of anxiety and depression.[1,14–20]

Intoxication with caffeine (Chapter 11) and any of the classical stimulants described in Chapter 5, can produce symptoms of nervousness and anxiety. Thus, individuals taking these stimulants can temporarily be very nervous (resembling generalized anxiety disorder), can have repeated panic attacks (resembling panic disorder), and are likely to develop discomfort with crowds or at parties (resembling social phobia). Similarly, temporary anxiety symptoms that resemble the major DSM-IV anxiety disorders are seen in depressant withdrawal. Therefore, intoxication and withdrawal from a variety of substances are likely to produce temporary clinical conditions that resemble some major anxiety disorders, and the reader is referred to DSM-IV[2] for further information on the types of symptoms likely to be observed.

Intoxication with depressants, if intense and repetitive enough, will produce mood swings in almost anyone. Severe, long-lasting intoxication states can produce conditions that are (temporarily) virtually identical to major depressive disorders.[2] Withdrawal from stimulants, especially the amphetamines or cocaine, is associated with severe depressive symptoms for several days to several weeks for the majority of patients.

It is important to emphasize the *temporary* nature of alcohol and other drug-induced anxiety and depressive states. Although these conditions can last as long as an individual continues to take the substance, symptoms of anxiety and depression are likely to markedly improve within several days to perhaps a month of abstinence. Some problems with mood swings and anxiety can still be observed for up to 3–6 months after abstinence, but these are not likely to be intense enough to resemble DSM-IV major anxiety or depressive disorders. These lingering symptoms represent a protracted withdrawal or a continued resolution of symptoms with time.[1]

13.7.2. Differential Diagnosis

Each chapter describes the importance of obtaining a careful chronological history of an individual in order to establish the differential diagnosis between drug-induced (temporary) psychiatric symptoms on the one hand, and independent (often lifelong) major psychiatric disorders such as schizophrenia on the other.[2,15,21] The first step in this "time-line" approach is to establish the age at which the individual was likely to have first met the criteria for substance dependence (e.g., as defined by DSM-IV). Second, any extended periods of abstinence since the onset of dependence should be noted. The third step is to determine whether an individual fulfills the criteria for a major psychiatric disorder (not just some related symptoms) as outlined in DSM-IV. Then, the clinician can establish whether the person ever met the criteria for the major psychiatric disorder either before the onset of drug dependence or during an extended period of abstinence.[1,2] In the absence of evidence indicating an independent course of the psychiatric syndrome, there is perhaps a 90% or higher chance that the psychiatric symptoms are drug induced and will disappear with time.[1,21] An additional step requires that patients be observed over time with abstinence. Obviously, if a month or so of abstinence has passed but the individual is still so symptomatic as to meet criteria for a major DSM-IV psychiatric disorder, the clinician must consider an independent psychiatric disorder and institute the appropriate therapy.

13.7.3. Treatment

All clinically relevant psychiatric symptoms *must* be addressed, regardless of whether they are drug induced or related to an independent psychiatric disorder. For example, a patient who is suicidal is likely to require inpatient psychiatric hospitalization with suicide precautions.[14,15] Such hospitalization is especially important for individuals who are at high suicide risk, such as those who have had a recent loss, patients with a specific plan for the suicide, and individuals with a means to carry out the plan (e.g., the presence of a gun in the home).

Similarly, patients with drug-related panic attacks or those reporting additional intense anxiety symptoms must be educated and reassured regarding the temporary nature of the current anxiety problems. Whether it is a drug-induced anxiety disorder or an independent major anxiety syndrome (with the latter tending to be a lifelong condition), education, cognitive treatment, and behavioral approaches developing relaxation techniques and desensitizing an individual to any feared situations are important.

However, it is the chronological history indicating an independent psychiatric disorder and/or the persistence of severe psychiatric symptoms beyond a month or so of abstinence that indicate the potential existence of an independent psychiatric disorder. Obviously, true independent severe major depressive disorders might require antidepressant medications [i.e., manic–depressive disorder usually necessitates the use of lithium or valproic acid (Depakote)] and a variety of pharmacological approaches (as well as behavioral and cognitive treatments) are relevant for many of the major anxiety disorders.[22,23] Although it is important that clinicians not jump to the erroneous conclusion that temporary drug-induced psychiatric symptoms represent an independent psychiatric disorder, it is equally important to recognize those independent psychiatric disorders when they are present and to treat them appropriately.

REFERENCES

1. Schuckit, M. A. *Educating Yourself About Alcohol and Drugs.* New York: Plenum Publishing Co., 1998.
2. American Psychiatric Association. *The Diagnostic and Statistical Manual of Mental Disorders* (4th ed., text revision, DSM-IV TR). Washington, DC: American Psychiatric Press, 2000.
3. Fillmore, K. M., Kerr, W. C., & Bostrom, A. Changes in drinking status, serious illness and mortality. *Journal of Studies on Alcohol 64:*278–285, 2003.
4. Romero-Gomez, M., Grande, L., Nogales, M. C., Fernandez, M., Chavez, M., & Castro, M. Chronic alcohol use enhances the hepatitis C virus load in the liver. *Alcohol Research 7:*66, 2002.
5. Samet, J. H., Horton, N. J., Traphagen, E. T., Lyon, S. M., & Freedberg, K. A. Alcohol consumption and HIV disease progression: Are they related? *Alcoholism: Clinical and Experimental Research 27:*862–867, 2003.
6. Chang, G., & Kosten, T. R. Detoxification. In J. H. Lowinson, P. Ruiz, R. B. Millman, & J. G. Langrod (Eds.), *Substance Abuse: A Comprehensive Textbook* (4th ed.). Baltimore, MD: Lippincott, Williams & Wilkins, 2004, pp. 579–587.

7. Ma, O. J., & Kline, D. M. (Eds.). *Emergency Medicine Manual* (6th ed.). New York: McGraw-Hill Publishers, 2004.
8. Gutstein, H. B., & Akil, H. Opioid analgesics. In J. G. Hardman, L. E. Limbird, & A. G. Goodman (Eds.), *The Pharmacological Basis of Therapeutics* (10th ed.). New York: McGraw-Hill, 2001, pp. 569–620.
9. Charney, D. S., Mihic, J., & Harris, R. A. Hypnotics and sedatives. In J. G. Hardman, L. E. Limbird, & A. G. Goodman (Eds.), *The Pharmacological Basis of Therapeutics* (10th ed.). New York: McGraw-Hill, 2001, pp. 399–427.
10. Mausner, K. L. Sedatives and hypnotics. In O. J. Ma & D. M. Cline (Eds.), *Emergency Medicine Manual* (6th ed.). New York: McGraw-Hill Publishers, 2004, pp. 489–493.
11. D'Souza, D. C., Perry, E., MacDougal, L., Ammerman, Y., Cooper, T., Wu, Y.-T, Braley, G., Gueorguieva, R., & Krystal, J. H. The psychotomimetic effects of intravenous delta-9-tetrahydrocannabinol in healthy individuals: Implications for psychosis. *Neuropsychopharmacology 29:*1158–1172, 2004.
12. Sekine, Y., Iyo, M., Ouchi, Y., Matsunaga, T., Tsukada, H., Okada, H., Yoshikawa, E., Futatsubashi, M., Takei, N., & Mori, N. Methamphetamine-related psychiatric symptoms and reduced brain dopamine transporters studied with PET. *American Journal of Psychiatry 158:*1206–1214, 2001.
13. Curran, H. V., & Monaghan, L. In and out of the K-hole: A comparison of the acute and residual effects of ketamine in frequent and infrequent ketamine users. *Addiction 96:*749–760, 2001.
14. Preuss, U. W., Schuckit, M. A., Smith, T. L., Danko, G. P., Bucholz, K. K., Hesselbrock, M. N., Hesselbrock, V., & Kramer, J. R. Predictors and correlates of suicide attempts over 5 years in 1,237 alcohol-dependent men and women. *American Journal of Psychiatry 160:*56–63, 2003.
15. Preuss, U. W., Schuckit, M. A., Smith, T. L., Danko, G. P., Dasher, A. C., Hesselbrock, M. N., Hesselbrock, V. M., & Nurnberger, J. I., Jr. A comparison of alcohol-induced and independent depression in alcoholics with histories of suicide attempts. *Journal of Studies on Alcohol 63:*498–502, 2002.
16. Brook, D. W., Brook, J. S., Zhang, E., Cohen, P., & Whiteman, M. Drug use and the risk of major depressive disorder, alcohol dependence, and substance use disorders. *Archives of General Psychiatry 59:*1039–1044, 2002.
17. Gonzalez, G., Feingold, A., Oliveto, A., Gonsai, K., & Kosten, T. R. Comorbid major depressive disorder as a prognostic factor in cocaine-abusing buprenorphine-maintained patients treated with desipramine and contingency management. *The American Journal of Drug and Alcohol Abuse 29:*497–514, 2003.
18. Goodwin, R. D., Fergusson, D. M., & Horwood, L. J. Association between anxiety disorders and substance use disorders among young persons: Results of a 21-year longitudinal study. *Journal of Psychiatric Research 38:*295–304, 2004.
19. Hernandez-Avila, C. A., Modesto-Lowe, V., Feinn, R., & Kranzler, H. R. Nefazodone treatment of comorbid alcohol dependence and major depression. *Alcoholism: Clinical and Experimental Research 28:*433–440, 2004.
20. Kelly, J. F., McKellar, J. D., & Moos, R. Major depression in patients with substance use disorders: Relationship to 12-step self-help involvement and substance use outcomes. *Addiction 98:*499–508, 2003.
21. Schuckit, M. A., Tipp, J. E., Bergman, M., Reich, W., Hesselbrock, V. M., & Smith, T. L. Comparison of induced and independent major depressive disorders in 2,945 alcoholics. *American Journal of Psychiatry 154:*948–957, 1997.
22. Mason, B. J., Kocsis, J. H., Ritvo, E. C., & Cutler, R. B. A double-blind placebo-controlled trial of desipramine in primary alcoholics stratified on the presence or absence of major depression. *Journal of the American Medical Association 275:*1–7, 1996.
23. Cornelius, J. R., Salloum, I. M., Ehler, J. G., Jarrett, P. J., Cornelius, M. D., Perel, J. M., Thase, M. E., & Black, A. Fluoxetine in depressed alcoholics. *Archives of General Psychiatry 54:*700–705, 1997.

CHAPTER 14

Rehabilitation

14.1. INTRODUCTION

The steps required to enter recovery for substance dependence are straightforward.[1–3] The process is similar to that encountered with any long-term and potentially life-threatening disorder such as diabetes or hypertension. The person must recognize that his or her functioning is impaired, admit that the use of substances has either caused the problems or has significantly exacerbated them, and reach a point where he or she realizes that all possible steps must be taken to correct the situation. Treatment strives to help the person learn how to change the pattern of life functioning, to maximize the chance that compliance (i.e., abstinence) will continue, and to prevent relapses or to minimize their duration and adverse impact if they occur.[1,4] Each of these steps is described for patients or clients and for their families in the companion book entitled *Educating Yourself about Alcohol and Drugs*.[1]

In viewing this process, it is important to remember that most people who seek recovery from substance-use disorders do very well.[5] As one might guess, the best chances of achieving and maintaining abstinence (similar to the best chances for gaining control of blood sugar in diabetes or keeping blood pressures within the normal range) are seen for the people who are the most highly motivated and for those who have the highest level of functioning despite their chronic disorder. So, it should not be surprising that men and women who are alcohol or drug dependent who have jobs to go back to and family support (a group that represents the *majority* of people with substance dependence) have a 60% or higher chance of maintaining at least 1 year of abstinence if they complete the intensive several weeks to 1-month portion of a treatment program.[1,6,7] Other evaluations report similar high levels of 1-year abstinence, and even programs dealing with the public inebriate show marked improvements on follow-up.[8] Although most studies only carry out 1-year follow-ups, additional data indicate that 1 year of abstinence is predictive of abstinence at 2 and 5 years.[9]

Perhaps the most challenging part of substance-use disorder rehabilitation, or rehab, is catching the attention of the patient or client. Treatment programs talk about the necessity of "bottoming out," a process that I interpret to mean that a person has come to the conclusion that some crisis has convinced him that he is not willing to tolerate a continuation of substance-related life problems. For one of my patients, a prominent physician, this "hitting bottom" occurred when he was so intoxicated one day that he could not remember having picked up his 10-year-old daughter from school and bringing her home. Some level of recognition that the status quo cannot continue is an important step in beginning to address the need for help. However, the decision to seek care is complicated.[10]

All health-care providers have a key role in this recognition and intervention step. For example, physicians need to recognize the high prevalence of alcohol and drug dependence, keeping vigilant for signs and symptoms of the problems. Interventions by a health-care provider can go a long way in helping an individual to decide to enter care.[11,12] Often, the initial stages of treatment can take place in the office of a physician, a nurse, a psychologist, or other health-care provider, even before referral to any specialized program.

For all the substance dependencies, the process of encouraging change and maintaining sobriety uses counseling and education, as well as cognitive and behavioral approaches.[1,13–15] Although these can be effectively delivered one-on-one, even when given in a group setting these messages are as effective, and can be less costly.[16] This intervention is followed by more intensive 2–4 weeks of either inpatient or outpatient rehabilitation, where group counseling sessions are offered daily with a focus placed on helping people to remember the liabilities of continuing to use substances and to actively plan for how to optimize functioning and minimize the possibility of a relapse.[1,8]

Most alcohol and drug programs reach out to family members to optimize their level of understanding of the processes required for recovery.[1,17] Patients and clients are also urged to develop a supportive, abstinent peer group through 12-step-like programs such as Alcoholics Anonymous (AA), Cocaine Anonymous (CA), and so on.[18,19]

Once the process of treating withdrawal (detoxification or detox) has been completed (a procedure potentially relevant to depressants, stimulants, and opioids), medications can be helpful, but their role is limited for most substance-use disorders. For example, few pharmacological treatments have yet been proven through double-blind trials to be effective for stimulant-dependence rehabilitation. However, some medications can be an important part of rehab efforts for opioid dependence (e.g., methadone maintenance), alcohol dependence, and for the treatment of nicotine dependence (e.g., nicotine replacement therapies).

This chapter serves as an introduction to the concept of rehabilitation for alcohol and for other substance abuse and dependence, but it is not a definitive discussion of all aspects of care. It can be read for general knowledge, for guidelines to the appropriate referral of patients, as a framework for the critical evaluation of programs, or as a basis for developing your own treatment efforts. It is hoped that you will want to turn to some of the references for more information.

The following sections present a series of general rules that (with modifications) fit rehabilitation for most substance misusers. These are followed by a discussion of guidelines specifically tailored to particular drug approaches.

14.1.1. Some General Rules

The same basic guidelines apply to all types of rehabilitation efforts with substance misusers. Each is stated only briefly in the following section, and most are discussed in more detail in the subsections on rehab of alcohol dependence (Section 14.2) and of other drugs (Sections 14.3–14.5).

14.1.1.1. Justify Your Actions

Coming to see us in the midst of crises, our patients may be prepared to "do almost anything" to make things improve. However, doing something and then observing how well a patient does is not enough to show that the treatment caused the outcome.[10,20] This is because substance-related problems tend to fluctuate in intensity, with the result that one can see temporary improvement with time alone. There is also a 20% higher rate of "spontaneous remission" with no intervention at all. The key questions to be addressed in judging any treatments are "Did the improvement occur *because of* the treatment?" and "Were the therapeutic efforts those with the greatest chance of success and lowest potential for doing harm?" The therapist must constantly justify his actions, both within a financial cost–benefit framework, and in a manner that considers patient and staff time, physical or emotional dangers to the patient, and the trauma of separation from job and family.[3,21–23]

14.1.1.2. Know the Natural Course of the Disorder

It is only through knowledge of the probable course of substance-use disorder that one can make adequate treatment plans and determine if the treatment is justified, while educating patients and their families of the consequences likely to occur if the substance use continues.[24] The usual course of alcoholism is discussed in Chapter 3.

14.1.1.3. Guard Against the Overzealous Acceptance of New Treatments

Most treatment efforts "make sense" in some theoretical framework, and most patients improve at least temporarily with time alone, while many get "well," no matter what treatment is used. This improvement can be the result of the fluctuating nature of the disorder and of spontaneous remission. Therefore, demand good, controlled investigations before accepting a newer treatment approach as valid.

14.1.1.4. Keep It Simple

In evaluating treatment efforts or adopting new therapies, a sensible approach is to stay with the least costly, potentially least harmful, and simplest maneuvers until there are good data to justify more complex procedures.

14.1.1.5. Apply Objective Diagnostic Criteria

It is not enough to accept a patient into a program because he or she appears at the door of a treatment center. To make use of knowledge of the natural course and to predict future problems, as well as to justify treatment efforts, standard diagnostic criteria must be applied.[25] An individual may, however, be given a "probable" diagnosis and treated as if he or she had a definite disorder, but with extra care taken to reevaluate the label at a future date. Of course, all patients must be evaluated for major preexisting psychiatric disorders that require treatment or affect the prognosis (e.g., an independent major depressive disorder or the antisocial personality, as described in Section 3.1.2.3).

14.1.1.6. Establish Realistic Goals

In treating substance-use disorders, we rarely achieve immediate "magical cures." I attempt to maximize the chances for recovery, to encourage abstinence at an earlier age than it might have been achieved with no therapeutic intervention, to offer good medical care, to help the people close to the patient better understand what is happening, and to educate patients so that they can make informed decisions about treatment goals. Although health-care practitioners can and must offer their best efforts, the patient's motivation and level of "readiness" for recovery have a great impact on outcome.[26]

Different therapeutic interventions have different goals. For instance, a detoxification facility established in an area with many homeless people attempts to offer the best possible medical care and general social supports along with detox.[27] However, while treatment personnel will encourage permanent abstinence, the lower probable long-term abstention for patients seeking only detox might not justify abstinence as the only marker of success. On the other hand, an alcohol rehabilitation program established within an industry, the military, or with married and working patients does focus more on rehabilitation and less on immediate medical care, as with adequate rehab two thirds of the patients are likely to be dry a year later, and most abstinent people will be functioning as well as their nonalcoholic peers.

14.1.1.7. Know the Goals of Your Patients

In establishing patients' goals, it is important to understand the patient's reasons for entering treatment: Was it to detox only? To deal with a crisis? Or actually to aim at long-term abstinence? Working with this patient and considering their desires is also a key element in motivating them to enter and complete the recommended treatment.[28]

14.1.1.8. Attempt to Match Your Patients' Goals and Characteristics with the Specific Treatment

For several decades, clinicians and researchers in the substance-related disorders field have hypothesized that treatment effectiveness would increase if we could identify specific characteristics of patients that correlated with their specific treatment needs.[29,30] It has been difficult to gather adequate data to test this common-sense assumption, at least in part because of differences between programs and research projects in the definitions and methods used.

In the early 1990s, the National Institute of Alcoholism and Alcohol Abuse established a Project MATCH program testing the relationships between specific treatment characteristics and the goals of patients.[29] The good news from this project is that the large majority of these men and women demonstrated marked improvement at the 1-year follow-up. The results also indicated that those individuals who had previously been in an inpatient program did better than those who had only received outpatient care, a finding consistent with additional research that the more intensive the treatment, the better the outcome. However, there were very few client characteristics that indicated which individuals would be most likely to respond to which of the three types of therapies offered.

I interpret the latter findings to indicate that health-care providers do not need to search for the "perfect" program for each patient or client. Rather, it is the general helping mechanisms associated with the programs, not highly specific components, that matter. However, it is possible that other types of treatments are best matched with additional patient or client characteristics, and there is a need for further study of the matching hypothesis.

14.1.1.9. Make a Long-Term Commitment

Because there is no "magic cure" in these areas, recovery is usually a long-term process that requires some counseling and a therapeutic relationship for at least 6 months to 1 year after the more intensive first several weeks of rehab.[31]

14.1.1.10. Use All Available Resources

The patient's substance dependence does not operate in a vacuum. Part of the therapeutic effort should be directed at encouraging the family, friends, and, if appropriate, the employer to increase their level of understanding of the problem; to be available to help whenever necessary; to make realistic future plans for themselves as they relate to the patient; and, in specific instances, to function as "ancillary therapists," helping to carry out your treatment efforts in the home setting.

A second important resource can be found in the workplace. Many employment settings have developed specific programs aimed at identifying and helping workers with various forms of impairment, including those related to alcohol and other drugs.[32] These Employee Assistance Programs (EAPs) are more likely to be found in larger industries that are self-insured and have affiliated unions. Not only can such programs screen for individuals with substance use and related problems, but also they can help monitor recovery and optimize the chances that the employee will return to work in the best and most supportive environment.

14.1.1.11. When Appropriate, Notify All Involved Physicians and Pharmacists

When dealing with a substance dependent person who is obtaining inappropriate drugs from physicians or pharmacists, it is my preference to make all possible efforts to cut off the patient's supply. This must be done with tact, with understanding, and with empathy for the ego of the prescribing physician or the dispensing pharmacist and only with the patient's permission, to avoid infringing on his legal rights.

14.1.1.12. Do Not Take Final Responsibility for the Patient's Actions

Although I do everything within my power to help, in the final analysis the decision to achieve and maintain abstinence is the patient's responsibility.[1] If I do not follow this rule and the patient allows me to assume the responsibility or stops only to please me, he will soon find an excuse to get angry with me and return to alcohol and/or to drugs.

14.1.2. A "General" Substance Dependence Treatment Program

Because there are patients and clients in need and money is available for care, there is usually a great deal of pressure to "do anything as long as you do it now," but that is not always the best course. With some forethought, it is possible to establish a rehabilitation program that will probably do the best with the least harm. The *usual* rehabilitation program would do the following:

1. Attempt to accomplish four basic goals:
   a. Maximize physical and mental health, as patients will find it difficult to achieve abstinence if chronic medical problems have not been adequately treated.

   b. Enhance motivation toward abstinence through educating the patient and his family about the usual course of the disorder, employing appropriate medications to stop the patient from returning to substance misuse on the spur of the moment—for example, opioid antagonists like naltrexone (Trexan) for people who are heroin dependent—and using cognitive and behavior modification approaches. The ability to change a person's view regarding the need to continue to comply with treatment (i.e., cognitive therapies) is the core of treating chronic relapsing disorders.
   c. Help the patient to rebuild a life without the substance through advising, group therapy, vocational and avocational counseling, family counseling, by helping him develop a substance-free peer group, by showing him how to use free time, and so on.
   d. Teach techniques for avoiding relapses and for minimizing their duration if they occur.[33,34]
2. Whenever possible, begin with outpatient rehabilitation rather than inpatient, as the former costs less and teaches the patient how to adjust to a life without the substance while he is functioning in the "real world." However, inpatient care makes the most sense and is likely to be cost-effective for more severely impaired people and for those who failed in outpatient rehabilitation efforts.[23,35,36] Candidates for inpatient rehabilitation include patients who have not responded to outpatient counseling, those with medical or psychiatric problems severe enough to warrant hospitalization, people who live a great distance from the hospital and cannot regularly attend outpatient groups, and patients whose lives are in such chaos that it is difficult or impossible to deal with them on an outpatient basis.[37]
3. If inpatient rehabilitation is used, keep it as short as possible (usually 2–4 weeks), as longer inpatient care and other more intensive interventions have not been demonstrated to be more effective than short-term care for the average patient, as long as the shorter course is followed by 6- to 12-months of aftercare.
4. Avoid using medications in the treatment of substance dependence after withdrawal is completed, unless there are good data to support this step. Exceptions are methadone or naltrexone for opioid dependence, and naltrexone or acamprosate (Campral) for alcoholism.[38]
5. Use group more than individual counseling, as the former costs less and is probably equally effective.
6. Use self-help groups such as AA, Narcotics Anonymous (NA), and CA, as they can be quite helpful and they cost nothing.[18,39,40] They offer the patient a model that may be important in his achieving

and maintaining recovery. These programs are discussed in more detail below.

7. Recognize that there is no evidence that any one specialized and expensive form of psychotherapy (e.g., gestalt or transactional analysis) is any more effective than general "day-to-day" life counseling for the person with a substance-use disorder.
8. Incorporate formal relapse prevention procedures into the treatment and the aftercare phases of rehabilitation.[33,34,41] This approach helps patients to avoid or take control of situations in which relapse is likely. There are several mechanisms for teaching relapse prevention, including asking the patient to imagine situations in which relapse is likely to occur and to practice the steps to be taken if a relapse actually develops. For the latter, the goal is to learn to not use a "slip" as an excuse for returning to a full-blown episode of substance use. Most of the relapse-prevention approaches place an emphasis on the need to recognize that the person is responsible for his or her own actions, such as placing himself in a situation in which return to use is more likely (e.g., a bar or a neighborhood in which drugs used to be purchased). Relapse prevention groups ideally should be used as an integral part of either the intensive outpatient or the inpatient first phase of rehabilitation, and then continued throughout aftercare.
9. Reach out to the social support group, including family members and friends to educate them about what can be expected as part of a treatment program[17]. These efforts can also decrease miscommunication regarding treatment goals that might be carried to the family by the patient, and they can help friends and relatives to become invested in the most important phase of rehabilitation, aftercare.[42]
10. Maintain continued contact with the patient for at least 6–12 months. All efforts should be used to decrease attrition. For example, letters and/or phone calls noting your desire to continue to help should be used to try to get patients to come back after they have missed even one aftercare or outpatient counseling session.
11. Incorporate nondegreed (paraprofessional) counseling staff into your program if they are supervised by people with more formal training in counseling, as there is little evidence that treatment can be successfully carried out only by individuals with advanced degrees.
12. For men and women with few social supports or with chaotic life situations, consider using a halfway or recovery home for 3–6 months while continuing aftercare and self-help group participation.
13. The basic treatment approach for any disorder requires that common-sense modifications be made for the specific patient. Therefore, while the same cognitive behavioral-based rehab approach is used

for men and women, it is important that the clinician consider specific elements of care more appropriate for females, including issues related to drinking during pregnancy, child care, problems associated with being a single parent, feelings of vulnerability and the need for support from other women, and so on.[43,44] Similarly, while the same basic approach is used in the rehabilitation of a 25-year old and a 70-year old, older patients require more careful attention to medical problems, may benefit from the involvement of their grown children, are more likely to have lingering levels of temporary confusion following detoxification, and may require efforts to help them feel more intellectually and emotionally fulfilled despite retirement.[45,46] Similar suggestions for flexibility apply to adolescents versus adults, individuals being treated in rural versus urban settings, plumbers versus physicians, and so on.

14.2. A SPECIAL CASE: ALCOHOL ABUSE AND DEPENDENCE (305.00 AND 303.90 IN DSM-IV)

Because alcohol is the most common substance of abuse, I have used rehabilitation of the person with alcoholism as the prototype. The discussion is written assuming you have already reviewed Chapter 3 and recognize that the average person with alcoholism is a middle-class man or woman with a family who is most likely to come into your office with rather nonspecific complaints, and rarely appears intoxicated or in withdrawal. The diagnosis is made by realizing that one in five patients is alcoholic and through observing the pattern of medical problems (e.g., substance-induced mild hypertension, cancers of the esophagus, the stomach, or the head and neck, or impotence) and the pattern of psychological complaints (e.g., substance-induced depression, anxiety, or insomnia) most closely associated with alcoholism. Diagnosis is aided by carefully observing the pattern of laboratory results, especially mild elevations in the MCV, uric acid, triglycerides, and especially CDT or GGT, as explained in Chapter 3. With these points in mind, this section reviews general treatment philosophy, the process of intervention, and rehabilitation.

To maximize the resources available and thereby reach the greatest possible number of patients, I emphasize outpatient rehabilitation. This costs 5–10 times less than inpatient care and may be just as effective for the average patient.[1,4]

Even with inpatient approaches, the types of interventions offered should follow the general rules offered in Section 14.1.2, as the most direct and least complex schemes may be as good as or even superior to the more costly ones. Figure 14.1 gives a *simplified* flow of the steps generally followed in identifying and treating a person with substance dependence. The diagnosis is established from the history given by the patient and by his family as

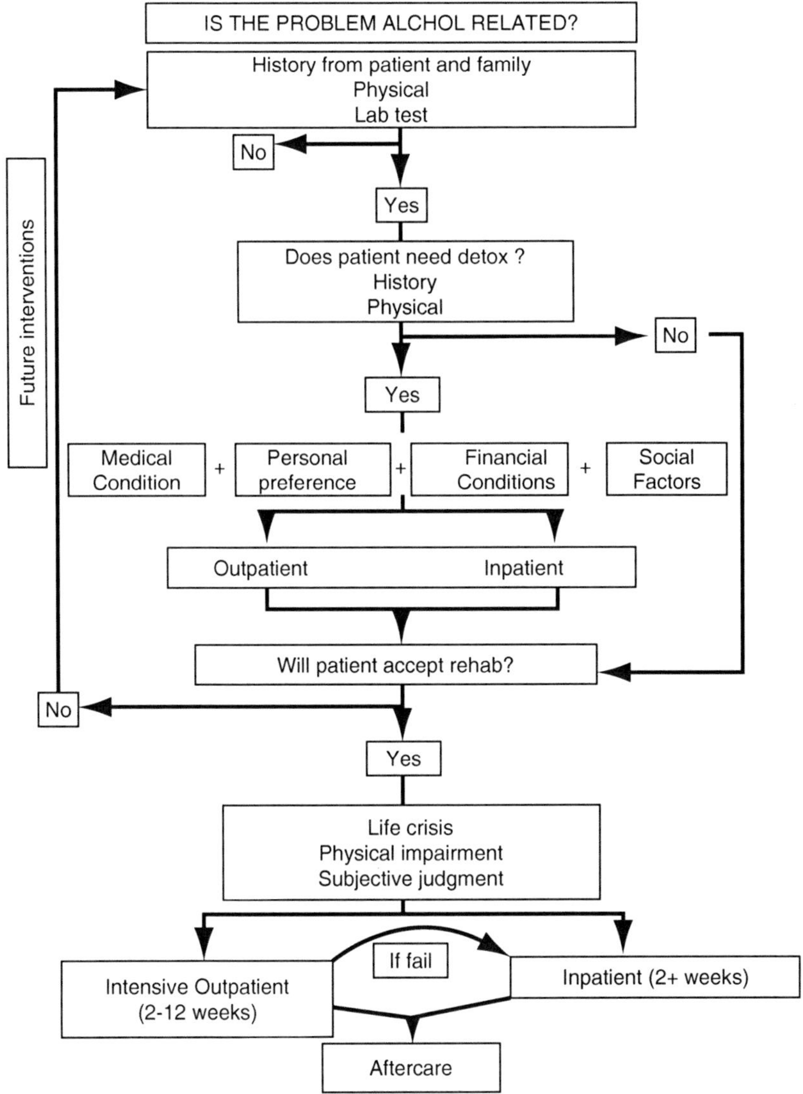

Figure 14.1. Discussions in alcoholism treatment.

well as from the physical examination and the laboratory tests. Once you decide that the patient is alcohol dependent, you face the decision about detoxification, remembering that if you miss potentially important withdrawal signs, the patient may lose faith because of the rigors of withdrawal and dropout of treatment. Detoxification can be carried out in either an inpatient or an outpatient setting, with inpatient care preferred for individuals who have serious medical difficulties, those who have had withdrawal seizures in the past, as well as for older people or patients who are debilitated (see Section 4.2.6). Finally, rehabilitation, whether inpatient or an outpatient, must be followed with extended aftercare for 6–12 months for all patients.

14.2.1. The Process of Intervention

The pattern of laboratory tests, physical findings, history of life problems, and information gathered from family members may help you to recognize the patient or client with alcohol abuse or dependence. Once this is accomplished, the next step is to share your findings with him or her in an attempt to enhance recognition of the problem and to encourage action from that recognition.[1]

The patient is responsible for his actions; your responsibility is to do all that is possible to raise his level of motivation. Whether your efforts "take" or not may be beyond your control, but you can use aspects of motivational interviewing to carry out interventions that enhance the probability of compliance.[28,47,48]

A first step in the intervention is to utilize the patient's area of concern and to demonstrate, in an empathic way, how alcohol ties in to the worries. Here, health-care providers such as physicians and nurse practitioners have a big role.[49,50] For instance, you can begin to motivate an individual coming in complaining of just "not feeling well" or of insomnia, high blood pressure, and so on by telling him that he has good reason for concern. You might then go on to share the relevant laboratory tests and physical findings and to state: "There is one way I have of pulling all of these findings together. I believe you have reached a point in life where alcohol is causing more trouble than it's worth."

Then, you might teach him about the difficulties he can expect in the future unless he stops drinking. It may not be necessary at this point to use the term *alcoholism*; rather, in this initial confrontation, alcohol-related life problems can be the focus.

Next, discuss the probable future course of the alcohol-related problems and explore possible avenues for treatment. If he accepts help, determine whether detoxification is required, and either begins counseling or refer him to an alcohol-treatment facility (either outpatient or inpatient) or, if he or she refuses formal treatment, use AA.

Many patients will not respond to your initial efforts. Most individuals recognize that they are having alcohol-related problems, but they have been aggressively denying this both to themselves and to others. You might best tell the individual who refuses to respond to your first intervention that you respect his need to make his own decisions, but would like to know more about why he is reluctant to get help. You can then work with him or her to change their unrealistic fears or to modify your treatment plan in a way that they find more acceptable. If he continues to be reluctant, you might maintain contact by saying that you need to evaluate some things further, and that he should return to you in several weeks (hoping that in the interim he will decrease his level of denial and be more likely to cooperate). In effect, you are also trying to gauge his readiness for change while keeping the door open for future efforts. If he refuses to come back or continues to deny problems, I tell him that I am willing to treat him for general problems and will do all I can to help him maximize his functioning despite his alcohol-related difficulties. I do warn him, however, that I will not be able to fully treat his medical and psychological problems until he stops drinking. I hope that he will see me as a reasonable and caring physician, and that he will return to me as his alcohol problems escalate. I generally arrange with the patient for a "checkup" at least every 3 months to try to maximize the chance that he will come back.

Some patients respond to the initial (or 17th) intervention by admitting that alcohol might be a problem and that they should "cut down." As is apparent in the natural history of alcoholism outlined in Section 3.4, cutting down is not usually a problem; it is staying cut down that becomes so difficult.[1] I do all I can to persuade the patient not just to cut down but to abstain. If he or she resists, I set up a meeting with the patient and the patient's close relative (e.g., usually the spouse). This approach might be most helpful for men and women with abuse but not with severe dependence.[51] Here, I continue to try to discourage "controlled drinking," pointing out that it is not likely to work for any period of time, but I will yield if the patient insists. Next, I establish a regimen that, if followed, will stop the patient from ever becoming intoxicated. For instance, the patient's intake of alcohol should be limited to two drinks per 24 h; a drink is defined as 12 oz of beer, 4 oz of nonfortified wine, or 1.5 oz of 80-proof beverage. The 24 h is also defined as a magical clock that begins ticking the moment the first sip of a beverage is taken. However, the dependent patient's drinking almost inevitably escalates beyond this regimen, and problems develop. At that point, I hope that the patient will come back to me for help.

It can be seen that intervention is rarely a "one-shot" phenomenon. Rather, my attempts to increase motivation frequently involve multiple contacts with the patient (always keeping the responsibility for his behavior with him, not me), outreach to the family, and various stages of general support, until the patient finally decides not to drink. Once the patient has agreed to abstain, I evaluate the need for detoxification (see Section 4.2.2) and enter him in either an outpatient or an inpatient rehabilitation program. Attempts to rehabilitate people with alcoholism consist of long-term contact aimed at enhancing motivation and increasing the ease of readjustment to life without alcohol.

Some clinicians recommend a more structured and intensive intervention plan.[52] Using what is often described as the Johnson Institute approach, the clinician helps members of the patient's social network to organize a meeting where important relatives and friends have the opportunity to tell the patient or client exactly which behaviors have concerned them and the fears they have regarding the future should he continue to drink or take drugs. This confrontation by multiple important persons in the patient's life appears to increase the probability that an individual will enter treatment, although it is more difficult to show whether such patients are more likely to remain in care or are less likely to relapse than those who enter treatment through alternative mechanisms. A less complex variation on this approach, known as ARISE, has also been described.

A variation of this process of intervention has been described for health-care providers.[11,49] Finally, an expanded process of intervention by the health-care provider can also be helpful. Recent articles have described how physicians can implement between 2 and 7 visits of perhaps 10–15 min during which they use a detailed manual to guide them in attempting to enhance the patient's motivation and to decrease substance-related problems.[47–50] These appear to be cost-effective ways to both enhance abstinence, and for those who continue to drink, decrease levels of alcohol intake and associated problems.

14.2.2. Enhancing Motivation

These maneuvers are used during the process of intervention and through rehabilitation in either the outpatient or the inpatient setting. The steps in this area include the following:

1. Educating the patient and his or her family about the natural course of alcoholism and about the problems they can expect in the future. The family can be very important, as the spouse and other family members can impact favorably on the patient's success with continued abstinence.
2. Emphasizing the patient's responsibility for his own actions. For example, the family should never protect the patient from the actions of his drinking by putting him to bed when he is drunk (they should let him fall asleep in front of the television set and go up to bed themselves) or rescuing him from jail (he should spend the evening in jail if necessary). In your interactions, any "Yes, but," should be met with "You can make decisions about what you wish to do and the consequences you're willing to accept."

14.2.3. Helping the Person with Alcoholism Readjust to a Life Without Alcohol

By the time you have established a diagnosis, the average person with alcoholism has had serious life problems for 10 years or more. Once he has entered rehabilitation, he has recognized (on some level) that alcohol is causing more troubles than it is worth and has agreed that he should stop drinking. However, because alcohol has been such a central part of his life for so long, there are many life situations that decrease his chance of continued abstinence. These must be carefully addressed.

Alcohol treatment programs utilize group counseling for the patient *and for the family*, vocational rehabilitation for the patient, sessions that center on the proper use of free time, and the establishment of a group of abstinent peers.[1] They also do everything else possible to enhance a smooth readjustment to life without alcohol. These programs may be begun in an inpatient setting, but the day-to-day emphasis on group counseling should continue for many months in an outpatient or aftercare mode so that the patient can receive support and counseling while he is actually attempting to function in his real-life situation.

14.2.4. The Role of Alcoholics Anonymous (AA) and Other Self-Help Groups

AA is an excellent resource for treatment.[18,53] It is also referred to as a "12-step" program, a name that comes from the series of steps prescribed for the individual by AA and by similar organizations to optimize the chance of developing and maintaining abstinence while rebuilding a more functional and sober lifestyle. This group, composed of individuals who are themselves recovering from alcoholism (many of whom have been "dry" for years), establishes a milieu in which help is available 24 h a day, 7 days a week. At meetings, members share their own recovery experiences, demonstrating to the patient that he is not alone and that a better lifestyle is possible. AA also offers additional help in the form of groups that discuss the special problems of the children of people with alcoholism (Alateen) and of their spouses (Al-Anon). In fact, the core of 12-step programs can be seen as helping to change a person's view of using alcohol and other drugs while working to decrease the risk for relapse (cognitive components), helping the person to reestablish key interpersonal relationships and rebuild their lives without alcohol (behavioral components).

AA can be used as a referral resource where no other outpatient service is either available or acceptable to the patient. It can also be utilized as an adjunct to outpatient or to inpatient treatment efforts. Each AA group has its own personality, and it is important to choose a meeting in which the individual patient is likely to feel most comfortable. Factors to consider include the educational level of the average member, the male-to-female ratio of the group, smoking policies, and degrees of emphasis on religion or spirituality.[40,54] While the latter elements can be a strength during recovery, a belief in God is not required in order to derive benefit from these groups. The agnostic person or atheist can be advised to translate references to a "higher power" or God into terms meaningful to them, such as aspects of life or the Universe that are beyond their understanding. Although self-help group participation is of greatest help in outpatient settings, it is essential that the patient or client be introduced to AA or to similar programs during the initial intensive phase of care to optimize the probability that he or she will actively participate.

Data are still developing regarding the actual contribution to recovery for these self-help groups. Most studies of AA have shown levels of improvement that approach those expected from more formal counseling, although the optimal outcome appears to be associated with a combination of both formal treatment and active AA participation. The greater the intensity of exposure to AA and the greater the amount of continued participation, the better the outcome.[18,55]

Although AA is the most widely known and best studied of these self-help groups, representing the best example of what is known as a 12-step program, alternate approaches are available. These include Rational Recovery, which places less intense emphasis on spirituality or religion while using more behavioral approaches, as well as the Secular Organization for Sobriety (SOS), and Women for Sobriety (WFS).

14.2.5. The Role of Medications in Alcoholism Rehabilitation

Over the years many medications have been evaluated for their possible role in alcoholism rehabilitation. These have included brain-depressant drugs such as diazepam (Valium), antipsychotic medications such as olanzapine (Zyprexa), lithium, anticonvulsants, and antidepressants. In fact, almost all types of psychiatric medications have been touted at one time or other.[56–60]

Complicating the evaluation of these pharmacological treatments is the fact that the course of alcohol dependence is so variable. Thus, the intensity of drinking and related problems fluctuate over time, temporary periods of abstinence are commonly observed in the course of any substance-use disorder, and there is a 20–30% rate of permanent spontaneous remission.[1,24,61] This makes it difficult to determine whether a good outcome is the result of the medication itself or just a reflection of the natural course of alcoholism over time. Therefore, the only way to determine whether a medication works is to carry out controlled studies where the outcome associated with the active drug is compared to that observed with placebo.

Such controlled studies are important for a number of reasons. First, the continued use of a medication that is not actually beneficial takes up scarce health-care dollars that would be better invested elsewhere. Second, all medications have side effects and dangers, and these problems are likely to be amplified by the concurrent use of these medications in the context of continued heavy drinking. Therefore, medications that do not actively contribute to recovery carry unnecessary dangers.

While reading the following sections regarding medications, it is important to remember that no drug has been shown to be sufficient on its own in causing recovery from any substance dependence. Rather, medications are used as part of a more holistic approach to treatment and are combined with behavioral and cognitive therapies, outreach to family and friends, education, AA, and so on.[62] With these thoughts in mind, I present an updated overview of the possible medications for use in the treatment of alcohol dependence, discussing those that appear most promising first.

14.2.5.1. Acamprosate (Campral)

This drug (known as calcium acetylhomotaurinate) has been widely tested in Europe since about 1990 and became available in the US in 2004.[63–66] Structurally, acamprosate resembles the sedating brain neurotransmitter GABA, and part of its hypothesized mechanism of action might occur through enhancement of GABA-like brain effects. A more likely explanation rests with the observation that this medication is also an antagonist of some of the stimulating actions of another brain neurotransmitter system involving the amino acid glutamate and the associated NMDA receptor system.[67,68]

Studies in animals support potential calming effects of acamprosate during alcohol withdrawal and its ability to produce a lower level of preference for alcohol. Human research has been carried out with thousands of individuals in diverse alcohol treatment programs where they usually received placebo or between 1,300 and 3,000 mg of acamprosate per day over periods up to 12 months. Most, but not all, of these clinical trials support a modest impact for this drug on a variety of alcohol outcome measures. Serious side effects are relatively uncommon, with the most frequently reported difficulties involving headache and diarrhea.

In summary, acamprosate is a promising medication that appears to offer a modest but significant level of improved outcome compared to placebo in most studies. The evaluations of this drug are most impressive for the large number of subjects who were studied for 6–12 months to observe both short-term and moderate-term effects of the medication.

14.2.5.2. Naltrexone (Revia or Trexan)

This is the second promising and more extensively studied medication for alcohol dependence, prescribed at 50–100 mg/day or 150 mg every 3 days.[69–73] However, the studies of naltrexone have been much smaller in size and have usually been limited to only 12 weeks of active drug administration. These characteristics make it difficult to determine the overall efficacy or the long-term safety and to be certain that tolerance does not develop to the beneficial effects. An injectable depot form of the drug (150 mg IM every month) is currently being evaluated and holds promise.[74,75]

Although the mechanisms of action of opiate antagonists such as naltrexone, or its cousin nalmephene, are well understood, the attributes that contribute most directly to helping men and women with alcoholism is less certain.[70,76] It is hypothesized that the opioid antagonists might decrease the intensity of reinforcement that occurs with drinking, might diminish craving for alcohol, and, at least in animals, might contribute to a taste aversion associated with alcoholic beverages.[77,78] Regarding reinforcement, alcohol has been shown to produce a release of the body's own endorphins, a phenomenon that might be blocked with opioid antagonists, which might also impact on the complex relationships among opioid receptors and the dopamine-rich ventral tegmental reward systems in the brain, as discussed in Chapter 3.

Research in animals supports a diminution of alcohol intake when they are treated with naltrexone. The effect appears to be maximal at moderate naltrexone doses (e.g., between 50 and 100 mg/day), but there are reports that the impact on alcohol intake might be relatively temporary and that some subgroups of animals might actually increase alcohol intake while being administered naltrexone.[79]

Most studies reveal that the side effect profile for naltrexone is relatively modest.[80] In one recent investigation, headaches were reported by 10%, nausea by approximately 10%, and only 15% of patients stopped the medication because of side effects. As with any medication, it is important that the clinician work to optimize compliance.[81] Clinical protocols have not observed prominent elevations in the usual liver function tests, findings that had previously been reported with higher doses of naltrexone.

In summary, animal studies suggest a probable effect for this drug regarding alcohol intake, and most evaluations of alcohol consumption in people without alcoholism support at least a mild decrease in alcohol intake associated with naltrexone. The evaluations with naltrexone in the alcoholics indicate a significant but modest benefit. However, more studies will be required evaluating larger numbers of individuals over a longer period of time before final conclusions can be drawn regarding the general applicability of opioid antagonists in treating alcohol dependence.

14.2.5.3. Naltrexone–Acamprosate Combination

Several recent studies have addressed the possibility that acamprosate and naltrexone may be more effective in combination than they are when used alone. This question is important because the hypothesized mechanisms of these two drugs are quite different, raising the possibility that the combined effect might be better than one would predict from the results associated with either drug alone.

The process began with evaluations to determine that the combination had the predicted effect in animals, and was relatively safe in humans.[38,68,82,83] Subsequently, a modest-sized three-month clinical trial in Germany indicated a potential superiority of the combination of medications using 50 mg of naltrexone and about 3,000 mg of acamprosate daily.[84] A large-scale longer term investigation has also been carried out in the United States, with results revealing a modest improvement when the drugs are used together over the effect of either drug alone. The combination was well tolerated by patients from Project COMBINE.[83]

14.2.5.4. Disulfiram (Antabuse)

Disulfiram has been used for many years for the treatment of alcoholism, and it is usually given at a daily oral dose of 250 mg/day, over an extended period of time, perhaps up to 1 year.[81,85–87] The drug works by causing an irreversible blockade of the actions of aldehyde dehydrogenase, the enzyme responsible for the metabolism of acetaldehyde, the first major breakdown product of ethanol (see Section 3.2). As a result, after drinking, acetaldehyde builds up in the blood and symptoms develop. The intensity of the disulfiram–ethanol reaction depends on the blood-alcohol level (and thus on the amount and rapidity of drinking), as well as on poorly understood individual characteristics of patients. Although disulfiram does not decrease the "drive" to drink, the hope is that the patient's knowledge of a possible severe physical reaction following drinking while on disulfiram will be associated with an improved recovery rate.

In the midst of an alcohol–disulfiram reaction, the most frequent symptoms include facial flushing, palpitations and a rapid heart rate, difficulty in breathing, a potentially serious drop in blood pressure, and nausea and vomiting. The most usual reaction begins within minutes to half an hour after drinking and may last for 30–60 min. Once it has begun, no specific mode of treatment is greatly effective, and most authors advocate general supportive care, antihistamines (to block the effects of acetaldehyde-medicated histamine release), and vitamin C (to possibly enhance acetaldehyde oxidation). Although a healthy person is likely to tolerate the ethanol–disulfiram interaction well, it could be quite dangerous for individuals with a history of serious heart disease, stroke, serious hypertension, or diabetes.

Even without alcohol, disulfiram carries potential dangers. These include precipitating a serious neuritis (including an optic neuritis), possibly exacerbating a peripheral neuropathy, inducing a life-threatening and possibly irreversible hepatitis, and, through its active metabolite, carbon disulfide, might increase the risk of atherosclerotic heart disease, although the risk for these problems is probably quite low.[88]

The efficacy of this drug is difficult to prove.[87] Controlled studies comparing disulfiram with no medication show a higher rate of abstinence with disulfiram. However, other studies comparing disulfiram with a placebo have not always shown that fewer patients on the active drug returned to drinking.[87,89] Thus, the clinician is placed in a dilemma, because if a placebo is prescribed to all patients with alcoholism, eventually no one will believe that he is getting the active drug, and any placebo effect (i.e., fear of a reaction when he drinks) will be lost.

Another difficulty with disulfiram is the need to take the drug daily. Investigators are currently working on the development of a long-lasting implant, but although there have been some promising developments, some methods have not been successful in maintaining adequate blood levels of the drug. Finally, disulfiram is *not* an effective agent for aversive conditioning, because the time lag between the ingestion of alcohol and the reaction is often up to 30 min, and the intensity of the reaction is unpredictable.

The optimum response to disulfiram requires that the drug be used as part of a full and comprehensive alcohol treatment program.[62,88] Furthermore, the medication is most likely to be effective if it is taken daily under the supervision of a family member, a health-care provider, or a pharmacist.[89] One study has also suggested that disulfiram might be especially useful for individuals who are dependent on both alcohol and cocaine.[90]

Several additional medications have been evaluated as alternative approaches to disulfiram. Both metronidazole (Flagyl) and calcium carbamide inhibit aldehyde dehydrogenase and thus have potential promise in the treatment of alcoholism. Although each of these drugs is likely to produce a level of psychological deterrence, as with disulfiram there is likely to be a relatively high dropout rate, and definitive data regarding efficacy in appropriately controlled trials are difficult to establish.

14.2.5.5. Drugs that Affect Brain Levels of the Neurotransmitter Serotonin (5-HT)

There are many indications that the levels of 5-HT activity in the brain affect alcohol consumption in animals and humans.[91] Boosting 5-HT levels is associated with as much as a 10% decrease in alcohol intake, while lowering 5-HT can increase drinking, and there are several reports of levels of drinking relating to genes that affect levels of 5-HT in the synaptic space between neurons.[92–94] However, despite the implications of these results, data do not consistently support the conclusion that medications that increase 5-HT levels in the brain (e.g., selective serotonin reuptake inhibiting [SSRI] antidepressants) are significantly better than placebo in helping alcoholics to achieve and maintain abstinence. The potential usefulness of these drugs has also led to speculation that SSRIs might be particularly useful in alcoholic individuals with independent depressive episodes.[95] However, even this hypothesis has not been consistently supported by studies, and it is possible that the use of SSRIs in an alcohol-dependent individual might actually impair the response to cognitive or behavioral therapies.[96] It is also important to remember that these drugs can have potent side effects including anxiety, insomnia, and agitation, and may not be safely mixed with alcohol.

A medication with more focused effects on serotonin is the 5-HT_3 antagonist, ondansetron (Zofran). Several studies have reported the potential usefulness of this drug in alcoholics with an early onset of problems associated with other drugs as well as alcohol, along with antisocial behaviors.[57,97–99] Used in oral doses of 1–4 μg/kg twice daily, this drug may contribute to a decreased number of drinks per day, although it is not clear whether the medication is of use to the usual alcoholic with a later onset, trials to date have been relatively short term and involved a limited number of patients, and side effects including fatigue, headache, and dizziness are not always well tolerated.

A third type of drug that impacts on serotonin systems is the 5-HT_{1A} partial agonist buspirone (Buspar). This agent is marketed for its impact on general feelings of anxiety, although it does not have sedative properties and effects do not resemble those seen with the benzodiazepines such as diazepam (Valium). Despite initial promising results from uncontrolled trials, more rigorous evaluations do not indicate a likelihood that buspirone is superior to placebo in treating the usual alcoholic.

14.2.5.6. Some Additional Potential Medications

The classical tricyclic-type *antidepressant medications*, such as desipramine (Norpramin), have also been discussed as possible treatments for alcohol dependence. Although there are some suggestions that these drugs might be useful in treating depressions observed concomitant with alcoholism, especially if they are shown to be independent major depressive disorders, there are few studies that support the routine use of antidepressant medication in people with alcoholism.[100–102]

Perhaps reflecting sensitization of several neurochemical systems to repeated doses of alcohol or its withdrawal, specifically changes in GABA and glutamate–NMDA systems, other authors have recommended the possible usefulness of *anticonvulsants*, such as topiramate (Topamax), in alcohol rehabilitation. Although some studies have reported some improvement in drinking behaviors, data are relatively scarce.[103–105] This and similar anticonvulsant medications carry significant side effects including sedation, problems with thinking, and potentially life-threatening decreases in the functioning of the blood-producing systems as well as problems with liver functioning.

The importance of *dopamine* in the reinforcement of drug ingestion has raised the possibility that drugs that affect the activity levels of this neurochemical might help recovering alcoholics to maintain sobriety.[106] Despite preliminary reports from earlier uncontrolled or less well-controlled investigations, more recent studies indicate no general usefulness of drugs such as bromocriptine (Parlodel) in the treatment of alcoholism.[107] Nor is there evidence to support the routine use of the classical antipsychotics in the treatment of alcohol-use disorders.[58,108] One recent study proposed possible benefits to stimulating dopamine with transcranial magnetic stimulation, but this has not yet been evaluated clinically.[109]

While other GABA boosting drugs are theoretically attractive,[59] *sleeping pills* and *antianxiety drugs*, even though the patient may demand them, have *no place* in alcoholic *rehabilitation* (after withdrawal is completed) for the average person with alcoholism. These medications produce dangers of dependence, adverse reactions with other depressant drugs such as alcohol, and, for some hypnotics, the potential for over-dosage. Several over-the-counter drugs have been suggested as useful, including melatonin (to synchronize sleep/awake patterns), and the 5-HT boosting amino acid, L-tryptophan (not currently available in the US). Perhaps the best approach to dealing with lingering anxiety and insomnia, possibly reflecting a protracted abstinence syndrome, is to use cognitive-behavioral interventions dealing with establishing and maintaining regular sleep habits and altering frustration when temporary nervousness or sleep problems develop.[110]

I use such a cognitive-behavioral approach in dealing with complaints of insomnia and/or anxiety in alcoholics.[111] First, I let them know that I understand the intensity of their discomfort and that I will try to help them. Second, I tell them that many of their problems are a physiological response to the long-term use of a brain-depressing drug, and that these physical changes can persist for up to 6 months or longer, although at decreasing intensity. Third, I emphasize that sleeping pills or antianxiety drugs might help them for a week or two but will then make their problems worse and that they will inevitably have to face the day when their bodies must adjust to living without CNS-depressing medications.

To help them deal with their sleep difficulties, I prescribe a regimen of going to bed at the same time every night (getting up and reading or watching television, if necessary) and awakening at the same time every morning, even if they have had only 15 min of good sleep. This regimen is coupled with a rule against caffeinated beverages after noon and against naps during the day. All these measures combine to force the patient's sleep cycle into a more normal pattern after several days. Problems with anxiety are handled with similar types of explanation and a search, carried out jointly with the patient, to find nonmedicinal avenues for release of tension. Possibilities range from church work to developing a hobby to learning to play a musical instrument to yoga to physical exercise, and so on.

Finally, some additional potential treatments have recently come to light. These include plant derivatives such as kudzu.[112]

14.2.6. Treatment Programs

14.2.6.1. Inpatient Treatment

If patients fulfill the criteria for inpatient rehabilitation outlined in Section 14.1.2, you will choose either to hospitalize them yourself or to refer them to an established program.[1,8] Either way, there is no single best treatment element for alcoholism. Rather, because of the general helping nature of rehabilitation, most patients are offered programs with many components aimed at enhancing motivation and increasing the ease of readjustment to a life without drinking.

The selection of a specific inpatient or an outpatient treatment mode is based on the preferences of the patient or client and of his family, financial considerations, and your prior experiences. Although there are no absolute indications for hospitalization after detoxification, patients with serious medical or emotional problems, or those who face severe crises, will probably function best in a structured environment.[4] Also, many health-care providers feel that a short "time out" from life stresses is an important part of treating the average person with alcoholism.

There are no data to support a hospitalization of more than 2–4 weeks for the *average* patient.[1] Of course, common sense dictates that individuals with severe medical problems, or with persistent confusion or cognitive deficits, and those with very unstable life situations might require longer care. It is important, however, to recognize the potential dangers associated with inpatient care, which include risks of treatment-center-acquired infections, physical or emotional harm by patients or by staff, decreased income or loss of job, feelings of embarrassment, and family disruption through separation at a time of crisis. In addition, the patient is treated in an artificial environment where the lessons learned may not readily generalize to everyday living. Although inpatient care is a potentially important part of the rehabilitation spectrum, final decisions should depend on a calculated balance between the negative and positive aspects of any program.

14.2.6.1.1. The Facility

Good detoxification and rehabilitation for alcohol dependence can be carried out in a dedicated program or on a general medical ward, the latter being especially important when you are dealing with a patient who has serious medical problems or who refuses care from anyone other than his primary physician. In such instances, an element of treatment is medical, but the counselor can work with the treatment staff to carry out adequate detoxification, if needed, and to enhance the patient's receptivity to rehabilitation.

In a similar manner, the patient with concomitant independent major psychiatric disorders and alcoholism (see Section 3.1.2.3) may be best treated by a psychiatrist, or programs that specialize in helping patients with multiple disorders.[113] If these men and women have active suicidal ideation, care should be given in a psychiatric facility, where suicide precautions can be taken. After detoxification, active pharmacological treatment of the psychiatric disorder can be carried out. For patients presenting with independent major depressions who have no history of mania, this usually entails the same treatment given to any patient with unipolar affective disorders, usually SSRIs or tricyclic-type antidepressants. Patients who have both mania and depression are likely to respond best to lithium. However, in the absence of such independent disorders, there are few data that justify the routine use of antidepressants or lithium for the average alcoholic.[114] The rare person with alcoholism with an independent schizophrenia will require relatively high doses of antipsychotic medications such as risperidone (Risperdal). The clinician must take special care to not misdiagnose an alcohol-induced psychosis as schizophrenia (see Section 4.2.4).

For patients without serious medical or psychiatric problems, the treatment facility can be chosen with other considerations in mind. Because the characteristics of the patient rather than those of the treatment program best predict outcome, a particular facility can be selected considering the cost, convenience to the patient, and other patient-related issues. Usually, a treatment program established in a freestanding facility located near a hospital can offer many of the same benefits as a hospital-based inpatient program, and care can be carried out at less cost (because of decreased overhead).

14.2.6.1.2. The Daily Schedule

Rehabilitation includes good education, counseling for the patient *and for the family*, and a long-term commitment to help with life adjustment.[1] The usual inpatient schedule offers daily educational lectures and/or films along with daily counseling and, in some centers, behavior modification therapy. Most programs favor a busy schedule.

14.2.6.1.3. Counseling or Psychotherapy

The patient usually meets daily with a counselor in a group setting to clarify life adjustment issues and to set the stage for outpatient follow-up visits.[1,62] The family should be included in some sessions to help them deal with the life problems and to increase their understanding of alcoholism. Many of these issues, including the role of the family, are also described in a book similar to this one but written specifically to fit the needs of the patients themselves and their families.[1]

Therapy generally centers on the "here and now" of the patient's life, giving him a chance to discuss his adjustment to a life without alcohol and to dealing with the stresses of job, friends, and family. The focus is on the reactions of those around him and on how to handle the situations in which he is most likely to return to drinking.[1] In addition, lecture/discussion sessions can emphasize the dangers of alcohol and can help the patient understand the course and effects of his disease. Along with other forms of therapy, patients should be encouraged to take part in AA.

Comparisons of group and individual counseling for alcoholism reveal that group therapy is as effective as individual therapy. Some authors believe that group therapy has specific *advantages*, such as allowing the patient to share his feelings with a number of other people and teaching him social skills. However, there is little evidence to back up this belief. The group session is an excellent place to begin an interdisciplinary approach, with the psychiatrist or psychologist functioning primarily as supervisor of other therapists.

14.2.6.1.4. Behavioral Approaches

Some alcoholism treatment programs use several specific behavioral approaches for dealing with their patients. This may include the offering of supports such as biofeedback to help with anxiety and with sleep problems, teaching the patient how to relax and handle stress, and exercise programs.[115] Another behaviorally oriented intervention, assertiveness training, is based on the premise that in the midst of their alcoholism (or perhaps because of some original problem existing before the alcoholism began), most patients do not learn how to express their desires and frustrations. The training sessions usually involve education about recognizing situations in which resentment occurs and practicing a variety of methods for handling them.

Behavioral approaches can also form a core resource in the treatment of alcoholism. The behavioral modification procedures are usually added to the regular education and counseling as previously described. Most often, this treatment involves attempts to "teach" the patient *not* to drink by coupling the sight, scent, or taste of alcohol with an unpleasant event, such as vomiting or receiving a mild electric shock to the skin.[116] Chemical aversion treatments, aimed at inducing vomiting in the presence of alcohol, usually utilize such substances as emetine or apomorphine and are generally felt to be more effective than electrical aversion. These treatments are usually offered in hospitals that have special experience with them, and controlled studies indicate that this approach is as effective as any other in dealing with alcoholism. Although it is possible that a specific type of person responds preferentially to behavioral interventions, there are no data to help us choose the appropriate patients.

One modification of the electrical aversion treatment attempts to teach people with alcoholism how to drink in a moderate, controlled manner. This approach may have some potential for persons with isolated problems or abuse, but at present, there are *no* data to justify its use in any clinical setting treating patients with dependence.[1,6] Any use outside the experimental laboratory must await clear demonstration that the assets of such a treatment outweigh the liabilities.

14.2.6.1.5. Addressing Nicotine Dependence

Approximately 65% of men and women who are alcohol dependent are current smokers, and almost 20% are former consumers of nicotine products, usually cigarettes.[117] Among those with alcohol dependence who have had experience with nicotine, between 70 and 80% fulfilled criteria for nicotine dependence. Those people with alcoholism who currently smoke cigarettes are likely to have more severe alcohol dependence, including a higher maximum number of drinks per day and a larger number of alcohol-related life problems, with even higher drinking parameters for alcoholics with nicotine dependence. It is also important to note that the cessation of smoking in nicotine dependence is likely to be associated with higher levels of mood disorders among alcoholics than are observed with alcoholism alone.[118]

The close relationship between these syndromes, along with the high rate of morbidity and mortality associated with each drug, raises the question of whether alcohol treatment programs should incorporate nicotine dependence treatment. Further supporting this possibility are data that indicate that the co-occurrence of the two syndromes might be associated with a slightly worse prognosis among people with alcoholism, and reports that among those who have been dependent on both, lighting up a cigarette might produce an increased craving for alcohol. At the very least, studies indicate that adding a nicotine cessation component to an alcohol dependence program is not likely to diminish the alcohol-related outcomes.[119] Thus, it appears appropriate to incorporate nicotine cessation groups as a routine part of the treatment of substance-use disorders.

14.2.6.2. Outpatient Programs

Inpatient programs have the assets of enhanced intensity of intervention, but cost more and do not treat patients in their real-life settings. In fact, the distinction between inpatient and outpatient approaches is somewhat specious because most inpatient programs are followed by a minimum of 3–6 months of outpatient aftercare, and many patients originally given outpatient care subsequently find themselves as inpatients. Outpatient programs offer the same components as inpatient venues, but do so anywhere from daily to once or twice a week through scheduled group meetings.

Outpatient rehab programs include private care, clinics, day hospital approaches, and the outpatient extensions of inpatient programs.[62] Special type outpatient "interventions" are job-based, and reach out to troubled employees, a large percentage of whom have substance-related problems. In the workplace, the counselor may be able to make an accurate diagnosis and to refer to outpatient or to inpatient therapy. In any setting the patient is counseled about day-to-day life adjustments and is helped to deal with crisis situations. Usually, counseling is begun several times a week, but then it is slowly decreased, so that by the end of a year, the patient is seen about once a month. If problems with drinking or life adjustment occur, the frequency of meeting can be increased to meet the acute need.

For alcohol-dependent men and women who have independent psychiatric disorders (see Section 3.1.2.3) and who do not require inpatient care, referral to a mental-health specialist should be considered. If the diagnosis is an independent depressive disorder, but the patient is *not* felt to be severely incapacitated or suicidal (if suicidal, he should be hospitalized), outpatient treatment with antidepressants is possible. In such instances, the patient should be referred either to a psychiatric clinic or to a psychiatrist for evaluation in addition to his alcoholic rehabilitation.

In delivering care to the person with alcoholism and the *antisocial personality* (ASPD), it is necessary to recognize the high rates of concomitant drug dependence and the elevated risk for the commission of serious crimes by these individuals.[1,120] There is no highly effective treatment for ASPD, but some authors favor more structured group sessions following a therapeutic community model. Outpatient referral to an experienced health specialist is advisable, as there is no evidence that inpatient care is routinely justified.

14.2.7. An Overview

In summary, alcoholic rehabilitation consists of a series of general maneuvers aimed at increasing and maintaining high motivation toward abstinence, helping the individual to reestablish a lifestyle without alcohol (and reaching out to the family), and maximizing physical and mental functioning. Inpatient rehabilitation has not been shown to be essential, although individuals with specific needs may be best reached in the more intensive setting.

Whether in an inpatient or an outpatient mode, most patients are offered group counseling sessions centering on day-to-day living. These cover such problems as reestablishing meaningful relationships with the spouse and with other family members, handling oneself at parties and with friends when alcohol is offered, reestablishing free-time activities and peer groups free of ethanol, adjusting job or avocational activities so they are consistent with abstinence, and so on.

Thus, therapy involves a common-sense approach to group counseling, long-term follow-up, and working with the patient and the family together.

14.3. A SPECIAL CASE: OPIOID ABUSE OR DEPENDENCE (305.50 AND 304.00 IN DSM-IV)

The usual opioid dependent person is younger, may have serious antisocial problems, and is likely to misuse more types of drugs than the usual person with alcoholism. Even with these differences, however, the same general rules for rehab offered above apply. These "basics" include detoxification, reaching out to the family, carefully evaluating efforts, establishing clear patient goals, drug education, and using self-help groups such as NA.

The best predictors of the outcome following treatment for opioid dependence are similar to those discussed for alcohol.[31,121] Men and women entering care with a job, relatively good health, a stable address, and fewer legal problems are more likely to complete treatment and to be abstinent several years later. Such individuals are likely to report lower levels of drug use, fewer arrests, and increased psychological functioning.

While the cognitive-behavioral core of treatment is similar to that offered to alcoholics, the medications used in rehab of the opioid-dependent person are different. The next section discusses some relevant drugs.

14.3.1. Methadone and L-Alpha-Acetyl Methadol (LAAM) and Other Maintenance Approaches

Methadone and LLAM maintenance can be given only in licensed clinics that offer a breadth of counseling and outreach to the social support group, and that have safeguards to minimize the flow of these opioids into illegal channels.[122–124] The patient or client must have been opioid dependent for a year or more and must have been unresponsive to drug-free treatment approaches.

14.3.1.1. Goals

Methadone and other maintenance approaches (e.g., buprenorphene as discussed below) can help people with opioid dependence who are motivated but cannot stay clean to improve functioning. The programs substitute a legal and longer acting drug (e.g., methadone) for the dependence on a shorter acting drug such as heroin. Therefore, they do not go into withdrawal every 4–8 h, can work and maintain family relationships, have less craving for street drugs, better health, are less likely to use needles, and get significantly less feelings of reward if they do take heroin.

Methadone or LAAM should be given only as part of an approach that incorporates all the other aspects of rehabilitation described above.[123,125,126] These include outreach to families, job counseling, legal advice, referral to NA, as well as the "here and now" focused cognitive and supportive psychotherapies. One study of methadone reported abstinence from other drugs in about 60% of people in 6 months and 55% in 1 year when a comprehensive program was used,[127] and another noted 40% were abstinent in 2–3 years.[128] Almost all evaluations note a significant reduction in IV drug use, and a marked decrease in criminality, with impressive cost savings when program expenses are compared to improvements in health, work, and the decrease in legal problems.[129]

14.3.1.2. Methadone Treatment Programs

Methadone is a long-acting opioid that shares almost all of the physiological properties of heroin, including producing physiological dependence, sedation, respiratory depression, and effects on the heart and on muscle. The person who is dependent who has been carefully evaluated may be maintained on a relatively low-dose (30–40 mg/day) or a higher dose (60–120 mg/day) methadone schedule, the former giving fewer side effects but not the same degree of hypothetical "blockade" against the effects of heroin. Higher doses (e.g., 60 mg or more per day) result in higher levels of retention in treatment and in consequent lower levels of arrest, use of street drugs, and health problems.

The drug is administered in an oral liquid given once a day at the treatment facility, with weekend doses taken by the patient at home. To minimize the dropout rate, it is probably best to initiate medication as soon as possible after evaluating the patient. The average methadone maintenance patient stays on the drug for 2 years, although, perhaps reflecting persistent changes in opioid brain systems, many individuals continue to take methadone for very long periods of time.[125,128] This treatment approach can be useful to a wide range of individuals with various ethnic and socioeconomic backgrounds, and improves functioning even in people who have a concomitant dependence on alcohol or cocaine.[130]

After the period of maintenance (usually a year, or longer), the clinician should work closely with the patient to regulate the rate of drug decrease. Anecdotally, some authors recommend very long-term use, but most studies suggest that the dose be lowered within a limited period of time, but as slowly as 3% of the maximum dose a week.

Care must be taken to avoid toxic reactions during the first several weeks of treatment, while clinicians are adjusting the dose. On the other hand, the drug appears to be relatively safe for use during pregnancy, and pregnant women who, while on methadone, do not also engage in the concomitant use of heroin show less birth-related problems than those on street drugs. Methadone-type drugs have been taken by some individuals for over 10 years and are felt by clinicians to be relatively safe and effective.[121] However, the additional problems associated with these drugs include the relatively benign side effect of constipation (seen in 17%), a potentially serious depression, and the possibility that the drug will find its way into illegal channels. Another special problem (seen in as many as one-fourth of methadone maintenance patients) is misuse of drugs like cocaine, Bzs, and alcohol, especially for those individuals who misused other substances before opioids or who took alcohol or drugs concomitantly with them. These problems are discussed in greater depth in Section 6.1.4.

14.3.1.3. LAAM Treatment Programs

Introduced in the 1970s, LAAM is an analogue of methadone that has a 72- to 96-h half-life.[126] Because of its long-lasting effects, it can be given orally every 3 days with a usual dose of 20–30 mg up to 100 mg. The dosing schedule offers an advantage in more rural or sparsely populated areas where it might be more difficult to travel to the clinic. The every third day treatment schedule also saves staff time, and it minimizes potential problems from hanging out with other people who are opioid dependent every day at the clinical. The outcomes for LAAM and methadone are generally similar, but might be a bit better with methadone.

14.3.1.4. Buprenorphene Maintenance Programs

The favorable results observed with methadone and with LAAM have spawned a search for other, possibly safer (e.g., regarding toxic reactions) types of maintenance programs for opioid-dependent persons.[131–133] Recent evaluations have focused on buprenorphene, a mixed agonist-antagonist opioid prescribed IM for pain, with doses of about 0.3 mg being the equivalent of 10 mg of morphine and serving as an effective analgesic over a 6-h period. The half-life of the drug is estimated to be about 2.2 h.

When used as a maintenance approach in people who are opioid dependent, most programs prescribe about 8 mg/day sublingually (held under the tongue for 5 min to facilitate absorption), or as an oral pill, whereas some use 16 mg on Mondays and Wednesdays, along with 32 mg on Fridays. Compared to placebo, buprenorphene is associated with higher rates of program retention, lower proportions of opioid-positive urines, and decreased self-reports of craving. However, the results with buprenorphene may not be quite as good as those observed with 80 mg of methadone.[134,135] Efforts are currently underway to develop a depot form.[136] The most frequently used form of this drug in recent years combines 2–8 mg buprenorphene with 0.5–2 mg of the opioid antagonist naltrexone in a sublingual pill, using the mixture (of Suboxone) to deter patients from crushing the pills and injecting them IV.[133] Buprenorphene maintenance programs should incorporate all of the cognitive-behavioral counseling and relapse prevention groups and other services described above for alcohol treatment and for methadone.

14.3.1.5. Other Maintenance Approaches

Historically, *heroin maintenance* has been used in Great Britain to improve levels of functioning and to decrease relatively dangerous self-injecting behaviors among people who are opioid dependent.[137] However, in a recent survey, few individuals actually receive heroin maintenance, and it is difficult to marshal evidence regarding the efficacy or the safety of this approach. The fact that so few clinicians who are licensed to use heroin maintenance in Europe actually choose to do so might reflect the inherent problems.

At least one study has discussed the possibility of the use of 70 mg/day of *morphine* as a *maintenance approach*.[138] However, a review of that manuscript does not reveal any apparent advantages over methadone, LAAM, or buprenorphene.

14.3.2. Opiate Antagonists

These drugs occupy opiate receptors in the brain and block the effects of heroin and of other opioids.[123,139–141] These antagonists help in the treatment of opioid toxic reactions, and they can be used to test people who say that they are drug-free (the antagonist will precipitate withdrawal if dependence on opioids is present). In rehabilitation, however, the antagonists are administered over an extended period so the patient experiences less of a “high” if he takes opioids.

14.3.2.1. Specific Antagonists

There are a variety of opioid antagonists, which include the following:

1. *Naloxone* (Narcan) is an excellent narcotic antagonist that has no known morphine-like (agonistic) properties. Unfortunately, it is not well absorbed orally, and its action lasts no more than 2–3 h, so up to 3 g/day may be needed to block 15 mg of heroin over a 24-h period.[125]
2. *Nalorphine* (Nalline) was at one time primarily used to test for physical dependence on opioids. When 2–5 mg is administered, a person who is physically dependent will show pupillary dilatation within 15–30 min, whereas a non-dependent person will demonstrate pupillary constriction. If no reaction is noted, 5 mg and then 7 mg can be given at half-hour intervals. This drug has been replaced by naltrexone as a challenge agent.
3. *Naltrexone* (Trexan or Revia) is a widely used narcotic antagonist that can be given orally, has a length of action of approximately 24 h, and has modest side effects. A dose of 50 mg/day is effective in blocking 15 mg of heroin for 24 h, and higher doses (125–150 mg) of naltrexone are capable of blocking 25 mg of IV heroin for 72 h. This drug is free of agonistic properties (e.g., there is no associated high), and there are no known withdrawal symptoms when the medication is stopped. The side effects include mild GI distress, anxiety, and insomnia, all of which tend to disappear over a period of days. However, some patients report a mild sadness (or dysphoria) or impaired ability to feel joy, especially if doses are increased relatively abruptly, and some demonstrate a reversible hepatitis, especially at doses exceeding 300 mg/day. Because of the liver changes, it is unwise to use naltrexone in patients with hepatitis.

In the usual approach during rehabilitation, patients to be started on this antagonist should be relatively healthy and should be free of short-acting opioids for a minimum of 5 days, and longer periods if on methadone. They can then be challenged with 0.8 mg of naloxone to be certain that they will be able to tolerate the longer acting antagonist naltrexone. If patients have not been properly screened and administration of naltrexone precipitates relatively severe withdrawal symptoms, which can last up to 48 h, it may be necessary to give a fairly fast-acting opioid agonist with minimal respiratory depression and minimal histamine release.

Assuming that the challenge dose results in few if any withdrawal symptoms, a 10 mg dose of naltrexone can be given, and over the next 10 days, the daily dose might be increased up to 100 mg on Mondays and Wednesdays and to 150 mg on Fridays.[141,142] Most programs then carry out periodic blood or urine screens for opioid use. The recent development of a depot injectable one per month form of naltrexone may prove useful in enhancing compliance.[73]

Of course, treatment with an antagonist alone is inadequate. Patients will benefit from a close relationship with treatment personnel, and they may also gain from behavioral techniques that help them to learn how to handle anxiety and to cope with life situations. While some opiod dependent persons are reluctant to stay with narcotic antagonist treatment, some do, and this drug may contribute significantly to a better outcome.[143] Although rates of dropout are greater than those observed with methadone maintenance in similar patients, those who do remain in treatment with antagonists might be less likely than methadone patients to take other drugs.

Another potential use of opioid antagonists relates to rapid opioid withdrawal in a hospital setting and in the context of heavy sedation.[144,145] There are few data to support the ability of this approach to contribute subsequent good outcomes in rehabilitation.

14.3.3. Other Possible Treatments

The treatment of opioid dependence is one of the more theoretically sound potential uses of *acupuncture*, as this procedure decreases pain and mobilizes the body's own opioid peptides.[146] Although few well-controlled trials of acupuncture for opioid dependence have been published, there are persistent perceptions that this approach is significantly better than placebo, at least during opioid detoxification.

Similarly, a few trials have reported that low levels of electrical activity administered to the skull in the process of *transcranial neuroelectric stimulation* might have some benefit in the treatment of individuals who are opioid dependent. However, adequate data are not available.[147] Antidepressants have also been considered for opioid treatment,[148] but controlled data are lacking.

Potentially interesting approaches have also developed from *folk medicine.* For example, the herb henantos has been used by Vietnamese opioid-dependent persons who live in poppy-growing areas and who must learn to cope with withdrawal at times of crop failures.[149] Anecdotal reports indicate that the consumption of a half liter per day for 4 days of a brew made from this herb, followed by lower doses ingested through capsules for 6 months, helps people function despite the lack of readily available opioids.

14.3.4. Drug-Free Programs

Most residential treatments offered to the person who is opioid dependent utilize modifications of the therapeutic community (TC) concept first proposed by Maxwell Jones.[150,151] This is an exception to the general rule of short-term live-in rehabilitation. Although some programs last a month or less, some require participation for a year or more where the dependent person is taken out of the street culture and given a new view of life within the group. In this structure, group members, including recovering dependent leaders, constantly confront each behavior in an attempt to help the participants gain insight and find a new and more successful lifestyle for coping with problems. Most large cities in the United States have programs run on these Synanon or Day Top models.

It is difficult to compare results from TCs with those seen with methadone maintenance, as the patients in the former tend to be young and Caucasian, whereas those in the latter tend to be older and are more often minority group members. However, individuals assigned to methadone maintenance are more likely to follow through and to appear at the clinic for care and may be more likely to stay in treatment for 1 year. As is true in other approaches, the best prognosis for people in TCs is for those who are employed, have high school diplomas, have had less intense involvement with heroin, have less extensive jail records, and who stay in treatment for 2 months or longer. The most usual retention rate in a TC is approximately 50% at 12 months, but some studies reveal figures of less than 20%.

14.3.5. The Person with Dependence on Prescribed Opioids

The middle-class individual who is primarily dependent on prescription opioids may be more similar to the person with alcoholism in general life outlook and in history than to the person who is dependent on "street" opioids. There is little good information on the best rehabilitation mode for this population, and the final program should be tailored to the specific patient or client, perhaps using the same approach applied to the person with alcoholism.

An important variation is the individual who developed his or her opioid dependence in the context of chronic pain.[152] In viewing the optimal care of these challenging patients, it is important to recognize that although many blame the pain syndrome as the initial cause of their dependence, the best data sometimes indicate otherwise.[153] The chronic self-administration of opioids is likely to produce tolerance to the painkilling effects of these drugs, and during periods of withdrawal (which will occur daily for short-acting drugs) the feelings of pain are likely to markedly escalate.

Regardless of the causes, treatment of individuals with both chronic pain syndromes and with opioid dependence who seek out the drugs in larger doses than prescribed is quite complex. Although it would not be appropriate for a brief text such as this to review the treatment of such syndromes in detail, there is an excellent publication to which the readers can turn.[154]

14.4. A SPECIAL CASE: REHABILITATION OF STIMULANT ABUSE OR DEPENDENCE (305.70, 304.40, 305.60, AND 304.20 IN DSM-IV)

Amphetamines and cocaine produce powerful feelings of craving, which, along with a protracted abstinence syndrome, can make abstinence difficult to maintain.[155] The protracted withdrawal can persist for many months, during which the patient is likely to demonstrate intermittent moodiness, problems concentrating, and high levels of craving. Associated drug-seeking can be intense.

Rehabilitation efforts aimed at people who are stimulant dependent follow the same general principles outlined in preceding sections.[156,157] The need for early identification, gathering information from resource persons as well as from patients, and the importance of careful physical examinations must be emphasized. As is true of all substance-related problems, the mainstay of rehabilitation efforts often boils down to using cognitive, behavioral, and psychological approaches that increase and maintain high levels of motivation for abstinence, while working closely with patients to help them rebuild their lives without abusing any substances.[122,158,159] Although the specific implementation of these general rules differs with each individual, a careful rereading of Section 14.2 can be most helpful, because issues similar to those experienced in alcoholic rehabilitation are experienced with patients entering rehabilitation for cocaine or for amphetamine dependence.

As is true for other substances, patients will often respond well to outpatient rehabilitation efforts.[160] Indications to hospitalize for detoxification and for rehabilitation have not been carefully established, but some suggestions have been offered. Similar to the guidelines used for alcoholism, hospitalization would seem appropriate for patients with severe psychiatric disturbances (e.g., psychoses or suicidal depressions) whether substance induced or independent of their drug dependence, for those dependent on multiple drugs, and for individuals with such severe social impairment that their survival on a day-to-day basis could be jeopardized, as well as those who, in their outpatient participation, seemed unable or unwilling to stop their stimulant dependence. It is also probable that individuals with histories of more intensive drug problems might require at least short-term hospitalization.

14.4.1. Cognitive, Behavioral, and Counseling Approaches

Counseling and brief, relatively superficial, forms of psychotherapy are also important in the treatment of people who are stimulant dependent, with evidence that the more hours of therapy, the better the outcome. This treatment most usually takes the form of discussing issues such as relationships with relatives and friends, the need to establish a drug-free peer group, the importance of structuring and using active free time, and so on. A more intense form of interpersonal psychotherapy, often used in conjunction with relapse prevention, has also been proposed. The latter focuses on the need to decrease impulsiveness by carefully thinking about events before acting, the need to recognize the context in which craving is most likely to be intense, and the need to recognize the identifying cues that stimulate the craving so these situations can be avoided.

Several behavioral approaches are also potentially useful. One involves contingency contracting, where the patient or client agrees to perform certain behaviors and to accept both rewards and potentially adverse results. The latter, often invoked as a result of a "dirty" urine test, can include giving money to charity or, for physicians who are dependent, a potential loss of license. Another behavioral approach offers vouchers that can be exchanged for money, with the value of each voucher increasing with each consecutive negative urine test.

While offering general supports, it is important to recognize the potential role of self-help groups.[156] CA, or similar groups such as NA or AA, can complement other treatment efforts. Because many people who are stimulant dependent are also dependent on alcohol and on other drugs, the selection of the specific type of organization often reflects the individual's own wishes as well as the specific groups available. A point similar to that made in Section 14.2.4 is that through such groups, people who are cocaine dependent are likely to meet others who are willing to help them 24 h a day, are able to develop a cohort of drug- and alcohol-free friends, and to learn that it is possible to enjoy oneself while free of drugs and of alcohol. For individuals seeking such additional supports, these groups can also offer a structured series of steps to follow in maintaining abstinence and freedom from drugs while offering a belief system that for some can be quite comforting. Formal treatment approaches that facilitate these 12-step self-help groups have been shown to be more effective than general supportive psychotherapy in individuals dependent on both alcohol and cocaine.

14.4.2. The Limited Role of Medications in Rehabilitation from Stimulants

No medication has been shown by adequate double-blind, controlled trials to add significantly to cognitive, behavioral, or general counseling techniques during the rehabilitation phase of the treatment of men and women who are stimulant dependent.[161] Many pharmacological approaches have been touted over the years, only to turn out to be no better than placebo when more carefully evaluated.

Numerous different types of medications have been proposed to help amphetamine and cocaine dependent individuals maintain sobriety or decrease their intensity of involvement with stimulants. Antidepressant medications are at least theoretically attractive as potential adjuncts to controlling mood problems, and, therefore, optimizing sobriety. However, most controlled evaluations of these drugs do not support their superiority to placebo, and at least one study raised the possibility of enhanced toxicity for stimulants among patients taking antidepressants.[162]

Disulfiram (Antabuse) might be useful in cocaine-dependent men and women.[26,163] The mechanism of action of this aldehyde dehydrogenase inhibitor in stimulant dependent individuals is not known, although perhaps concomitant abstinence from alcohol might help control amphetamine and cocaine use.

Several anticonvulsant drugs, each of which directly or indirectly increase levels of GABA have been described as potentially useful in the treatment of stimulant dependence, but most studies are fairly short term and incorporate relatively few subjects.[164–166] The observation that stimulant-dependent individuals may have at least temporary periods of cognitive dysfunction, have also led to the proposal of using either aspirin or calcium channel antagonists to decrease the intensity of the cognitive problems and, presumably, increase the effectiveness of cognitive and behavioral treatments.[167,168] However, there are no impressive clinical data to support this contention.

Some pharmacological treatment approaches have been developed on the basis of the impact that stimulants have on dopamine receptor systems.[169] These have included agonist-like treatments with amphetamines, methylphenidate (Ritalin), and modafinil (Provigil).[161,170] However, while these and other dopamine-boosting drugs [e.g., amantidine (Symmetrel) 100 mg TID[171]] were worth considering in the treatment of stimulant dependence, there are few convincing controlled data to support their use, or to override concerns regarding the potential misuse of the medications. Nor are there double-blind controlled data that support the potential usefulness of acupuncture for stimulant-related syndromes.[172]

Finally, researchers have been able to produce proteins that can attach to the cocaine molecule and stimulate the production of antibodies that then markedly diminish the ability of subsequent doses of cocaine to cross the blood–brain barrier and cause intoxication.[173] Although animals and humans thus "immunized" against cocaine showed few additional ill effects of the procedure, a great deal of work still needs to be done to evaluate the efficacy and safety of this approach.

14.4.3. A Recap

Efforts aimed at rehabilitation of people who are stimulant dependent follow the same general supportive and commonsense approaches suggested for rehabilitation of people dependent on other types of drugs. As is true of dependence on substances in the two other categories known to be physically addicting (brain depressants and opioids), rehabilitation efforts are jeopardized by the probability of a protracted, less intense abstinence phase likely to last many months and even up to 1 year. At present, clinicians should focus on general supports, supportive psychotherapy, outreach to families, and the use of self-help groups such as CA. Until more impressive data accrue, medications should probably not be used in usual clinical practice.

14.5 A SPECIAL CASE: NICOTINE DEPENDENCE (305.10 IN DSM-IV)

14.5.1. Some General Comments

The treatment of people who are nicotine dependent involves blending many of the efforts outlined in earlier sections of this chapter.[174,175] The goal, as always, is to alleviate withdrawal symptoms, use counseling and education to enhance and maintain high levels of motivation, and use cognitive and behavioral therapies. As discussed below, several pharmacological approaches are also useful.

Intervention and rehabilitation efforts with men and women who are nicotine dependent should focus on abstinence, although smoking reduction is a step in the right direction.[176] Some cigarette users will try changing to other forms of tobacco, but because they will probably continue to inhale, it may do little good to advise them to switch to a pipe or a cigar. Others may turn to low-yield or smaller cigarettes, might attempt to smoke only part of a cigarette, or might use filters that mix more air with the smoke. Unfortunately, this approach rarely works to the patient's advantage because he or she is likely to inhale more deeply or use more of the low-yield brands than of the high-yield ones.

14.5.2. Behavioral Approaches

Although many cigarette users seem to be able to stop at least temporarily on their own, and some actually achieve and maintain abstinence without help, a significant percentage turn to specialized smoking clinics that incorporate behavioral approaches. Treatment can be expected to result in some fairly rapid level of improvement (if abstinence is used as a measure), but it is unlikely that this level will be maintained for extended periods unless the patient is given "refresher" courses. Some variation on these clinics using phone or mailed feedback are being evaluated.[177,178]

One type of behavior modification involves self-control strategies. Here, the smoker is asked to keep reminding himself why he wants to stop and to smoke in the least pleasurable way possible. For instance, he may be told never to smoke after meals, always to smoke alone, or to begin smoking his least-preferred brand.

Other behavioral approaches center on aversive conditioning, coupling an unpleasant event with the nicotine intake. The use of mild electric shocks to the hands while smoking does not appear to be as effective as aversions more directly related to the smoking itself. Many programs use a forced consumption of two to three times the usual amount of tobacco, having stale and warm smoke blown in the smoker's face, or enforced rapid chain smoking. Cognitive restructuring and self-hypnosis can also be of potential use. As is true with all forms of behavior modification, the results are probably enhanced when the patient has a positive relationship with the counselor.

14.5.3. Pharmacological Approaches

14.5.3.1. Nicotine Replacement

Although some individuals can stop smoking without medications, this process is especially difficult for men and women who have failed in prior attempts to stop nicotine, those who complain of withdrawal symptoms, or individuals who demonstrate more intense signs of nicotine dependence (for example, usually smoking a cigarette soon after waking up). For these people it is likely that the more acute and protracted symptoms of withdrawal are contributing to relapse. Therefore, several different methods have been developed to help the individual cope with the discomfort through diminishing levels of nicotine replacement. While special care must be used in the context of some other conditions, the approach can be helpful.[179] When used in the context of a cognitive and behavioral program, these approaches are likely to improve the chance of successful smoking cessation by between 1.6- and 2.4-fold.

The most established treatment over the years has used *nicotine gum*.[176] This is available OTC as 2 or 4 mg of nicotine polacrilex, a form of the drug that promotes the buccal absorption and inhibits destruction in the GI tract. A 2 mg piece of gum produces approximately 30% of the blood steady-state level of nicotine seen after smoking, with peak levels at approximately 30 min. The drug is usually prescribed as one piece to be chewed every 15–30 min as needed to deal with craving, with most patients taking between 10 and 20 pieces per day over 3 months or so. Nicotine gum seems to be well tolerated by most individuals, although some report difficulty in chewing the substance, and others complain of a burning sensation in the mouth or throat. This form of treatment should not be used by people with preexisting mouth inflammation, esophagitis, or people with peptic ulcer disease.

The *nicotine skin patch* may be more popular for treating nicotine dependence.[175,180] There are multiple preparations of the patch including three that produce clinically relevant blood levels for 24 h, and one (to facilitate sleep) that works for 16 h. The 24-h patches come in 21 or 22 mg doses, whereas the shorter duration patch has 15 mg. These are applied to the skin every morning, with a resulting peak nicotine blood level within 6–10 h, after which the levels stay at a steady state for hours. After 4–6 weeks, the dose is usually decreased to a 14 mg patch for 24 h or a 10 mg patch for 16 h, which after 2–4 more weeks is replaced by 7- and 5-mg patches, respectively.

The third preparation is the nicotine *inhaler*, which has the advantage of more rapid absorption. There is also a nicotine *nasal spray* that delivers approximately 1 mg per administration.[181] The spray, when used regularly, gives nicotine blood levels that are lower than those usually associated with smoking, and might produce throat irritation, sneezing, and coughing.

14.5.3.2. Antidepressants

There is a complex but interesting potential relationship between smoking, smoking cessation, and major depressive episodes.[182] Therefore, it is easy to understand why several studies have evaluated the potential usefulness of various types of antidepressants as part of smoking cessation programs, even for patients who do not have an independent major mood disorder. While, overall, there is an absence of convincing data regarding antidepressants in general, there are some exceptions,[175,183,184] especially when medications are used in the context of cognitive and behavioral therapy. The effects of these drugs could rest with mood stabilization, but might also reflect changes in neurochemistry, especially in dopamine.

The most consistent data support the effectiveness of an antidepressant medication known to also affect dopamine functioning.[185] Bupropion is marketed as an antidepressant under the name Wellbutrin, and for smoking cessation as Zyban, although it is still the same drug despite the two names. Studies have consistently demonstrated that this drug (used in doses of 100–300 mg/day—levels similar to those used for major depressive episodes) is superior to placebo when used as part of a smoking cessation program.[185,186] Interesting data are also available regarding the potential usefulness of another type of an antidepressant, selective monoamine oxidase B inhibitors such as selegiline (Eldepryl).[187,188] Smokers have been reported to have lower levels of MAO B brain activity, and the prescription of an MAO B inhibitor such as selegiline (e.g., 5 mg twice per day) has been reported to reduce craving and enhance abstinence when used as part of a broader smoking cessation treatment approach.[188] These are doses similar to those used for the treatment of parkinsonism. There are other studies suggesting the usefulness of additional antidepressants including nortriptyline (Pamelor) in doses comparable to those used for depressive disorders.[189] Thus, antidepressant medication is worth considering in the treatment of smoking cessation, with the most plentiful data available regarding bupropion.

14.5.3.3. Clonidine (Catapres)

Another type of drug has been discussed for helping alleviate withdrawal and perhaps helping patients achieve abstinence.[190] Clonidine has been reported to significantly decrease feelings of tension, anxiety, irritability, and restlessness as well as to decrease feelings of craving during smoking cessation. Clonidine can be given orally as 0.1 mg several times a day, or as a skin patch of 0.1–0.4 mg/day.[190] However, although some reports are promising, there is debate about the effectiveness of this drug in smoking cessation and a lack of data on the optimal length of treatment. Also, the potentially significant side effect profile of this drug argues against its prescription until more data accumulate.

14.5.3.4. Other Treatments

There has been much interest over the years in the potential usefulness of *acupuncture* in the treatment of smoking cessation. A recent meta-analysis of nine trials involving 2,707 patients showed a modest 1.5-fold increase in the odds ratio of abstinence at 6–12 months.

Other pharmacological-like approaches that have been touted over the years include *appetite suppressants* and *antianxiety medications*, although the results have not been promising.[190] Some OTC preparations contain a nicotine-like substance, *lobeline*, but the higher dose of this medication (8 mg) is associated with prominent side effects of dizziness and digestive disturbances, and the data regarding its efficacy are not very convincing.[190] Another drug that affects the body's nicotine receptors is *mechanmylamine*, but this agent has not been shown to be highly effective, and is associated with dry mouth, headache, and GI problems.[190] A cannabinoid antagonist, rimonabant (Acomplia), has recently been proposed for smoking cessation, and for obesity and perhaps other substance dependence rehab treatment. The double blind short term trials for this drug in smoking cessation are promising.[191] Finally, similar to the case with cocaine, efforts are underway to develop a vaccine for nicotine.[192]

14.5.4. A Summary

Considering the morbidity and mortality associated with tobacco use (see Section 11.3), treatment of heavy smokers and users of smokeless tobacco appears to be warranted. Much of the general information regarding rehabilitation applies here because the most prominent therapeutic efforts involve treatment of withdrawal along with education, behavioral techniques, and the judicious use of medications. Tobacco users should first be encouraged to stop on their own, and physicians as well as other health-care deliverers should do all they can to help them achieve and maintain abstinence. However, for those individuals for whom these approaches are not enough, referral to a specialized smoking clinic is worth consideration. Such clinics do seem to have enhanced levels of effectiveness over efforts given in the physician's office. Nicotine replacement therapy is also appropriate when needed, and, although not recommended for general use at present, some antidepressants, especially bupropion, might prove to be useful.

REFERENCES

1. Schuckit, M. A. *Educating Yourself About Alcohol and Drugs.* New York: Plenum Publishing Co., 1998.
2. McLellan, A. T. Have we evaluated addiction treatment correctly? Implications from a chronic care perspective (editorial). *Addiction 97:*249–252, 2002.
3. Watkins, K., Pincus, H. A., Tanielian, T. L., & Lloyd, J. Using the chronic care model to improve treatment of alcohol use disorders in primary care settings. *Journal of Studies on Alcohol 64:*209–218, 2003.

4. Cox, W. M., Rosenberg, H., Hodgins, A. H. A., McCartney, J. I., & Maurer, K. A. United Kingdom and United States healthcare providers recommendations of abstinence versus controlled drinking. *Alcohol & Alcoholism 39:*130–134, 2004.
5. Schuckit, M. A. Penny-wise, ton-foolish? The recent movement to abolish inpatient alcohol and drug treatment. *Journal of Studies on Alcohol 59:*5–7, 1998.
6. Simpson, D. D., Joe, G. W., & Broome, K. M. A national 5-year follow-up of treatment outcomes for cocaine dependence. *Archives of General Psychiatry 59:*538–544, 2002.
7. Gossop, M., Marsden, J., Stewart, D., & Kidd, T. The National Treatment Outcome Research Study (NTORS): 4–5 year follow-up results. *Addiction 98:*291–303, 2003.
8. Long, C. G., Williams, M., & Hollin, C. R. Treating alcohol problems: A study of programme effectiveness and cost effectiveness according to length and delivery of treatment. *Addiction 93:*561–571, 1998.
9. Weisner, C., Ray, G. T., Mertens, J. R., Satre, D. D., & Moore, C. Short-term alcohol and drug treatment outcomes predict long-term outcome. *Drug and Alcohol Dependence 71:*281–294, 2003.
10. Tucker, J. A., Vuchinich, R. E., & Rippens, P. D. Environmental contexts surrounding resolution of drinking problems among problem drinkers with different help-seeking experiences. *Journal of Studies on Alcohol 63:*334–341, 2002.
11. Fleming, M. F., Mundt, M. P., French, M. T., Baier Manwell, L., Stauffacher, E. A., & Lawton Barry, K. Brief physician advice for problem drinkers: Long-term efficacy and benefit–cost analyses. *Alcoholism: Clinical and Experimental Research 26:*36–43, 2002.
12. Moyer, A., Finney, J. W., Swearingen, C. E., & Vergun, P. Brief interventions for alcohol problems: A meta-analytic review of controlled investigations in treatment-seeking and non-treatment-seeking populations. *Addiction 97:*279–292, 2002.
13. Anderson, P., Laurant, M., Kaner, E., Wensing, M., & Grol, R. Engaging general practitioners in the management of hazardous and harmful alcohol consumption: Results of a meta-analysis. *Journal of Studies on Alcohol 65:*191–199, 2004.
14. Berglund, M. A better widget? Three lessons for improving addiction treatment from a meta-analytical study. *Addiction 100:*742–750, 2005.
15. McCrady, B. S., Hayaki, J., Epstein, E. E., & Hirsch, L. S. Testing hypothesized predictors of change in conjoint behavioral alcoholism treatment for men. *Alcoholism: Clinical and Experimental Research 26:*463–470, 2002.
16. Marques, A. C. P. R., & Formigoni, M. L. O. S. Comparison of individual and group cognitive-behavioral therapy for alcohol and/or drug-dependent patients. *Addiction 96:*835–846, 2001.
17. McAweeney, M. J., Zucker, R. A., Fitzgerald, H. E., Puttler, L. I., & Wong, M. M. Individual and partner predictors of recovery from alcohol use disorder over a nine year interval: Findings from a community sample of alcoholic married men. *Journal of Studies on Alcohol 66:*220–228, 2005.
18. Bond, J., Kaskutas, L. A., & Weisner, C. The persistent influence of social networks and Alcohol Anonymous on abstinence. *Journal of Studies on Alcohol 64:*579–588, 2003.
19. Tonigan, J. S., Miller, W. R., & Schermer, C. Atheists, agnostics and Alcoholics Anonymous. *Journal of Studies on Alcohol 63:*534–541, 2002.
20. Sobell, L. C., Sobell, M. B., Leo, G. I., Agrawall, S., Johnson-Young, L., & Cunningham, J. A. Promotion self-change with alcohol abusers: A community-level mail intervention based on natural recovery studies. *Alcoholism: Clinical and Experimental Research 26:*936–948, 2002.
21. Anzai, Y., Kuriyama, S., Nishino, Y., Takahashi, K., Ohkubo, T., Ohmori, K., Tsubono, Y., & Tsuji, I. Impact of alcohol consumption upon medical care utilization and costs in men: 4-year observation of National Health Insurance Beneficiaries in Japan. *Addiction 100:*19–27, 2005.
22. Godfrey, C., Stewart, D., & Gossop, M. Economic analysis of costs and consequences of the treatment of drug misuse: 2-year outcome data from the National Treatment Outcome Research Study (NTORS). *Addiction 99:*697–707, 2004.

23. Corry, J., Sanderson, K., Issakidis, C., Andrews, G., & Lapsley, H. Evidence-based care for alcohol use disorders is affordable. *Journal of Studies on Alcohol 65:*521–529, 2004.
24. Schuckit, M. A., Danko, G. P., Smith, T. L., Hesselbrock, V., Kramer, J., & Bucholz, K. A 5-year prospective evaluation of DSM-IV alcohol dependence with and without a physiological component. *Alcoholism: Clinical and Experimental Research 27:*818–825, 2003.
25. American Psychiatric Association. *Diagnostic and Statistical Manual of Mental Disorders* (4th ed., text revision, DSM-IV-TR). Washington, DC: American Psychiatric Association, 2000.
26. Carroll, K. M., Fenton, L. R., Ball, S. A., Nich, C., Frankforter, T. L., Shi, J., & Rounsaville, B. J. Efficacy of disulfiram and cognitive behavior therapy in cocaine-dependent outpatients: Randomized placebo-controlled trial. *Archives of General Psychiatry 61:*264–272, 2004.
27. Kashner, T. M., Rosenheck, R., Campinell, A. B., Suris, A., and the CWT Study Team. Impact of work therapy on health status among homeless, substance-dependent veterans: A randomized controlled trial. *Archives of General Psychiatry 59:*938–944, 2002.
28. McCambridge, J., & Strang, J. The efficacy of single-session motivational interviewing in reducing drug consumption and perceptions of drug-related risk and harm among young people: Results from a multi-site cluster randomized trial. *Addiction 99:*39–52, 2004.
29. Project MATCH Research Group. Matching alcoholism treatments to client heterogeneity: Project MATCH three-year drinking outcomes. *Alcoholism: Clinical and Experimental Research 22:*1300–1311, 1998.
30. Sterling, R. C., Gottheil, E., Weinstein, S. P., & Serota, R. The effect of therapist/patient race- and sex-matching in individual treatment. *Addiction 96:*1015–1022, 2001.
31. Moos, R. H., & Moos, B. S. Long-term influence of duration and intensity of treatment on previously untreated individuals with alcohol use disorders. *Addiction 98:*325–327, 2003.
32. Spicer, R. S. & Miller, T. R. Impact of a workplace peer-focused substance abuse prevention and early intervention program. *Alcoholism: Clinical and Experimental Research 29:*609-611, 2005.
33. Brown, T. G., Seraganian, P., Tremblay, J., & Annis, H. Process and outcome changes with relapse prevention versus 12-step aftercare programs for substance abusers. *Addiction 97:*677–689, 2002.
34. Witkiewitz, K., & Marlatt, G. A. Relapse prevention for alcohol and drug problems. That was Zen, this is Tao. *American Psychologist 59:*224–235, 2004.
35. Finney, J. W., Hahn, A. C., & Moos, R. H. The effectiveness of inpatient and outpatient treatment for alcohol abuse: The need to focus on mediators and moderators of setting effects. *Addiction 91:*1773–1796, 1996.
36. Zhang, Z., Friedmann, P. D., & Gerstein, D. R. Does retention matter? Treatment duration and improvement in drug use. *Addiction 98:*673–684, 2003.
37. Magura, S., Staines, G., Kosanke, N., Rosenblum, A., Foote, J., DeLuca, A., & Bali, P. Predictive validity of the ASAM patient placement criteria for naturalistically matched vs. mismatched alcoholism patients. *The American Journal of Addictions 12:*386–397, 2003.
38. Carmen, B., Angeles, M., Ana, M., & Maria, A. J. Efficacy and safety of naltrexone and acamprosate in the treatment of alcohol dependence: A systematic review. *Addiction 99:*811–828, 2004.
39. Gossop, M., Harris, J., Best, D., Man, L.-H., Manning, V., Marshall, J., & Strang, J. Is attendance at Alcoholics Anonymous meetings after inpatient treatment related to improved outcomes? A 6-month follow-up study. *Alcohol & Alcoholism 38:*421–426, 2003.
40. Zemore, S. E., & Kaskutas, L. A. Helping, spirituality and Alcoholics Anonymous in recovery. *Journal of Studies on Alcohol 65:*383–391, 2004.
41. Daley, D. C., & Marlatt, G. A. Relapse prevention. In J. H. Lowinson, P. Ruiz, R. B. Millman, & J. G. Langrod (Eds.), *Substance Abuse: A Comprehensive Textbook* (4th ed.). Baltimore, MD: Lippincott, Williams & Wilkins, 2004, pp. 772–785.
42. Weisner, C., Delucchi, K., Matzger, H., & Schmidt, L. The role of community services and informal support on five-year drinking trajectories of alcohol dependent and problem drinkers. *Journal of Studies on Alcohol 64:*862–873, 2003.
43. Wiesbeck, G. A. Gender-specific issues in alcoholism—introduction. *Archives of Women's Mental Health 6:223*–224, 2003.

44. Kaskutas, L. A., Zhang, L., French, M. T., & Witbrodt, J. Women's programs versus mixed-gender day treatment: Results from a randomized study. *Addiction 100:*60–69, 2005.
45. Lynskey, M. T., Day, C., & Hall, W. Alcohol and other drug use disorders among older-aged people. *Drug and Alcohol Review 22:*125–133, 2003.
46. Schutte, K. K., Nichols, K. A., Brennan, P. L., & Moos, R. H. A ten-year follow-up of older former problem drinkers: Risk of relapse and implications of successfully sustained remission. *Journal of Studies on Alcohol 64:*367–374, 2003.
47. Cuijpers, P., Riper, H., & Lemmers, L. The effects on mortality of brief interventions for problem drinking: A meta-analysis. *Addiction 99:*839–845, 2004.
48. Ballesteros, J., Duffy, J. C., Querejeta, I., Arino, J., & Gonzalez-Pinto, A. Efficacy of brief interventions for hazardous drinkers in primary care: Systematic review and meta-analyses. *Alcoholism: Clinical and Experimental Research 28:*608–618, 2004.
49. Zarkin, G. A., Bray, J. W., Davis, K. L., Babor, T. F., & Higgins-Biddle, J. C. The costs of screening and brief intervention for risky alcohol use. *Journal of Studies on Alcohol 64:*849–857, 2003.
50. Wutzke, S. E., Conigrave, K. M., Saunders, J. B., & Hall, W. D. The long-term effectiveness of brief interventions for unsafe alcohol consumption: A 10-year follow-up. *Addiction 97:*665–675, 2002.
51. Rosenberg, H., Devine, E. G., & Rothrock, N. Acceptance of moderate drinking by alcoholism treatment services in Canada. *Journal of Studies on Alcohol 57:*559–562, 1996.
52. Loneck, B., Garrett, J. A., & Banks, S. M. A comparison of the Johnson Intervention with four other methods of referral to outpatient treatment. *American Journal of Drug and Alcohol Abuse 22:*233–246, 1996.
53. Morgenstern, J., Bux, D., Labouvie, E., Blanchard, K. A., & Morgan, T. J. Examining mechanisms of action in 12-step treatment: The role of 12-step cognitions. *Journal of Studies on Alcohol 63:*665–672, 2002.
54. Cook, C. C. H. Addiction and spirituality. *Addiction 99:*539–551, 2004.
55. Pagano, M. E., Friend, K. B., Tonigan, J. S., & Stout, R. L. Helping other alcoholics in Alcoholics Anonymous and drinking outcomes: Findings from Project MATCH. *Journal of Studies on Alcohol 65:*766–773. 2004.
56. He, D.-Y., McGough, N. N. H., Ravindranathan, A., Jeanblanc, J., Logrip, M. L., Phamluong, K., Janak, P. H., & Ron, D. Glial cell line-derived neurotrophic factor mediates the desirable actions of the anti-addiction drug ibogaine against alcohol consumption. *The Journal of Neuroscience 25:*619–628, 2005.
57. Dundon, W., Lynch, K. G., Pettinati, H. M., & Lipkin, C. Treatment outcomes in Type A and B alcohol dependence 6 months after serotonergic pharmacotherapy. *Alcoholism: Clinical and Experimental Research 28:*1065–1073, 2004.
58. Guardia, J., Segura, L., Gonzalvo, B., Iglesias, L., Roncero, C., Caardus, M., & Casas, M. A double-blind, placebo-controlled study of olanzapine in the treatment of alcohol-dependence disorder. *Alcoholism: Clinical and Experimental Research 28:*736–745, 2004.
59. Flannery, B. A., Garbutt, J. C., Cody, M. W., Renn, W., Grace, K., Osborne, M., Crosby, K., Morreale, M., & Trivette, A. Baclofen for alcohol dependence: A preliminary open-label study. *Alcoholism: Clinical and Experimental Research 28:*1517–1523, 2004.
60. Johnson, B. A., Swift, R. M., Ait-Daoud, N., DiClemente, C. C., Javors, M. A., & Malcolm, R. J., Jr. Development of novel pharmacotherapies for the treatment of alcohol dependence: Focus on antiepileptics. *Alcoholism: Clinical and Experimental Research 28:* 295–301, 2004.
61. Bischof, G., Rumpf, H.-J., Hapke, U., Meyer, C., & John, U. Remission from alcohol dependence without help: How restrictive should our definition of treatment be? *Journal of Studies on Alcohol 63:*229–236, 2002.
62. American Psychiatric Association, Work Group on Substance Use Disorders. Practice guideline for the treatment of patients with substance use disorders: Alcohol, cocaine, opioids. *American Journal of Psychiatry 153:*1–59, 1995.

63. Namkoong, K., Lee, B.-O., Lee, P.-G., Choi, M.-J., Lee, E., & Korean Acamprosate Clinical Trial Investigators. Acamprosate in Korean alcohol-dependent patients: A multi-centre randomized, double-blind, placebo-controlled study. *Alcohol & Alcoholism 38:*135–141, 2003.
64. Kranzler, H. R., & Van Kirk, J. Efficacy of naltrexone and acamprosate for alcoholism treatment: A meta-analysis. *Alcoholism: Clinical and Experimental Research 25:*1335–1341, 2001.
65. Mann, K., Lehert, P., & Morgan, M. Y. The efficacy of acamprosate in the maintenance of abstinence in alcohol-dependent individuals: Results of a meta-analysis. *Alcoholism: Clinical and Experimental Research 28:*51–63, 2004.
66. Brasser, S. M., McCaul, M. E., & Houtsmuller, E. J. Alcohol effects during acamprosate treatment: A dose–response study in humans. *Alcoholism: Clinical and Experimental Research 28:*1074–1083, 2004.
67. al Qatari, M., Khan, S., Harris, B., & Littleton, J. Acamprosate is neuroprotective against glutamate-induced excitotoxicity when enhanced by ethanol withdrawal in neocortical cultures of fetal rat brain. *Alcoholism: Clinical and Experimental Research 25:*1383–1392, 2001.
68. Heyser, C. J., Moc, K., & Koob, G. F. Effects of naltrexone alone and in combination with acamprosate on the alcohol deprivation effect in rats. *Neuropsychopharmacology 28:*1463–1471, 2003.
69. Rubio, G., Ponce, G., Rodriguez-Jimenez, R., Jimenez-Arriero, M. A., Hoenicka, J., & Palomo, T. Clinical predictors of response to naltrexone in alcoholic patients: Who benefits most from treatment with naltrexone? *Alcohol & Alcoholism 40:*227–233, 2005.
70. O'Malley, S. S., Rounsaville, B. J., Farren, C., Namkoong, K., Wu, R., Robinson, J., & O'Connor, P. G. Initial and maintenance naltrexone treatment for alcohol dependence using primary care vs specialty care: A nested sequence of 3 randomized trials. *Archives of Internal Medicine 163:*1695–1704, 2003.
71. Krystal, J. H., Cramer, J. A., Krol, W. F., Kirk, G. F., & Rosenheck, R. A. Naltrexone in the treatment of alcohol dependence. *The New England Journal of Medicine 345:*1734–1739, 2001.
72. Rohsenow, D. J. What place does naltrexone have in the treatment of alcoholism? *CNS Drugs 18:*547–560, 2004.
73. Srisurapanont, M. & Jarusuraisin, N. Naltrexone for the treatment of alcoholism: A meta-analysis of randomized controlled trials. *International Journal of Neuropsychopharmacology 8:*267–280, 2005.
74. Kranzler, H. R., Wesson, D. R., & Billot, L., for the Drug Abuse Sciences Naltrexone Depot Study Group. Naltrexone depot for treatment of alcohol dependence: A multicenter, randomized, placebo-controlled clinical trial. *Alcoholism: Clinical and Experimental Research 28:*1051–1059, 2004.
75. Johnson, B. A., Ait-Daoud, N., Aubin, H.-J., van den Brink, W., Guzzetta, R., Loewy, J., Silverman, B., & Ehrich, E. A pilot evaluation of the safety and tolerability of repeat dose administration of long-acting injectable naltrexone (Vivitrex®) in patients with alcohol dependence. *Alcoholism: Clinical and Experimental Research 28:*1356–1361, 2004.
76. Drobes, D. J., Anton, R. F., Thomas, S. E., & Voronin, K. A clinical laboratory paradigm for evaluating medication effects on alcohol consumption: Naltrexone and nalmefene. *Neuropsychopharmacology 28:*755–764, 2003.
77. O'Malley, S. S., Krishnan-Sarin, S., Farren, C., Sinha, R., & Kreek, M. J. Naltrexone decreases craving and alcohol self-administration in alcohol-dependent subjects and activates the hypothalamo-pituitary-adrenocortical axis. *Psychopharmacology 160:*19–29, 2002.
78. Drobes, D. J., Anton, R. F., Thomas, S. E., & Voronin, K. Effects of naltrexone and nalmefene on subjective response to alcohol among non-treatment-seeking alcoholics and social drinkers. *Alcoholism: Clinical and Experimental Research 28:*1362–1370, 2004.
79. Boyle, A. E. L., Stewart, R. B., Macenski, M. J., Spiga, R., Johnson, B. A., & Meisch, R. A. Effects of acute and chronic doses of naltrexone on ethanol self-administration in Rhesus monkeys. *Alcoholism: Clinical and Experimental Research 22:*359–366, 1998.

80. Croop, R. S., Faulkner, E. G., & Labriola, D. F. The safety profile of naltrexone in the treatment of alcoholism. *Archives of General Psychiatry 54:*1130–1135, 1997.
81. Hermos, J. A., Young, M. M., Gagnon, D. R., & Fiore, L. D. Patterns of dispensed disulfiram and naltrexone for alcoholism treatment in a veteran patient population. *Alcoholism: Clinical and Experimental Research 28:*1229–1235, 2004.
82. Mason, B. J., Goodman, A. M., Dixon, R. M., Abdel Hameed, M. H., Hulot, T., Wesnes, K., Hunter, J. A., & Boyeson, M. G. A pharmacokinetic and pharmacodynamic drug interaction study of acamprosate and naltrexone. *Neuropsychopharmacology 27:*596–606, 2002.
83. Pettinati, H. M., Zweben, A., & Mattson, M. E. COMBINE Study: Conceptual, Methodological and Practical Issues in a Clinical Trial that Combined Medication and Behavioural Treatments, *Journal of Studies on Alcohol* (Supplement No.15), 2005.
84. Kiefer, F., Jahn, H., Tarnaske, T., Helwig, H., Briken, P., Holzbach, R., Kämpf, P., Stracke, R., Baehr, M., Naber, D., & Wiedemann, K. Comparing and combining naltrexone and acamprosate in relapse prevention of alcoholism: A double-blind, placebo-controlled study (*Presented at RSA Annual Meeting*, July 1, 2002, San Francisco, CA). *Archives of General Psychiatry 60:*92–99, 2003.
85. Martin, B., Clapp, L., Bialkowski, D., Bridgeford, D., Amponsah, A., Lyons, L., & Beresford, T. P. Compliance to supervised disulfiram therapy: A comparison of voluntary and court-ordered patients. *American Journal on Addictions 12:*137–143, 2003.
86. Petrakis, I. L., Poling, J., Levinson, C., Nich, C., Carroll, K., Rounsaville, B., & The VA New England VISN I MIRECC Study Group. Naltrexone and disulfiram in patients with alcohol dependence and comorbid psychiatric disorders. *Biological Psychiatry 57:*1128–1137, 2005.
87. Fuller, R. K., Branchey, L., Brightwell, D. R., Dermen, R. M., Emrick, C. D., Iber, F. L., James, K. E., Lacoursiere, R. B., Lee, K. K., & Lowenstam, I. Disulfiram treatment of alcoholism: A Veterans Administration cooperative study. *The Journal of the American Medical Association 256:*1449–1455, 1986.
88. Zorzon, M., Mase, G., Biasutti, E., Vitrani, B., & Cazzato, G. Acute encephalopathy and polyneuropathy after disulfiram intoxication. *Alcohol & Alcoholism 30:*629–631, 1995.
89. Kristenson, H. How to get the best out of antabuse. *Alcohol & Alcoholism 30:*775–783, 1995.
90. Carroll, K. M., Fenton, L. R., Ball, S. A., Nich, C., Frankforter, T. L., Shi, J., & Rounsaville, B. J. Efficacy of disulfiram and cognitive behavior therapy in cocaine-dependent outpatients: A randomized placebo-controlled trial. *Archives of General Psychiatry 61:* 264–272, 2004.
91. Kranzler, H. R., Modesto-Lowe, V., & Van Kirk, J. Naltrexone vs. nefazodone for treatment of alcohol dependence: A placebo-controlled trial. *Neuropsychopharmacology 22:*493–503, 2000.
92. Hu, X., Oroszi, G., Chun, J., Smith, T. L., Goldman, D. A., & Schuckit, M. A. An expanded evaluation of the relationship of four alleles to the level of response to alcohol and the alcoholism risk. *Alcoholism: Clinical and Experimental Research 29:*8–16, 2005.
93. Barr, C. S., Newman, T. K., Becker, M. L., Champoux, M., Lesch, K. P., Suomi, S. J., Goldman, D., & Higley, J. D. Serotonin transporter gene variation is associated with alcohol sensitivity in rhesus macaques exposed to early-life stress. *Alcoholism: Clinical and Experimental Research 27:*812–817, 2003.
94. Hu, X., Oroszi, G., Chun, J., Smith, T. L., Goldman, D., & Schuckit, M. A. An expanded evaluation of the relationship of four alleles to the LR to alcohol and the alcoholism risk. *Alcoholism: Clinical and Experimental Research 29:*8–16, 2005.
95. Cornelius, J. R., Salloum, I. M., Ehler, J. G., Jarrett, P. J., Cornelius, M. D., Perel, J. M., Thase, M. E., & Black, A. Fluoxetine in depressed alcoholics. *Archives of General Psychiatry 54:*700–705, 1997.
96. Kranzler, H. R., Burleson, J. A., Brown, J., & Babor, T. R. Fluoxetine treatment seems to reduce the beneficial effects of cognitive–behavioral therapy in Type B alcoholics. *Alcoholism: Clinical and Experimental Research 20:*1534–1541, 1996.
97. Kranzler, H. R., Pierucci-Lagha, A., Feinn, R., & Hernandez-Avila, C. Effects of ondansetron in early- versus late-onset alcoholics: A prospective, open-label study. *Alcoholism: Clinical and Experimental Research 27:*1150–1155, 2003.

98. Johnson, B. A., Ait-Daoud, N., Ma, J. Z., & Wang, Y. Ondansetron reduces mood disturbance among biologically predisposed, alcohol-dependent individuals. *Alcoholism: Clinical and Experimental Research 27:*1773–1779, 2003.
99. McBride, W. M., Lovinger, D. M., Machu, T., Thielen, R. J., Rodd, Z. A., Murphy, J. M., Roache, J. D., & Johnson, B. A. Serotonin-3 receptors in the actions of alcohol, alcohol reinforcement, and alcoholism. *Alcoholism: Clinical and Experimental Research 28:* 257–267, 2004.
100. Pettinati, H. M. Antidepressant treatment of co-occurring depression and alcohol dependence. *Biological Psychiatry 56:*785–792, 2004.
101. Nunes, E. V., & Levin, F. R. Treatment of depression in patients with alcohol or drug dependence: A meta-analysis. *The Journal of the American Medical Association 291:* 1887–1896, 2004.
102. Gual, A., Balcells, M., Torres, M., Madrigal, M., Diez, T., & Serrano, L. Sertraline for the prevention of relapse in detoxicated alcohol dependent patients with a cormorbid depressive disorder: A randomized controlled trial. *Alcohol & Alcoholism 38:*619–625, 2003.
103. Gabriel, K. I., & Cunningham, C. L. Effects of topiramate on ethanol and saccharin consumption and preferences in C57BL/6J mice. *Alcoholism: Clinical and Experimental Research 29:*75–80, 2005.
104. Johnson, B. A., Ait-Daoud, N., Bowden, C. L., DiClemente, C. C., Roache, J. D., Lawson, K., Javors, M. A., & Ma, J. A. Oral topiramate for treatment of alcohol dependence: A randomized controlled trial. *Lancet 361:*1677–1685, 2003.
105. Johnson, B. A. Progress in the development of topiramate for treating alcohol dependence: From a hypothesis to a proof-of-concept study. *Alcoholism: Clinical and Experimental Research 28:*1137–1144, 2004.
106. Marra, D., Warot, D., Berlin, I., Hispard, E., Notides, C., Tilikete, S., Payan, C., Lépine, J.-P., Dally, S., & Aubin, H.-J. Amisulpride does not prevent relapse in primary alcohol dependence: Results of a pilot randomized, placebo-controlled trial. *Alcoholism: Clinical and Experimental Research 26:*1545–1552, 2002.
107. Naranjo, C. A., Dongier, M., & Bremner, K. E. Long-acting injectable bromocriptine does not reduce relapse in alcoholics. *Addiction 92:*969–978, 1997.
108. Wiesbeck, G. A., Weijers, H.-G., Chick, J., & Boening, J. Ritanserin in relapse prevention in abstinent alcoholics: Results from a placebo-controlled double blind international multicenter trial. *Alcoholism: Clinical and Experimental Research 23:*230–235, 1999.
109. Erhardt, A., Sillaber, I., Welt, T., Muller, M. B., Singewald, N., & Keck, M. E. Repetitive transcranial magnetic stimulation increases the release of dopamine in the nucleus accumbens shell of morphine-sensitized rats during abstinence. *Neuropsychopharmacology 29:*2074–2080, 2004.
110. Currie, S. R., Clark, S., Hodgins, D. C., & el-Guebaly, N. Randomized controlled trial of brief cognitive-behavioural interventions for insomnia in recovering alcoholics. *Addiction 99:*1121–1132, 2004.
111. Schade, A., Marquenie, L. A., van Balkom, A. J. L. M., Koeter, M. W. J., de Beurs, E., van den Brink, W., & van Dyck, R. The effectiveness of anxiety treatment on alcohol-dependent patients with a comorbid phobic disorder: A randomized controlled trial. *Alcoholism: Clinical and Experimental Research 29:*794–800, 2005.
112. Lukas, S. E., Penetar, D., Berko, J., Vicens, L., Palmer, C., Mallya, G., Macklin, E. A., & Lee, D. Y.-W. An extract of the Chinese herbal root kudzu reduces alcohol drinking by heavy drinkers in a naturalistic setting. *Alcoholism: Clinical and Experimental Research 29:*756–762, 2005.
113. Moos, R. H., Finney, J. W., Federman, E. B., & Suchinsky, R. Specialty mental health care improves patients' outcomes: Findings from a nationwide program to monitor the quality of care for patients with substance use disorders. *Journal of Studies on Alcohol 61:*704–713, 2000.

114. Fawcett, J., Kravitz, H. M., McGuire, M., Easton, M., Ross, J., Pisani, V., Fogg, L. R., Clark, D., Whitney, M., Kravitz, G., Javaid, J., & Teas, G. Pharmacological treatments for alcoholism: Revisiting lithium and considering buspirone. *Alcoholism: Clinical and Experimental Research 24:*666–674, 2000.
115. Ussher, M., Sampuran, A. K., Doshi, R., West, R., & Drummond, D. C. Acute effect of a brief bout of exercise on alcohol urges. *Addiction 99:*1542–1547, 2004.
116. Howard, M. O. Pharmacological aversion treatment of alcohol dependence. I. Production and prediction of conditioned alcohol aversion. *American Journal of Drug and Alcohol Abuse 27:*561–585, 2001.
117. Jensen, M. K., Sorensen, T. I. A., Andersen, A. T., Thorsen, T., Tolstrup, J. S., Godtfredsen, N. S., & Gronbaek, M. A prospective study of the association between smoking and later alcohol drinking in the general population. *Addiction 98:*355–363, 2003.
118. Schmitz, N., Kruse, J., & Kugler, J. Disabilities, quality of life, and mental disorders associated with smoking and nicotine dependence. *American Journal of Psychiatry 160:*1670–1676, 2003.
119. Cooney, J. L., Cooney, N. L., Pilkey, D. T., Kranzler, H. R., & Oncken, C. A. Effects of nicotine deprivation on urges to drink and smoke in alcoholic smokers. *Addiction 98:* 913–921, 2003.
120. Schuckit, M. A. Vulnerability factors for alcoholism. In K. Davis (Ed.), *Neuropsychopharmacology: The Fifth Generation of Progress.* Baltimore: Lippincott, Williams & Wilkins, 2002, pp. 1399–1411.
121. Lowinson, J. H., Marion, I., Joseph, H., Langrod, J., Salsitz, E. A., Payte, J. T., & Dole, V. P. Methadone maintenance. In J. H. Lowinson, P. Ruiz, R. B. Millman, & J. G. Langrod (Eds.), *Substance Abuse: A Comprehensive Textbook* (4th ed.). Baltimore, MD: Lippincott, Williams & Wilkins, 2004, pp. 616–634.
122. Rawson, R. A., Huber, A., McCann, M., Shoptaw, S., Farabee, D., Reiber, C., & Ling, W. A comparison of contingency management and cognitive-behavioral approaches during methadone maintenance treatment for cocaine dependence. *Archives of General Psychiatry 59:*817–824, 2002.
123. Ling, W., Huber, A., & Rawson, R. A. New trends in opiate pharmacotherapy. *Drug and Alcohol Review 20:79*–94, 2001.
124. Herning, R. I., Better, W. E., Tate, K., Umbricht, A., Preston, K. L., & Cadet, J. L. Methadone treatment induced attenuation of cerebrovascular deficits associated with the prolonged abuse of cocaine and heroin. *Neuropsychopharmacology 28:*562–568, 2003.
125. Jaffe, J. H., & Strain, E. C. Opioid-related disorders. In B. J. Sadock & V. A. Sadock (Eds.), *Comprehensive Textbook of Psychiatry* (8th ed.). Baltimore, MD: Williams & Wilkins, 2004, pp. 1265–1290.
126. Ritter, A. J., Lintzeris, N., Clark, N., Kutin, J. J., Bammer, G., & Panjari, M. A randomized trial comparing levo-alpha acetylmethadol with methadone maintenance for patients in primary care settings in Australia. *Addiction 98:*1605–1613, 2003.
127. Kraft, M. K., Rothbard, A. B., Hadley, T. R., *et al.* Are supplementary services provided during methadone maintenance really cost-effective? *American Journal of Psychiatry 154:*1214–1219, 1997.
128. Magura, S., Nwakeze, P. C., & Demsky, S. Pre- and in-treatment predictors of retention in methadone treatment using survival analysis. *Addiction 93:*51–60, 1998.
129. Masson, C. L., Barnett, P. G., Sees, K. L., Delucchi, K. L., Rosen, A., Wong, W., & Hall, S. M. Cost and cost-effectiveness of standard methadone maintenance treatment compared to enriched 180-day methadone detoxification. *Addiction 99:*718–726, 2004.
130. Grabowski, J., Rhoades, H., Stotts, A., Cowan, K., Kopecky, C., Dougherty, A., Moeller, F. G., Hassan, S., & Schmitz, J. Agonist-like or antagonist-like treatment for cocaine dependence with methadone for heroin dependence: Two double-blind randomized clinical trials. *Neuropsychopharmacology 29:*969–981, 2004.

131. Greenwald, M. K., Johanson, C.-E., Moody, D. S., Woods, J. H., Kilbourn, M. R., Koeppe, R. A., Schuster, C. R., & Zubieta, J.-K. Effects of buprenorphine maintenance dose on mu-opioid receptor availability, plasma concentrations, and antagonist blockade in heroin-dependent volunteers. *Neuropsychopharmacology 28:*2000–2009, 2003.
132. Schottenfeld, R. S., Chawarski, M. C., Pakes, J. R., Pantalon, M. V., Carroll, K. M., & Kosten, T. R. Methadone versus buprenorphine with contingency management or performance feedback for cocaine and opioid dependence. *American Journal of Psychiatry 162:*340–349, 2005.
133. Johnson, R. E., Strain, E. C., & Amass, L. Buprenorphine: How to use it right. *Drug and Alcohol Dependence 70:*S59–S77, 2003.
134. Doran, C. M., Shanahan, M., Mattick, R. P., Ali, R., White, J., & Bell, J. Buprenorphine versus methadone maintenance: A cost-effectiveness analysis. *Drug and Alcohol Dependence 71:*295–302, 2003.
135. Giacomuzzi, S. M., Riemer, Y., Ertl, M., Kemmler, G., Rossler, H., Hinterhuber, H., & Kurz, M. Buprenorphine versus methadone maintenance treatment in an ambulant setting: A health-related quality of life assessment. *Addiction 98:*693–702, 2003.
136. Sobel, B.-F. X., Sigmon, S. C., Walsh, S. L., Johnson, R. E., Liebson, I. A., Nuwayser, E. S., Kerrigan, J. H., & Bigelow, G. E. Open-label trial of an injection depot formulation of buprenorphine in opioid detoxification. *Drug and Alcohol Dependence 73:*11–22, 2004.
137. Blanken, P., Hendriks, V. M., Koeter, M. W. J., van Ree, J. M., & van den Brink, W. Matching of treatment-resistant heroin-dependent patients to medical prescription of heroin or oral methadone treatment: Results from two randomized controlled trials. *Addiction 100:*89–95, 2005.
138. Moldovanyi, A., Ladewig, D., Affentranger, P., Natsch, C., & Stohler, R. Morphine maintenance treatment of opioid-dependent outpatients. *European Addiction Research 2:*208–212, 1996.
139. Farren, C. K., & O'Malley, S. A pilot double blind placebo controlled trial of sertraline with naltrexone in the treatment of opiate dependence. *American Journal on Addiction 11:*228–234, 2002.
140. Guardia, J., Caso, C., Arias, F., Gual, A., Sanahuja, J., Ramirez, M., Mengual, I., Gonzalvo, B., Segura, L., Trujois, J., & Casas, M. A double-blind, placebo-controlled study of naltrexone in the treatment of alcohol-dependence disorder: Results from a multicenter clinical trial. *Alcoholism: Clinical and Experimental Research 26:*1381–1387, 2002.
141. Kirchmayer, U., Davoli, M., Verster, A. D., Amato, L., Ferri, M., & Perucci, C. A. A systematic review on the efficacy of naltrexone maintenance treatment in opioid dependence. *Addiction 97:*1241–1249, 2002.
142. Mark, T. L., Kranzler, H. R., & Song, X. Understanding US addiction physicians' low rate of naltrexone prescription. *Drug and Alcohol Dependence 71:*219–228, 2003.
143. Moreno, R. M., & Rosado, T. D. Follow-up of a 12-month naltrexone maintenance programme. *Adicciones 8:*5–18, 1996.
144. Ali, R., Thomas, P., White, J., McGregor, C., Danz, C., Gowing, L., Stegink, A., & Athanasos, P. Antagonist-precipitated heroin withdrawal under anesthetic prior to maintenance naltrexone treatment: Determinants of withdrawal severity. *Drug and Alcohol Review 22:*425–431, 2003.
145. Wodak, A., Saunders, J. B., Mattick, R. P., & Hall, W. Rapid opiate detoxification and naltrexone treatment. Past, present and future. *Drug and Alcohol Review 20:*349–350, 2001.
146. Han, J.-S., Trachtenberg, A. I., & Lowinson, J. H. Acupuncture. In J. H. Lowinson, P. Ruiz, R. B. Millman, & J. G. Langrod (Eds.), *Substance Abuse: A Comprehensive Textbook* (4th ed.). Baltimore, MD: Lippincott, Williams & Wilkins, 2004, pp. 743–762.
147. Gariti, P., Auriacombe, M., Incmikoski, R., McLellan, A. T., Patterson, L., Dhopesh, V., Mezochow, J., Patterson, M., & O'Brien, C. A randomized double-blind study of neuroelectric therapy in opiate and cocaine detoxification. *Journal of Substance Abuse 4:*299–308, 1992.

148. Krupitsky, E. M., Burakov, A. M., Didenko, T. Y., Romanova, T. N., Grinenko, N. I., Slavina, T. Y., Grinenko, A. Y., & Tcheremissine, V. Effects of citalopram treatment of protracted withdrawal (syndrome of anhedonia) in patients with heroin addiction. *Addictive Disorders & Their Treatment 1:*29–33, 2002.
149. Stier, K. Nature's easier way down? *Asiaweek*, September 26, 1997.
150. O'Brien, W. B., & Perfas, F. B. The therapeutic community. In J. H. Lowinson, P. Ruiz, R. B. Millman, & J. G. Langrod (Eds.), *Substance Abuse: A Comprehensive Textbook* (4th ed.). Baltimore, MD: Lippincott, Williams & Wilkins, 2004, pp. 609–615.
151. De Leon, G. *The Therapeutic Community: Theory, Model and Method.* New York, NY: Springer Publishing Company, 2000.
152. Ohayon, M. M., & Schatzberg, A. F. Using chronic pain to predict depressive morbidity in the general population. *Archives of General Psychiatry 60:*39–47, 2003.
153. Atkinson, J. H., Slater, M. A., Patterson, T. L., Grant, I., & Garfin, S. R. Prevalence, onset, and risk of psychiatric disorders in men with chronic low back pain: A controlled study. *Pain 45:*111–121, 1991.
154. Portenoy, R. K., Payne, R., & Passik, S. D. Acute and chronic pain. In J. H. Lowinson, P. Ruiz, R. B. Millman, & J. G. Langrod (Eds.), *Substance Abuse: A Comprehensive Textbook* (4th ed.). Baltimore, MD: Lippincott, Williams & Wilkins, 2004, pp. 863–903.
155. Weiss, R. D., Griffin, M. L., Mazurick, C., Berkman, B., Gastfriend, D. R., Frank, A., Barber, J. P., Blaine, J., Salloum, I., & Moras, K. The relationship between cocaine craving, psychosocial treatment, and subsequent cocaine use. *American Journal of Psychiatry 160:*1320–1325, 2003.
156. McKay, J. R., Merikle, E., Mulvaney, F. D., Weiss, R. V., & Koppenhaver, J. M. Factors accounting for cocaine use two years following initiation of continuing care. *Addiction 96:*213–225, 2001.
157. Rawson, R. A., Marinelli-Casey, P., Anglin, M. D., Dickow, A., Frazier, Y., Gallagher, C., Galloway, G. P., Herrell, J., Huber, A., McCann, M. J., Obert, J., Pennell, S., Reiber, C., Vandersloot, D., Zweben, J., and the Methamphetamine Treatment Project Corporate Authors. A multi-site comparison of psychosocial approaches for the treatment of methamphetamine dependence. *Addiction 99:*708–717, 2004.
158. Higgins, S. T., Sigmon, S. C., Wong, C. J., Heil, S. H., Badger, G. J., Donham, R., Dantona, R. L., & Anthony, S. Community reinforcement therapy for cocaine-dependent outpatients. *Archives of General Psychiatry 60:*1043–1052, 2003.
159. Silva de Lima, M., Garcia de Oliveira Soares, B., Alves Pereira Reisser, A., & Farrell, M. Pharmacological treatment of cocaine dependence: A systematic review. *Addiction 97:*931–949, 2002.
160. Gottheil, E., Weinstein, S. P., Sterling, R. D., Lundy, A., & Serota, R. D. A randomized controlled study of the effectiveness of intensive outpatient treatment for cocaine dependence. *Psychiatric Services 49:*782–787, 1998.
161. Shearer, J., & Gowing, L. R. Pharmacotherapies for problematic psychostimulant use: A review of current research. *Drug and Alcohol Review 23:*203–211, 2004.
162. Campbell, J., Nickel, E. J., Penick, E. C., Wallace, D., Gabrielli, W. F., Rowe, C., Liskow, B., Powell, B. J., & Thomas, H. M. Comparison of desipramine or carbamazepine to placebo for crack cocaine-dependent patients. *American Journal on Addictions 12:* 122–136, 2003.
163. George, T. P., Chawarski, M. C., Pakes, J., Carroll, K. M., Kosten, T. R., & Schottenfeld, R. S. Disulfiram versus placebo for cocaine dependence in buprenorphine-maintained subjects. A preliminary trial. *Biological Psychiatry 47:*1080–1086, 2000.
164. Gonzalez, G., Sevarino, K., Sofuoglu, M., Poling, J., Oliveto, A., Gonsai, K., George, T. P., & Kosten, T. R. Tiagabine increases cocaine-free urines in cocaine-dependent methadone-treated patients: Results of a randomized pilot study. *Addiction 98:*1625–1632, 2003.

165. Halikas, J. A., Crosby, R. D., Pearson, V. L., & Graves, N. M. A randomized double-blind study of carbamazepine in the treatment of cocaine abuse. *Clinical Pharmacology and Therapeutics 62:*89–105, 1997.
166. DiCiano, P., & Everitt, B. J. The $GABA_B$ receptor agonist baclofen attenuates cocaine- and heroin-seeking behavior by rats. *Neuropsychopharmacology 28:*510–518, 2003.
167. Kosten, T. R., Gottschalk, P. C., Tucker, K., Rinder, C. S., Dey, H. M., & Rinder, H. J. Aspirin or amiloride for cerebral perfusion defects in cocaine dependence. *Drug and Alcohol Dependence 71:*187–194, 2003.
168. Johnson, B. A., Devous, M. D., Sr., Ruiz, P., & Ait-Daoud, N. Treatment advances for cocaine-induced ischemic stroke: Focus on dihydropyridine-class calcium channel antagonists. *American Journal of Psychiatry 158:*1191–1198, 2001.
169. Cervo, L., Carnovali, F., Stark, J. A., & Mennini, T. Cocaine-seeking behavior in response to drug-associated stimuli in rats: Involvement of D_3 and D_2 dopamine receptors. *Neuropsychopharmacology 28:*1150–1159, 2003.
170. Dackis, C. A., Kampman, K. M., Lynch, K. G., Pettinati, H. M., & O'Brien, C. P. A double-blind, placebo-controlled trial of modafinil for cocaine dependence. *Neuropsychopharmacology 30:*205–211, 2005.
171. Kampman, K. M., Volpicelli, J. R., Alterman, A. I., Cornish, J., O'Brien, C. P. Amantadine in the treatment of cocaine-dependent patients with severe withdrawal symptoms. *American Journal of Psychiatry 157:*2052–2054, 2000.
172. Margolin, A., Kleber, H. D., Avants, S. K., Konefal, J., Gawin, F., Stark, E., Sorensen, J., Midkiff, E., Wells, E., Jackson, T. R., Bullock, M., Culliton, P. D., Boles, S., & Vaughan, R. Acupuncture for the treatment of cocaine addiction: A randomized controlled trial. *The Journal of the American Medical Association 287:*55–63, 2002.
173. Carrera, M. R. A., Ashley, J. A., Wirsching, P., Koob, G. F., & Janda, K. D. A second-generation vaccine protects against the psychoactive effects of cocaine. *Proceedings of the National Academy of Sciences of the United States of America 98:*1988–1992, 2001.
174. Ebbert, J. O., Rowland, L. C., Montori, V. M., Vickers, K. S., Erwin, P. J., & Dale, L. C. Treatments for spit tobacco use: A quantitative systematic review. *Addiction 98:*569–583, 2003.
175. Hughes, J. R., & Burns, D. M. Impact of medications on smoking cessation. *Smoking and Tobacco Control Monograph* (Vol. 12). National Institute on Drug Abuse, 2001, pp. 155–164.
176. Wennike, P., Danielsson, T., Landfeldt, B., Westin, A., & Tonnesen, P. Smoking reduction promotes smoking cessation: Results from a double blind, randomized, placebo-controlled trial of nicotine gum with 2-year follow-up. *Addiction 98:*1395–1402, 2003.
177. Borland, R., Balmford, J., Segan, C., Livingston, P., & Owen, N. The effectiveness of personalized smoking cessation strategies for callers to a Quitline service. *Addiction 98:*837–846, 2003.
178. Collins, S. E., Carey, K. B., & Sliwinski, M. J. Mailed personalized normative feedback as a brief intervention for at-risk college drinkers. *Journal of Studies on Alcohol 63:*559–567, 2002.
179. Gariti, P., Alterman, A., Mulvaney, F., Mechanic, K., Dhopesh, V., Yu, E., Chychula, N., & Sacks, D. Nicotine intervention during detoxification and treatment for other substance use. *The American Journal of Drug and Alcohol Abuse 28:*671–679, 2002.
180. Shiffman, S., Hughes, J. R., DiMarino, M. E., & Sweeney, C. T. Patterns of over-the-counter nicotine gum use: Persistent use and concurrent smoking. *Addiction 98:*1747–1753, 2003.
181. Smith, R. C., Singh, A., Infante, M., Khandat, A., & Kloos, A. Effects of cigarette smoking and nicotine nasal spray on psychiatric symptoms and cognition in schizophrenia. *Neuropsychopharmacology 27:*479–497, 2002.
182. Dierker, L. C., Avenevoli, S., Stolar, M., & Merikangas, K. R. Smoking and depression: An examination of mechanisms of comorbidity. *American Journal of Psychiatry 1159:*947–953, 2002.

183. Wagena, E. J., Knipschild, P., & Zeegers, M. P. A. Should nortriptyline be used as a first-line aid to help smokers quit? Results from a systematic review and meta-analysis. *Addiction 100:*317–326, 2005.
184. Hall, S. M., Reus, B. I., Munoz, R. F., Sees, K. L., Humfleet, G., Hartz, D. T., Frederick, D., & Triffleman, E. Nortriptyline and cognitive-behavioral therapy in the treatment of cigarette smoking. *Archives of General Psychiatry 55:*683–690, 1998.
185. George, T. P., Vessicchio, J. C., Termine, A., Bregartner, T. A., Feingold, A., Rounsaville, B. J., & Kosten, T. R. A placebo controlled trial of bupropion for smoking cessation in schizophrenia. *Biological Psychiatry 52:*53–61, 2002.
186. Aubin, H. J., Lebargy, F., Berlin, I., Bidaut-Mazel, C., Chemali-Hurdry, J., & Lagrue, G. Efficacy of bupropion and predictors of successful outcome in a sample of French smokers: A randomized placebo-controlled trial. *Addiction 99:*1206–1218, 2004.
187. Berlin, I., Aubin, H.-J., Pedarriosse, A. M., & Rames, A. Lazabemide, a selective reversible monoamine oxidase B inhibitor, as an aid to smoking cessation. *Addiction 97:*1347–1354, 2002.
188. Biberman, R., Neumann, R., Katzir, I., & Gerber, Y. A randomized controlled trial of oral selegiline plus nicotine skin patch compared with placebo plus nicotine skin patch for smoking cessation. *Addiction 98:*1403–1407, 2003.
189. Hall, S. M., Humfleet, G. L., Reus, V. I., Muñoz, R. F., & Cullen, J. Extended nortriptyline and psychological treatment for cigarette smoking. *American Journal of Psychiatry 161:*2100–2107, 2004.
190. Hughes, J. R., Fiester, S., Goldstein, M., *et al.* Practice guideline for the treatment of patients with nicotine dependence. *American Journal of Psychiatry 153:*1–31, 1996.
191. LeFoll, B., & Goldberg, S. Rimonabant, a CB1 antagonist, blocks nicotine-conditioned place preferences. *NeuroReport 15:*2139–2143, 2004.
192. Carrera, M. R. A., Ashley, J. A., Hoffman, T. Z., Isomura, S., Wirsching, P., Koob, G. F., & Janda, K. D. Investigations using immunization to attenuate the psychoactive effects of nicotine. *Bioorganic & Medicinal Chemistry 12:*563–570, 2005.

Index

The page numbers with t indicates table.

Q

T

Breinigsville, PA USA
11 July 2010
241528BV00005B/180/A